Studies of Brain Function, Vol. 11

Studies of Brain Function

Volumes already published in the series:

1   *W. Heiligenberg*
    Principles of Electrolocation and Jamming Avoidance
    in Electric Fish
    A Neuroethological Approach

2   *W. Precht*
    Neuronal Operations in the Vestibular System

3   *J. T. Enright*
    The Timing of Sleep and Wakefulness
    On the Substructure and Dynamics of the Circadian
    Pacemakers Underlying the Wake-Sleep Cycle

4   *H. Braak*
    Architectonics of the Human Telencephalic Cortex

5   *H. Collewijn*
    The Oculomotor System of the Rabbit and Its
    Plasticity

6   *M. Abeles*
    Local Cortical Circuits
    An Electrophysiological Study

7   *G. Palm*
    Neural Assemblies
    An Alternative Approach to Artificial Intelligence

8   *J. Hyvärinen*
    The Parietal Cortex of Monkey and Man

9   *E. Zrenner*
    Neurophysiological Aspects of Color Vision
    in Primates

10 *U. Bässler*
    Neural Basis of Elementary Behavior
    in Stick Insects

11 *G. A. Orban*
    Neuronal Operations in the Visual Cortex

Guy A. Orban

Neuronal Operations in the Visual Cortex

With 188 Figures

Springer-Verlag
Berlin Heidelberg New York Tokyo 1984

Professor Dr. Guy A. Orban
Katholieke Universiteit Leuven, Faculteit der Geneeskunde
Laboratorium voor Neuro- en Psychofysiologie
Campus Gasthuisberg, Herestraat
3000 Leuven, Belgium

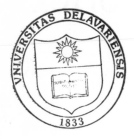

ISBN 3-540-11919-1 Springer-Verlag Berlin Heidelberg New York Tokyo
ISBN 0-387-11919-1 Springer-Verlag New York Heidelberg Berlin Tokyo

Library of Congress Cataloging in Publication Data Orban, Guy A., 1945 –
Neuronal operations in the visual cortex. (Studies of brain function ; vol. 11)
Includes bibliographical references and index. 1. Visual cortex. 2. Visual perception. 3. Cats – Physiology. 4. Monkeys – Physiology. I. Title. II. Series:
Studies of brain function ; v. 11. [DNLM: 1. Neurons – Physiology. 2. Visual
cortex – Physiology. W1 ST937KF v. 11 / WL307 0635n] QP382.022073 1984
599′.0188 83-20333

Media conversion: Daten- und Lichtsatz-Service, Würzburg
Offsetprinting and binding: Konrad Triltsch, Graphischer Betrieb, Würzburg
2131/3130-543210

Dedicated to Peter O. Bishop

Preface

The invitation by the editors of the series "studies of brain function" to contribute a monograph on the visual cortex gives me the opportunity to present in a concentrated manner much of the work I have done on the visual cortical areas of cat and monkey. However, the field of visual cortical physiology is so active and so diverse that the presentation of only my own work would have given a very incomplete view of visual cortical functioning. Therefore this monograph also reviews most of the studies carried out on the subject in the last two decades. Where possible I have tried not only to describe the cortical machinery but also its possible functional purpose regarding vision. In doing this I have expressed my personal views rather than just reviewing the experimental facts.

Much of the work presented in this monograph has been supported by the National Research Council of Belgium and the Research Council of the Catholic University of Leuven. I express my gratitude to them. I have enjoyed collaborating in these studies with P. O. Bishop, H. Kato, H. Kennedy, K. P. Hoffmann, H. Maes, J. Duysens, E. Vandenbussche, and H. van der Glas. I am much indebted to all those who have commented on earlier versions of this monograph: J. Allman, H. Barlow, J. Bullier, M. Callens, J. Duysens, O. J. Grüsser, P. Heggelund, H. Kennedy, L. C. Orban and L. Palmer. I would like to thank the many publishers who have given permission to reprint figures. Finally, it is a pleasure to acknowledge the help of G. Vanparrijs who drew the figures, J. Warmoeskerken who made the photographs, and Y. Celis who did the computerized typework.

Leuven, January 1984   GUY A. ORBAN

Contents

Introduction 1

Chapter 1   The Visual System of Cat and Monkey Compared 5

1.1 The Basic Layout of the Visual System in Cat, Owl Monkey,
and Rhesus Monkey. 7

    1.1.1 The Retina 7
    1.1.2 The Optic Chiasm and Optic Tract 11
    1.1.3 The Dorsal Lateral Geniculate Nucleus (dLGN) 13
    1.1.4 Visual Cortex 17
    1.1.5 Pulvinar 21
    1.1.6 Callosal Connections 23

1.2 Quantitative Aspects of the Retino-Geniculo-Cortical Projections 25

    1.2.1 The Overall Numbers of Cells in the Visual Pathway . . . 25
    1.2.2 Distribution of Retinal Cell Populations 27
    1.2.3 Magnification Factors 29

1.3 Conclusion 33

Chapter 2   The Visual Cortical Areas of the Cat 34

2.1 Description of the Visual Cortical Areas 34

    2.1.1 Area 17: The Prototype of Visual Cortical Areas 34
    2.1.2 Areas 18 and 19 39
    2.1.3 The Lateral Suprasylvian Areas 42
    2.1.4 Areas 20 and 21 47
    2.1.5 Additional Visual Areas? 47

2.2 The Levels of Processing in the Visual Cortical System of the Cat 47
2.3 Additional Observations on the Retinotopic Organization
in the Primary Complex 53

    2.3.1 Variability of the 3 Cortical Maps 53
    2.3.2 RF Scatter 55

2.3.3 The 17-18 Border and the Question of the Naso-Temporal
      Overlap   57
2.3.4 The 18-19 Border and the Question of the Visual Field Islands   62

2.4 Conclusion   62

**Chapter 3   Afferent Projections to Areas 17, 18, 19 of the Cat:
               Evidence for Parallel Input**   63

3.1 The Relay of Retinal Afferents: The Dorsal Lateral Geniculate
    Nuclear Complex   63
3.2 The Geniculocortical Projection   66
3.3 Functional Streams in the Retino-Geniculocortical Projection . .   68

    3.3.1 Functional Properties of Retinal and Geniculate X, Y, W
          Cells   69
    3.3.2 Correlation with Retinal Morphology   71
    3.3.3 Separation of Functional Streams at LGN Level   72
    3.3.4 Correlation with LGN Morphological Types   72
    3.3.5 Distribution of Functional Streams in dLGN Nuclear
          Complex   73
    3.3.6 Input to Different Areas of Primary Visual Complex . . .   74

3.4 Physiological Identification of the Functional Type of Afferents
    to Areas 17, 18 and 19   76
3.5 The Termination of Geniculate Afferents in the Visual Cortex .   80
3.6 Other Subcortical Afferents: Pulvinar-Lateralis Posterior
    Complex, Intralaminar Nuclei, Claustrum, and Brainstem . . .   83
3.7 The Ipsilateral Corticocortical Connections   84
3.8 The Connections Through the Corpus Callosum   85
3.9 Conclusion   86

**Chapter 4   Receptive Field Organization in Areas 17, 18 and 19
               of the Cat**   87

4.1 Twenty Years with the Simple-Complex-Hypercomplex Scheme .   88
4.2 Criteria for Classifying Cortical RFs   92

    4.2.1 The ON–OFF Overlap or the Parcellation of the RF into
          Subregions   94
    4.2.2 Position Test   97
    4.2.3 RF Dimensions   97
    4.2.4 End-Stopping or the Hypercomplex Property   104

4.3 The A, B, C, S Scheme   106

4.3.1 Properties and Distribution of Cell Types 107
4.3.2 The S and A Families 113
4.3.3 Responses to Other Stimuli 115

4.4 Correspondence of the A, B, C, S Scheme with Other Classification
    Schemes 117
4.5 Conclusion 123

**Chapter 5   Parameter Specificity of Visual Cortical Cells and Coding
              of Visual Parameters** 125

5.1 The Tuned Cells as Bandpass Filters: The Multichannel
    Representation of a Parameter 125
5.2 Are All Tuned Cells Simple (Passive) Bandpass Filters or Are Some
    of Them Active Filters? 131
5.3 Cells with Thresholds as High-Pass Filters: Single or Multichannel
    Representation of a Parameter 132
5.4 Conclusion 134

**Chapter 6   Influence of Luminance and Contrast on Cat Visual Cortical
              Neurons** 135

6.1 Contrast-Response Curves Obtained with Sinusoidal Gratings . . 135
6.2 Contrast-Response Curves Obtained with Slits 140
6.3 The Extreme Contrast Sensitivity at the 18–19 Border 144
6.4 Influence of Contrast and Luminance on Other Response
    Properties 147
6.5 Conclusion 148

**Chapter 7   Coding of Spatial Parameters by Cat Visual Cortical
              Neurons: Influence of Stimulus Orientation, Length, Width,
              and Spatial Frequency** 149

7.1 Orientation Tuning of Cortical Cells 150

    7.1.1 Definitions and Criteria 150
    7.1.2 Quantitative Determinations: Orientation-Response Curves. 151
    7.1.3 Qualitative Determination: Hand-Plotting 155
    7.1.4 Distribution of Preferred Orientations 157
    7.1.5 Orientation Columns 158
    7.1.6 Conclusion 161

7.2 Influence of Stimulus Length on Cortical Cells 161
7.3 Selectivity of Cortical Neurons for Spatial Frequency and Stimulus
    Width 165

7.3.1   Selectivity for Spatial Frequency 165
7.3.2   Spatial Frequency and Coding of Stimulus Dimensions . 169
7.3.3   Linearity of Cortical Cells 173
7.3.4   The Visual Cortex as a Fourier Analyzer 178
7.3.5   Spatial Frequency: Conclusion 181

7.4   Spatial Parameters: Conclusion 183

Chapter 8   Coding of Spatio-Temporal Parameters by Cat Visual Cortical Neurons: Influence of Stimulus Velocity Direction and Amplitude of Movement 184

8.1   Influence of Stimulus Velocity 184
8.2   Influence of the Direction of Movement 201
8.3   Influence of Stimulus Movement Amplitude 215
8.4   Conclusion 215

Chapter 9   Binocular Interactions in Cat Visual Cortical Cells and Coding of Parameters Involved in Static and Dynamic Depth Perception 218

9.1   The Binocularity of Cortical Cells and the Ocular Dominance Scheme 218
9.2   Position Disparity Tuning Curves and the Coding of Static Depth   226
9.3   Orientation Disparity, Another Mechanism for Static Depth Discrimination? 235
9.4   Neuronal Mechanisms Underlying Dynamic Depth Perception (Motion in Depth) 239
9.5   Conclusion 243

Chapter 10   The Output of the Cat Visual Cortex 244

10.1 The Projections of Layer V to the Superior Colliculus, Pons, Pretectum, and Pulvinar-LP Complex 244
10.2 The Projections of Layer VI to the dLGN and the Claustrum . 248
10.3 The Commissural Projections 250
10.4 The Associative Corticocortical Projections 252
10.5 Conclusion 255

Chapter 11   Correlation Between Geniculate Afferents and Visual Cortical Response Properties in the Cat 256

11.1 Electrical Stimulation of the Visual Pathways 256
11.2 The Question of ON or OFF Cell Input to Cortical S Cells . . 261
11.3 Other Attempts to Identify the LGN Input to Cortical Cells . . 268
11.4 Conclusion 271

Chapter 12   Intracortical Mechanisms Underlying Properties of Cat Visual Cortical Cells 272

12.1   The Role of Intracortical Inhibition 272

    12.1.1 Orientation Selectivity 272
    12.1.2 Direction Selectivity 276
    12.1.3 End-Stopping 279
    12.1.4 Ocular Dominance 282
    12.1.5 Velocity Upper Cut-Off 282
    12.1.6 Absence of Response to Two-Dimensional Noise . . . 283

12.2   Properties of the Intracortical Inhibitions 284
12.3   The Structural Counterpart of Inhibitions 296
12.4   Conclusion 298

Chapter 13   Non-Visual Influences on Cat Visual Cortex 300

13.1   Non-Visual Sensory Inputs to the Visual Cortex 300
13.2   Influence of Eye Movements on Visual Cortical Cells 303
13.3   The Influence of Sleep and Anesthesia 306

Chapter 14   Response Properties of Monkey Striate Neurons 308

14.1   Retinotopic Organization of Area 17 308
14.2   The Input-Output Relations of Monkey Striate Cortex 311
14.3   Receptive Field Organization and Size 311
14.4   Color Specificity in Monkey Striate Cortex 315
14.5   Influence of Light Intensity and Contrast on Monkey Striate Neurons 318
14.6   Influence of Spatial Parameters 320
14.7   Influence of Spatio-Temporal Parameters 321
14.8   Ocular Dominance Distribution and Depth Sensitivity 322
14.9   Columnar Organization and Functional Architecture of Striate Cortex 325
14.10 Correlation Between Response Properties and Afferent Input . 327
14.11 Conclusion 330

Chapter 15   Conclusion: Signification of Visual Cortical Function in Perception 331

15.1   Operating Principles in Cat Visual Cortex 331

    15.1.1 Retinotopic Organization 331
    15.1.2 Filtering 331
    15.1.3 ”Columnar” Organization 332

15.1.4 Distributed Processing in the Primary Complex 334
15.1.5 Changes with Eccentricity 335
15.1.6 Parallel Streams Within each Area 337

15.2 The Cat and Monkey Visual Cortex as a Model: The Question
of the Relationship Between Animal Physiology and Human
Visual Perception 337
15.3 The Role of the Primary Visual Cortex in Visual Perception: The
Significance of Parameter Specificities for Object Recognition . 339

References 343

Subject Index 365

List of Abbreviations

AC	area centralis	mm	millimeter
AEV	anterior ectosylvian visual area	μ	micron
ALLS	anterolateral lateral suprasylvian area	ms	millisecond
		MT	middle temporal area (primates)
AMLS	anteromedial lateral suprasylvian area	NDS	non-direction selective (cell)
		N_2O	nitrous oxide
c	contrast	NPD	non-preferred direction
CC	corpus callosum	ON	optic nerve
c/deg	cycles per degree	OR	optic radiations
cd/m^2	candles per square meter	OT	optic tract
CR	contrast-response (curve)	OX	optic chiasm
CRZ	cortico-recipient part of pulvinar-LP complex in the cat	PD	preferred direction
		PLLS	posterolateral later suprasylvian area
D	dimension	PMLS	posteromedial lateral suprasylvian area
DA	direction asymmetric (cell)		
DE	dark edge	PRZ	pretecto-recipient part of pulvinar-LP complex in the cat
deg	degrees		
deg/s	degrees per second	PSTH	post or peristimulus time histogram
DI	direction index	REM	rapid eye movement
DLS	dorsal lateral suprasylvian area	RF	receptive field
DS	direction selective (cell)	RRZ	retino-recipient zone of pulvinar-LP complex in the cat
GAD	glutamate decarboxylase		
GABA	gamma aminobutyric acid	SC	superior colliculus
GW	geniculate wing	S/M ratio	ratio between responses to stationnary flashed and moving slits
HM	horizontal meridian		
HRP	horseradish peroxydase	TRZ	tecto-recipient zone of pulvinar LP complex in the cat
IP	inferior pulvinar of the monkey		
jnd	just noticeable difference	V1	visual 1 (area)
LE	light edge	V2	visual 2 (area)
LGN	lateral geniculate nucleus	V3	visual 3 (area)
LP	lateral posterior nucleus of the cat thalamus	VBB	velocity broad-band (cell)
		VHP	velocity high-pass (cell)
	lateral pulvinar of the monkey	VLP	velocity low-pass (cell)
LR	length-response (curve)	VLS	ventral lateral suprasylvian area
LS	lateral suprasylvian area	VM	vertical meridian
M	magnification factor	VR	velocity-response (curve)
MDI	mean direction index	VT	velocity tuned (cell)
MIN	medial interlaminar nucleus		

Introduction

This monograph is an attempt to summarize and to put into perspective single unit studies of the visual cortex. The time for such an undertaking seems to be appropriate. The initial version of this study was written during the year in which Hubel and Wiesel were awarded the Nobel prize in Medicine for their pioneering studies of the visual cortex, which triggered most if not all the studies reviewed in this monograph. The vast number of these studies witnesses the importance of Hubel and Wiesel's contribution. After an initial rapid development following the first reports of Hubel and Wiesel in the early sixties, the electrophysiology of visual cortex now seems to progress at a steady if slower pace. Much of this maturation is due to a better evaluation of the neurophysiological techniques. Although qualitative studies of visual cortical cells with hand-held stimuli can reveal their basic properties such as orientation and binocularity, a precise assessment of their characteristics is only possible with *quantitative methods* such as post-stimulus time histograms and multihistograms pioneered by Bishop and the Canberra group. The use of computer-controlled stimuli and quantitative techniques has also shifted the emphasis in the explanation of many of the cortical properties from excitatory processes to *inhibitory mechanisms*. The recent iontophoretic studies of Sillito and his co-workers fully support the notion that visual cortical processing is largely inhibitory in nature, as is the one in the cerebellar cortex.

The visual scientist who has recorded from the visual thalamic relay nucleus (the lateral geniculate nucleus) and the visual cortex cannot help but be struck by the relative simplicity of the response of geniculate cells compared to that of cortical cells. It is indeed a very peculiar experience to record large stable action potentials from a cortical cell but be unable to elicit a reliable response. It is, however, just as striking that once the appropriate stimulus conditions are found, the same cell will respond in a regular manner. Therefore in addition to a computer, one of the best allies on the physiologist's side in his struggle to unravel cortical systems is a plotting table and patience. This *selectivity of cortical cells* and their precise stimulus requirements have been given two different interpretations: cells have been described as *feature detectors* (i.e., capable detecting the presence of a very specific configuration in the input) and as *filters*. To understand the difference between these two notions one has to consider the two complementary aspects

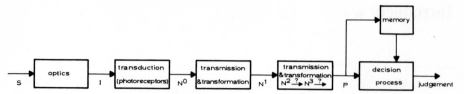

Fig. 0/1. Schematic model of a visual discrimination. S: stimulus; I: retinal image; Ni: neuronal representations at different levels; P: final neuronal representation.

of sensory information processing. Stimuli are first analyzed before a decision about the stimuli can be reached. These two steps are readily apparent in a flow diagram of visual processing in simple discrimination experiments in which the subject has to distinguish between two stimuli (Fig. 0/1). The stimuli are represented neuronally at different levels and a decision process acts on their final representation. These two steps can also be recognized in more complex tasks such as visual object recognition. According to Marr the visual scene is first represented as a primal sketch, a rich but primitive description of the scene. Different grouping algorithms are then performed on this representation in order to recognize the objects. In the psychophysical discrimination task as well as in the object recognition task, the second "synthetic" step supposes interactions between sensory processing and memory. Considering visual cortical cells as feature detectors means that the activity of a single cell identifies the presence of a given feature (e.g., an edge, a bar etc.). From this viewpoint visual cortical cells would then already be on the synthetic side of visual processing. Although Hubel and Wiesel never described cortical cells as edge or bar detectors, their reports on how the response of a simple cell could be predicted from its receptive field map, and on preferences of complex or hypercomplex cells for a particular edge or corner, paved the way for such an interpretation. Problems in connection with the view that cortical cells abstract features or seminaturalistic objects became readily apparent in the concept of the 'grandmother' cell.[1] An alternative view has developed from theories which consider the visual system as performing a Fourier-like analysis of the visual scene. Although it is unlikely that the visual system behaves as a Fourier analyser, these theories have stressed the importance of the decomposition of the visual scene by filtering. The particular parameter specificities of cortical cells enable them to act as filters[2] for different stimulus dimensions. From this viewpoint one of the major discoveries of Hubel and Wiesel is that cortical cells are filters for orientation. Also imbedded in theories of spatial frequency analysis is the

---

[1] The grandmother cell is the cell in the reader's visual cortex which identifies his (her) grandmother. Once this cell is lost, the reader would be unable to recognize his (her) grandmother.
[2] Used in a descriptive sense as in Regan (1982), see Chapter 5 for more elaboration on cortical cells as filters.

notion that an object is represented not by the activity of a single cell but by the distribution of activity *in a population of cells*. This is consistent with the observation that cortical cells discharge in response to any stimulus which shares the appropriate values of the parameters for which the cells are specific. From this alternative viewpoint cortical cells only represent visual objects and are still on the analytical side of sensory processing. Moreover, objects are only represented by their attributes and two objects can only be distinguished if they differ enough in at least one attribute to which the system is sensitive (i.e., for which it has filters). Recognition of the attribute of an object and even more so, recognition of the object itself, will always involve some combination of outputs of different filters (i.e., cells). The elegant work of Julesz, and of Ginsberg, has shown the power of spatial frequency filtering regarding the identification of stationary visual objects. Our own work suggests that the visual cortical cells may also be filters in the movement domain, direction and velocity possibly being the counterpart of orientation and spatial frequency in the spatial domain. Filtering in the velocity domain may well be as important for visual perception as spatial frequency filtering, especially in organisms which actively explore the visual scene.

Recent work on the cortical areas of all sensory systems has led to the discovery of *multiple representations* of peripheral receptor organs on the cortical surface. The work of Allman and Kaas in the owl monkey, of Zeki and Van Essen in the macaque and of Palmer, Rosenquist, and Tusa in the cat, has shown that there are numerous representations of the retina on the cerebral cortex (more than ten in each species). Such findings call for attention to visual areas other than area 17. In the cat, areas 17, 18, and 19 have been shown to contain only one retinal representation, while six representations have been described in the lateral suprasylvian area and two in each of areas 20 and 21. This monograph will deal primarily with areas 17, 18, and 19 of the cat which have recently been subjected to a comparative study in our laboratory. As will be argued in the second chapter, areas 17, 18, and 19 can be considered to be the *primary visual complex* of the cat. Comparison of neuronal properties in the 3 areas of the primary visual complex leads to the notion that there is a *distributed processing of visual information*, a conclusion also reached by Sprague and Berkley from behavioral studies of cats with lesions in these cortical areas.

The monograph will be divided into 4 unequal parts. In the first part, the visual system of cats and monkey will be compared, with particular emphasis on cortical representations. In addition, the position of areas 17, 18, and 19 among the visual cortical areas of the cat, as well as their retinotopic organization, will be described. In the second and largest part, the functional properties of cortical cells will be described using the cat as an experimental model. After a description of the receptive field organization of cortical cells, the principal parameters which the cortical cells filter will be described. In this description the differences between areas and changes with *eccentricity* will be stressed. In addition, the inputs to and the outputs from the visual cortex will be described, as well as the non-visual influences on cortical cells. The third part will be devoted to our knowledge of the mechanisms underlying the properties described in the second part. As far as possible, these "explanations" will not only be given in physiological, but also in neuro-anatomical and pharmacological terms. In the final section the properties of monkey visual cortical cells will be compared to those of their cat counter-parts and the relevance of these electrophysiological studies regarding the understanding of visual perception will be examined. Single unit studies are only one of the approaches to the study of vision and much can be learned from the confrontation of physiological data with behavioral and lesion studies. Indeed it is important to compare human and animal visual psycho-physics so as to decide to what extent the physiology of cat or monkey visual cortex can be of help in understanding normal and abnormal human vision.

Chapter 1. The Visual System of Cat and Monkey Compared

In this first chapter the visual system of the cat will be compared with that of two primates: the rhesus monkey (Macaca Mulatta), an Old World monkey, and the owl monkey (Aotus trivirgatus), a New World monkey. All these animals have frontally directed eyes with optical axes[1] that are nearly parallel. Primates (Fig. 1/1) have a large binocular visual field (130°–140° wide) (Allman, 1977). The cat is the non-primate with the largest binocular visual field (90–100°) (Allman, 1977; Hughes, 1977), for comparison the binocular field of the rabbit is only 30° wide.

Macaque Owl Monkey Cat

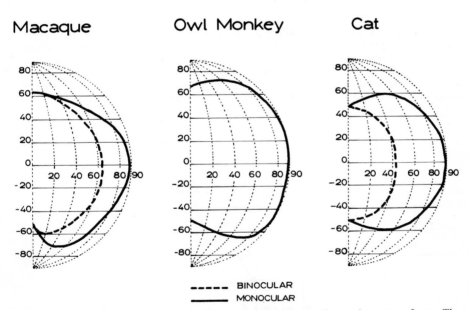

```
- - - - -  BINOCULAR
_____  MONOCULAR
```

Fig. 1/1. Visual hemifields in the three species compared. Zero indicates the center of gaze. The vertical through the center of gaze is the vertical meridian (VM) separating left and right hemifields. Numbers along the VM represent elevations (see Fig. 1/2) in degrees. The horizontal through the center of gaze is the horizontal meridian (HM). Numbers along the HM indicate azimuths (see Fig. 1/2). Macaque and cat data are from Bishop (1983). Owl monkey visual field has been estimated from the most peripheral receptive fields in V1 reported by Allman and Kaas (1971b).

---

[1] The optical axis of the eye is the line passing through the centers of rotation of the refractive optical media of the eye, the cornea, and the lens (Polyak, 1941).

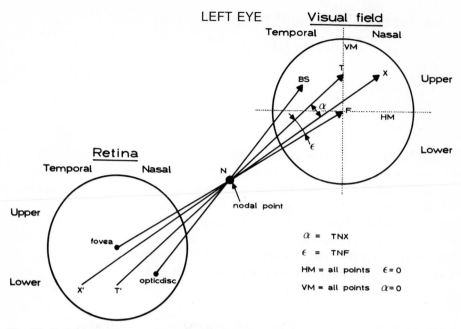

Fig. 1/2. Definition of the visual field coordinates (spherical polar scheme): azimuth and elevation. The fixation point (or center of gaze) is the point in the visual field projecting onto the fovea
(or area centralis) and the blind spot projects onto the optic disc (origin of the optic nerve). An
arbitrary point X in the visual field forms a retinal image in X'. Its position is defined by its
azimuth (α) and elevation (ε). Both are expressed in degrees of visual angle. The HM is the locus
where elevation is zero and the VM corresponds to all points with zero azimuth.

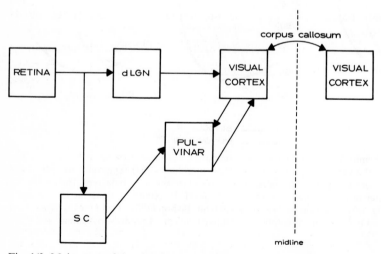

Fig. 1/3. Main parts of the visual system of higher mammals. dLGN: dorsal lateral geniculate
nucleus; SC: superior colliculus.

In the first part of this chapter it will be shown that the basic layout of the visual system is similar in the three species, although a number of important differences exist. In the second part the quantitative aspects of the retinogeniculo-striate projection, the main path from the eyes to the visual cortex (Fig. 1/3), will be described.

1.1 The Basic Layout of the Visual System in Cat, Owl Monkey, and Rhesus Monkey

1.1.1 The Retina

All three species have a duplex retina, containing a *mixture of rods and cones*. The more light sensitive rods subserve scotopic[2] vision while the cones subserve photopic vision. The owl monkey has a much larger rod/cone ratio than the rhesus monkey in agreement with their different life habit. While the owl monkey is a nocturnal animal, the macaque is a diurnal one. The rhesus monkey has three types of cones sensitive to different wavelengths, making it a trichomat with color vision similar to ours (De Valois et al., 1974 a). It was believed that the cat had only two types of cones with a maximum sensitivity at 556 and 450 nm respectively (Daw and Pearlman, 1969). Recent recordings from ganglion cells have provided evidence for a third type of cone with a maximum sensitivity at 500 nm (see Sterling, 1983 for review). It has however been shown that color vision in the cat is extremely reduced (see Hammond, 1978 for review). The owl monkey also has a rudimentary color vision. This species can however formally be classified as protanomolous trichromat (Jacobs, 1977 a).

All three species share the important feature of a central portion of the retina that contains *the maximum density of receptors and ganglion cells*[3] (Fig. 1/4 and 1/5). As a consequence most neural representations of the visual field in all three species have a disproportionally large part of these neural maps devoted to the central portion of the visual field. In all three species there is a clear increase in soma size of the ganglion cells with distance from

---

[2] Scotopic vision: vision under low background illumination, for man (assuming standard pupil size) $< 3.10^{-5}$ cd/m^2, for cat (assuming 1 mm^2 pupil) $< 5.10^{-1}$ cd/m^2 (Enroth-Cugell et al., 1977).
Photopic vision: vision under high background illumination for man (assuming standard pupil size) > 3 cd/m^2, for cat (assuming 1 mm^2 pupil) $> 2.10^2$ cd/m^2 (Enroth-Cugell et al., 1977).
[3] This point of maximal density corresponds to the fovea (depression in the retina due to absence of ganglion cells and inner plexiform layer) in the macaque and in the owl monkey (the depression in the owl monkey being quite variable), and to the area centralis (no depression but characteristic absence of retinal vessels) in the cat (Polyak, 1957; Rowe and Dreher, 1982).

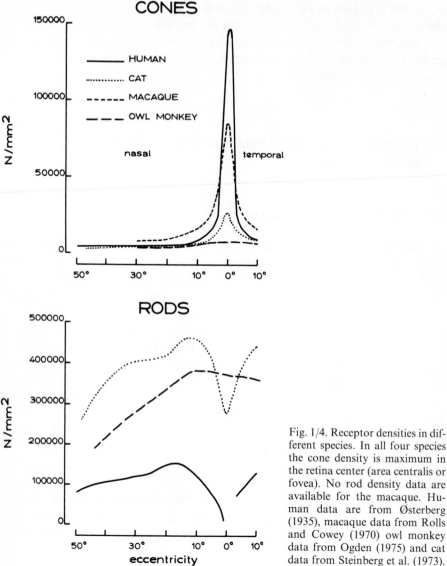

Fig. 1/4. Receptor densities in different species. In all four species the cone density is maximum in the retina center (area centralis or fovea). No rod density data are available for the macaque. Human data are from Østerberg (1935), macaque data from Rolls and Cowey (1970) owl monkey data from Ogden (1975) and cat data from Steinberg et al. (1973).

the area centralis or fovea (Stone, 1965, Webb and Kaas, 1976; Stone and Johnston, 1981). These changes are steeper in the macaque than in the other two species, probably due to larger packing density in the center of the retina (Fig. 1/6).

The ganglion cells, from which the axons project into the optic nerve, represent the output of the retina. In the cat the existence of *different functional classes* of ganglion cells has been clearly demonstrated (Enroth-Cugell and Robson, 1966; Cleland et al., 1971; Wilson et al., 1976). These classes will

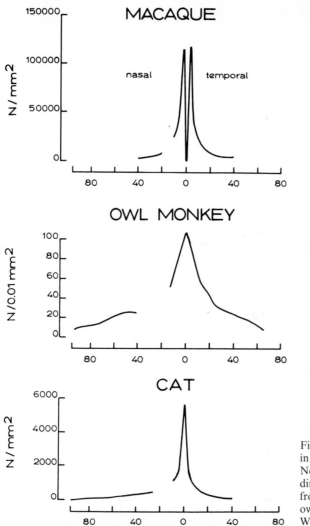

Fig. 1/5. Ganglion cell densities in the three species compared. Note the scale difference in ordinate. Macaque estimates are from Rolls and Cowey (1970), owl monkey estimates from Webb and Kaas (1976) and cat estimates from Stone (1965).

be described in more detail in Chapter 3. There is a correlation between the functional classes (X, Y, W)[4] and the three morphological types (α, β & γ)

---

[4] The terms X and Y cells were introduced by Enroth-Cugell and Robson (1966), who used "linearity of spatial summation" as criterion distinguishing between retinal X cells (linear) and Y cells (non-linear). Cleland et al. (1971), also studying retinal ganglion cells, introduced a different set of criteria and accordingly used a different terminology: sustained and transient cells. However in their study of LGN cells Hoffmann et al. (1972) used a set of criteria somewhat similar to that of Cleland et al. (1971), yet used the terminology of Enroth-Cugell and Robson (X and Y cells). Upon discovery of a third type of retinal ganglion cells these cells were called W cells by Stone and his coworkers (Stone and Hoffmann, 1972; Wilson et al., 1976), and sluggish cells by Cleland and Levick (1974a). The latter authors then renamed their sustained and transient cells, brisk sustained and brisk transient cells (see Chapter 3).

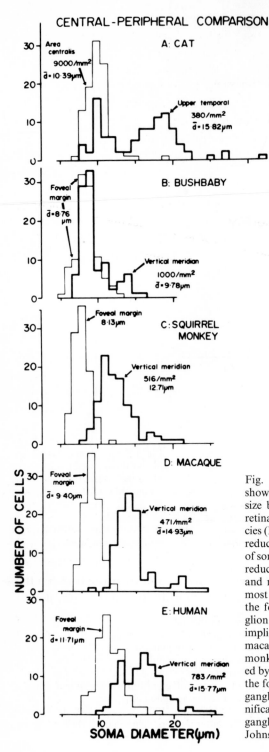

Fig. 1/6. Frequency/soma size histograms showing the difference in ganglion cell soma size between central and peripheral areas of retina in the cat (A) and in four primate species (B–E). In all four species there is a marked reduction in mean soma size, and in the range of soma size, at the area or fovea centralis. The reduction seems more marked in the primates, and most marked in the macaque, in which most of the cells identified as ganglion cells at the fovea are smaller than the smallest ganglion cells identified in peripheral retina. This implies that all classes of ganglion cells in the macaque retina, and probably in the squirrel monkey and human retinas as well, are affected by the packing constraint which operates at the fovea. In the cat, by contrast, the smallest ganglion cells at the area centralis are not significantly smaller than the smallest peripheral ganglion cell. With permission from Stone and Johnston (1981).

of Boycott and Wässle (1974). The correlation is excellent for Y-α, reasonably good for X-β and weak for W-γ. Similarly 3 functional classes have been described in the retina of the rhesus monkey (Gouras, 1969; De Monasterio and Gouras, 1975; De Monasterio, 1978; Schiller and Malpeli, 1977). Morphological correlates of some of these classes have been reported (Perry and Cowey, 1981). According to the recent work of these authors, 80% of the macaque ganglion cells are Pβ cells (resembling β cells of the cat) which project chiefly to the parvocellular layer of the LGN, and 10% are Pα cells (resembling α cells of the cat) which project mainly to the magnocellular layers of the LGN). The remaining ganglion cells are probably Pγ cells (resembling γ cells of cat, about 9–10%) which apparently only project to the midbrain (Perry and Cowey, 1983). Direct evidence for different functional classes of ganglion cells in owl monkey retina is still lacking. But in the view of the report of Sherman et al. (1976) on X and Y cells in the LGN of owl monkey it is likely that different functional classes exist among the owl monkey ganglion cells.

1.1.2 The Optic Chiasm and Optic Tract

In all three species there is a *partial decussation* of optic tract fibers: the fibers from the nasal retina cross the midline while those from the temporal retina do not.[5] Consequently the dorsal lateral geniculate nucleus (dLGN) of monkeys and cat receives a *topographic* projection[6] from the *contralateral* visual hemifield through both eyes (Fig. 1/8). There is however an important difference between primates and non-primates with respect to the retinal input into the superior colliculus (SC). In primates the optic tract fibers innervating the SC originate from the ipsilateral temporal retina and the contralateral nasal retina, resulting in a projection of the contralateral hemifield onto the SC. In the cat, as in all other non-primates (Allman, 1977), the SC receives input from the contralateral temporal and nasal hemiretinae, resulting in a projection of the whole visual field of the contralateral eye onto the SC[7] (Fig. 1/8). The proportion of optic tract fibers projecting to the LGN and SC is also different in primates and in the cat. In the cat about 50% of

---

[5] In lower species the optic fibers decussate completely, while in the cat at least some of the axons of γ cells still follow that pattern: same γ axons arising in the temporal retina do cross over (see Chapter 3).

[6] Topographic projection means that neighbouring LGN loci receive input from neighbouring retinal loci corresponding to neighbouring visual field loci (due to the lens the order of loci on the retina is the reverse from that in the visual field). This organization is called retino- or visuotopic organization (Fig. 1/7).

[7] In the cat the medial interlaminar nucleus (MIN), part of the LGN, also receives input from the contralateral nasal and temporal hemiretinae (see Chapter 3) and resembles in that respect the SC.

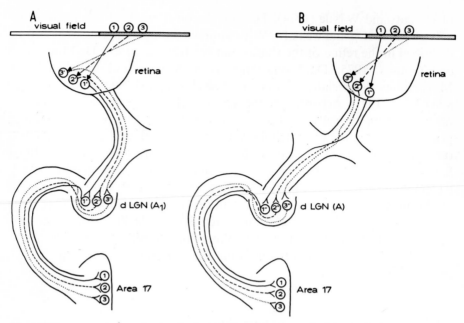

Fig. 1/7. Topographic organization in the visual cortex (first order transformation): A. projections from ipsilateral eye; B. projections from contralateral eye. Three neighbouring cells in the visual cortex (labelled 1, 2, 3) are connected to 3 neighbouring cells in the dLGN and indirectly to 3 neighbouring ganglion cells in each eye. Spatial sequences of cells in the cortex correspond to spatial sequences in the retina and hence in the visual field.

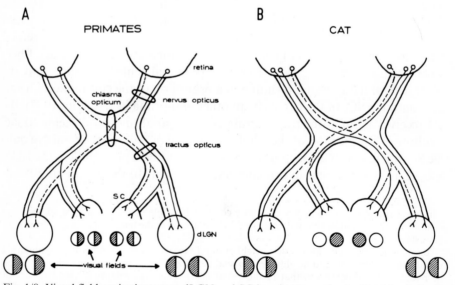

Fig. 1/8. Visual field projections onto dLGN and SC in primates and cats. Hatching indicates the part of the visual field represented in a nucleus. While in primates the contralateral hemifields of both eyes are represented in each SC, in cats the whole contralateral visual field is represented.

the retinal fibers project to SC (Wässle and Illing, 1980) while 10% do so in the macaque (Bunt et al., 1975). For comparison it is interesting to note that in the rabbit 100% of the retinal fibers project to the SC (Vaney et al., 1981).

There is a narrow vertical strip of retina passing through the area centralis or fovea which projects to the LGN *on both sides* and hence to both cortical hemispheres in cat (Stone, 1966; Leicester, 1968; Sanderson and Sherman, 1971, Illing and Wässle, 1981) and monkey (Stone et al., 1973; Bunt et al., 1977). The strip is narrower in the monkey (1° wide) than in the cat (2° wide). Consequently, in addition to a complete representation of the contralateral half of the visual field, the LGN and visual cortex also contain a representation of a narrow strip of the ipsilateral visual field adjoining the VM. It has been suggested (Blakemore, 1970) that this strip of naso-temporal overlap is important for binocular vision, ensuring that the neurons receiving projections from the fixation point, have neighbours connected to visual field loci adjoining the fixation point on both sides.

1.1.3 The Dorsal Lateral Geniculate Nucleus (dLGN)

In all three species the dorsal LGN is a *laminated* structure receiving afferents subserving the contralateral hemifield in a topographic fashion. The lamination pattern of the dLGN in cats and primates is different. The dLGN of the cat has 6 layers: 3 main layers (A, A1, & C) and three smaller ventral layers (C_{1-3}). This organization will be described in detail in Chapter 3. Suffice it to say that each layer, except C_3, receives afferents from one eye: A, C, and C_2 from the contralateral eye and A1 and C_1 from the ipsilateral eye (Fig. 3/1). Kaas et al. (1978) have suggested that the basic primate pattern of geniculate lamination consists of two parvocellular layers, two magnocellular layers, and two poorly developed and highly variable superficial layers which are ventrally located (Fig. 1/9). In the macaque the 2 parvocellular layers subdivide and interdigitate into 4 leaflets so as to give the appearance of 4 parvocellular layers. In the owl monkey the parvocellular layers are much less developed. The layers form pairs similar in cell types but different in ocular input.

In all three species each of the geniculate laminae receives a topographic projection from an hemiretina and projects to the cerebral cortex (see Fig. 1/10). The relay laminae are stacked in *visuotopic register* so that there is a direct continuity in visual field representation between adjacent laminae receiving input from different eyes. This organization, in which a column of cells orthogonal to the laminae represent one point in space seen through both eyes, has been called a projection column (Sanderson, 1971 b). The precise visuotopic alignment of input from both retinae is an important step toward binocular integration of visual input (Bishop, 1983, Allman, 1977).

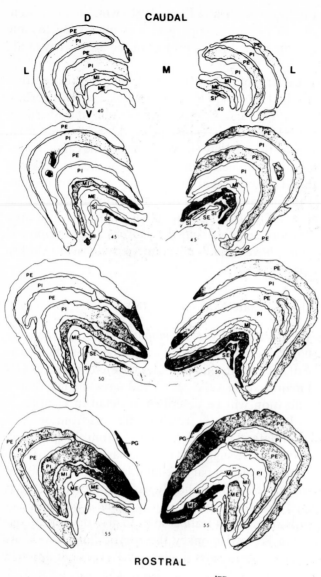

RHESUS 14   Fig. 1/9 A

Fig. 1/9. Lamination in the dorsal LGN of primates: series of line drawings illustrating the location of transported protein (dark stippled areas) within the dLGN of a rhesus monkey (A) and of a owl monkey (B) following intraocular injection of H³-proline. The brains were sectioned in the frontal plane. Ipsi and contra indicate ipsilateral and contralateral LGN with respect to the side of injection. Abbreviations: D dorsal, V ventral, L lateral, M medial; Ipm interlaminar zone between parvo and magnocellular layers; Ims interlaminar zone between magnocellular and superficial layers. PE external parvocellular layer; PI internal parvocellular layer; ME external magnocellular layer; MI internal magnocellular layer; SE external superficial layer; SI internal superficial layer; PG perigeniculate nucleus. With permission from Kaas et al. (1978).

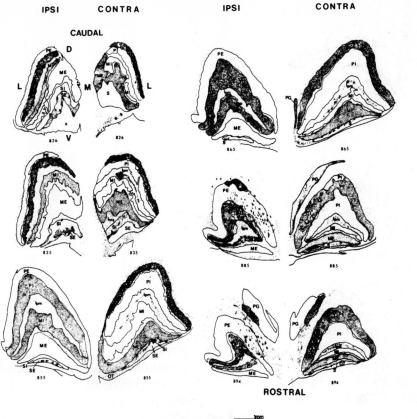

OWL MONKEY 74-79   Fig. 1/9. B

There is a distinct possibility that in all three species there is a correlation *between layers and functional types of cells.* In the cat the same three functional types can be distinguished among LGN cells and among ganglion cells (Cleland et al., 1971; Hoffmann et al., 1972; Wilson et al., 1976). As will be shown in Chapter 3 there is a good correlation between layers and functional types in the cat LGN. In rhesus monkey and owl monkey X- and Y-like cells have been described in the LGN (Dreher et al., 1976; Sherman et al., 1976; Kaplan and Shapley, 1982; Marrocco et al., 1982). Up to now there has been no agreement about the correlation between functional classes and layers in the rhesus monkey. Those who use linearity of spatial summation (Enroth-Cugell and Robson, 1966) as the main distinguishing feature between X and Y cells, consider that both X (linearly summating) and Y (non-linearly summating) cells occur in the magnocellular layers while all parvocellular cells are X cells (Kaplan and Shapley, 1982). Others have used the combination of criteria put forward by Hoffmann et al. (1972) (velocity sensitivity, conduc-

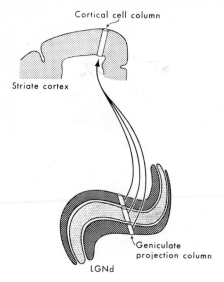

Cortical cell column

Striate cortex

Geniculate
projection column

LGNd

Fig. 1/10. Diagram showing the relationship between projection columns in the dLGN and the visual cortex. With permission from Sanderson (1971 b).

tion velocity, and RF size) to distinguish between X, Y, and W cells and have found a correlation between X- and Y-like cells and parvo- and magnocellular layers (Dreher et al., 1976). A possible explanation for these discrepancies has been suggested by Norton and Casagrande (1982): in bush-baby (a prosimian) Y cells distinguished by the set of 3 criteria of Hoffmann et al. (1972) mentioned above could be either linear or non-linear. In Norton and Casagrande's view non-linearity is due to non-linear subunits in the RF surround (probably due to some amacrine input in the retina) and is separate from other properties such as velocity sensitivity, RF size, or conduction velocity, which may be explained by morphological factors such as axon size and spread of dendritic tree. It so happens that in the species that was first studied (cat) the 2 classes of ganglion or geniculate cells from which one can record most easily (X and Y cells) could just as well be differentiated by linearity of spatial summation, as by the set of 3 criteria of Hoffmann et al. (1972), and that both classifications correlated well (Bullier and Norton, 1979 a). However, this correlation does not hold for the third type of ganglion and geniculate cells of the cat (W cells), which can be either linear or non-linear (Sur and Sherman, 1982; Levick and Thibos, 1980). Apparently, in primates this correlation falls apart for all types of cells. Another possibility is that while the magnocellular LGN cells of the rhesus monkey are comparable to cat LGN cells, and hence readily fit into the X and Y categories, the parvocellular LGN cells are quite different from cat LGN cells as indicated by their low contrast sensitivity (Kaplan and Shapley, 1982) and their color specificity.

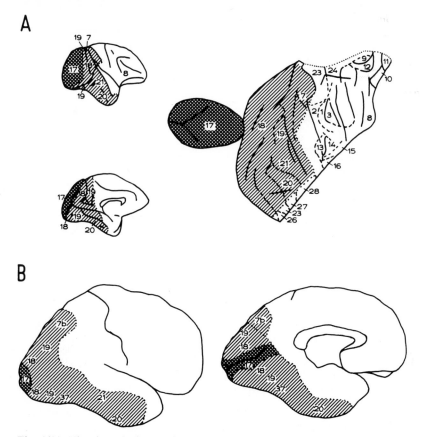

Fig. 1/11. Visual cortical areas in macaque (A) and human (B) compared. Heavy hatching indicates the primary visual cortex (area 17), light hatching the other visual cortical areas. In A the visual areas are indicated on a lateral and medial view of the hemisphere as well as on a flattened map (Van Essen and Maunsell, 1980). In B only a lateral and medial view of the hemisphere are shown. Area 37 was included among visual cortical areas following Iwai and Mishkin (1969) who demonstrated visual input to the transitional area between parietal and temporal cortex that can be considered as a precursor to area 37 in higher primates (Petr et al., 1949). Although the surface of area 17 in humans (2613 mm² – Filiminoff, 1932) is much larger than that in macaque (841 mm² – Colonnier and O'Kusky, 1981), proportionally the human striate cortex represents only 2.5% of the hemisphere (Van Economo, 1929), while the macaque striate cortex represents 10% (Popoff, 1929) or 17% (Van Essen and Maunsell, 1980). Overall all visual cortical areas represent 60% of an hemisphere in the macaque according to Van Essen and Maunsell (1980).

1.1.4 Visual Cortex (Fig. 1/11)

Following the pioneering studies of Allman and Kaas in the owl monkey (1971 a, b, 1974 a, b, 1975, 1976) it has been shown for all three species that there are *multiple representations of the retina on the cerebral surface*

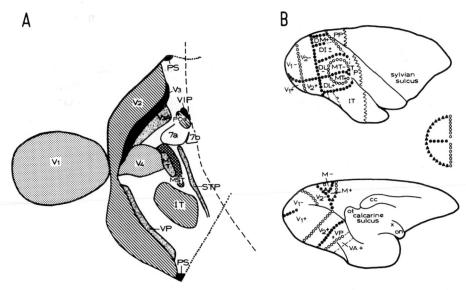

Fig. 1/12. Multiple visual cortical maps in the macaque (A) and owl monkey (B). In A the different visual cortical areas of the macaque are indicated on an unfolded cortical map (Van Essen, personal communication). In addition to V1, 13 other visual field representations have been reported. V2, V3, V4: second, third and fourth visual area; VP ventral posterior area; PS prostriate area; IT inferotemporal cortex; MT middle temporal area; MST middle superior temporal area; STP superior temporo-parietal cortex; PO parieto-occipital cortex; VIP: ventral inferior parietal cortex. In B the visual cortical maps in the owl monkey are represented in a dorsolateral (top) and ventromedial (bottom) view of the hemisphere (Newsome and Allman, 1980). The visual field symbols on the perimeter chart are superimposed on the cerebral cortex to illustrate the representation of the visual field in the individual areas. The open circles symbolize representation of the VM, filled circles denote representation of the HM, and the filled triangles locate representations of the periphery of the visual field. Pluses symbolize the upper visual field and minuses the lower field. Dashed lines are borders where visual field locations are represented other than the ones which are illustrated by the symbols on the perimeter chart. The row of V's on the dorsolateral view represents the approximate anterior border of the visual cortex and dotted lines broken by question marks are uncertain borders. For abbreviations see A, except PP posterior parietal cortex; DM dorsomedial and DI dorsointermediate area; DL dorsolateral crescent; M medial area; VA ventral anterior area; cc corpus callosum, on optic nerve, ot optic tract.

(Fig. 1/12). In addition to electrophysiological mapping techniques, other methods have been used to distinguish between different neural maps: cyto- or myeloarchitectonic features, e.g., the heavy myelination of areas 18 in the cat (Hubel and Wiesel, 1965) and of MT in the owl monkey (Allman and Kaas, 1971 a) and in the macaque (Van Essen et al., 1981), differences in input-output relationships (Tusa and Palmer, 1980), and patterns of termination of callosal afferents which correspond to vertical meridian projections and separate retinal representations (Zeki, 1970, Newsome and Allman, 1980). These studies have led to estimations that in the macaque 60% of the cerebral cortex processes visual information compared to 30% in the cat

(Van Essen and Maunsell, 1980). In the owl monkey the maps recently published by Newsome and Allman (1980) allow us to estimate the visual part of the cerebral cortex to be about 40%.

The full extent of the visual cortex is thus much larger than the primary visual cortex, which is defined as that part of the cortex receiving direct input from dLGN. In primates, the striate cortex or area 17 is the primary visual cortex (although a scant projection from LGN to prestriate cortex seems to exist, Yukie and Iwai, 1981; Benevento and Yoshida, 1981; Bullier and Kennedy, 1983) and contains a single, complete representation of the visual field (V1). Thus, in primates all 4 terms (primary visual cortex, area 17, striate cortex, and V1) are synonymous. In cat LGN projections are more wide spread. dLGN projects to areas 18 and 19 in addition to area 17 (Garey et al., 1968; Niimi and Sprague, 1970). As will be argued in Chapter 2, areas 17 (or striate cortex) 18, and 19, which each contain a representation of the visual field (V1, V2 and V3 respectively), represent a complex of 3 primary visual areas. In the cat in addition to V1, V2, and V3, 6 representations (AMLS, ALLS, PMLS, PLLS, VLS, DLS) have been described in the lateral suprasylvian sulcus by Palmer et al. (1978), 2 representations in area 20 (20 a, b) and 2 in area 21 (21 a, b) by Tusa and Palmer (1980), and one representation in the anterior ectosylvian sulcus by Olson and Graybiel (1981) and Mucke et al. (1982). Those maps will be considered in more detail in Chapter 2. In the owl monkey, Allman and Kaas have described 6 representations of the visual field in front of V1 [8]: V2 corresponding to area 18, and MT, DL, DI, DM, M all contained within area 19 (Fig. 1/12). There are hints (Allman and Kaas, unpublished quoted in Newsome and Allman, 1980) of 5 additional regions (VA, VP, PP, TP, IT) in this species. Similarly Zeki (1969), Van Essen and Zeki (1978), and Van Essen and colleagues (1980 a, b, 1981) have described several visual field representations anterior to V1 of the macaque (V2, V3, V3A, V4, VP, MT, MST, IT). In the macaque both areas 18 and 19 contain several representations (see Fig. 1/12). There is no reason to believe that in any of the 3 species the list of representations is closed.

With these different maps the representation of the visual field can be qualitatively and/or quantitatively different : there can be different orders of transformation of the visual hemifield (qualitative difference), the extent of the visual hemifield represented can differ and the disproportionate representation of the central portion of the visual field can be more or less accentuated (quantitative differences). Allman and Kaas (1974a) have distinguished between *first and second order transformation of the visual hemifield.* In the first order transformation neighbouring points on the hemiretina (and hence in the visual hemifield) project onto neighbouring points of the cortex (Fig. 1/7). The only distortion of the perimeter chart is that its representation

---

[8] All visual cortical areas in front of V1 are referred to as extrastriate areas.

is twisted and that portions are magnified. These first order transformations are typical of the dLGN and V1 in each of the three species (Tusa et al., 1978; Allman and Kaas, 1971 b; Van Essen, personal communication). They also occur in MT of owl monkey and possibly of the rhesus monkey (Allman and Kaas, 1971 a; Van Essen et al., 1981) and in AMLS, ALLS and 20a of the cat (Palmer et al., 1978; Tusa and Palmer, 1980). In the second order transformation of the visual field (Allman and Kaas, 1974 a) there is still a point to point projection but adjacent points in the hemiretina do not always project to adjacent points on the cortex. This transformation is typical for V2 of primates where there is a split representation of the horizontal meridian (Allman and Kaas, 1974 a; Allman, 1977). It also occurs in DL of the owl monkey, the pair of areas MT-DL being considered by Allman (1977) to be analogue with the pair V1–V2 (each pair having a disproportionately large representation of the vertical meridian as a border between its elements). A second order transformation seems also to be present in areas 18 and 19 of the cat. The second order transformation has been called field discontinuity by Van Essen et al. (1981). These authors described other types of irregularities (as map discontinuities, mosaic and repetitive representations) for which up to now there is no strong supportive evidence in the visual areas, although these irregularities have been demonstrated in somatosensory maps or cerebellar maps. In addition to first and second order transformations, which are both point to point projections, Palmer et al. (1978) have defined point to line projections (in DLS, VLS) and mixed projections in which both point to point and point to line projections occur (in PMLS, PLLS). Tusa and Palmer (1980) have shown that areas 20 b, 21 a, and 21 b all contain mixed types of transformation.

The *overrepresentation*[9] of the central portion of the visual field varies largely among the different maps. In V1 there is a large overrepresentation of the central visual field which is more accentuated in primates than in cats. It has been claimed that in the macaque 90% of the V1 is devoted to the central 10° of the visual field[10] compared to 50% in the cat (Tusa et al., 1978). A strong overrepresentation of the central visual field is also found in V2 and V3 of the cat (Albus and Beckmann, 1980) and MT of the macaque (Gattass and Gross, 1981). Among different areas within the same region the proportion of the area devoted to central versus peripheral parts of the visual field can differ widely: e.g. while 75% of DL in the owl monkey is devoted to the visual field within 10° of the center only 4% of the neighbouring area M is devoted to this part of the visual field (Allman and Kaas, 1976).

---

[9] Overrepresentation means that equal areas of the visual field project to unequal volumes of a neuronal structure: the central portion projects to a larger volume than an equally sized portion of the periphery of the visual field.
[10] According to more recent data from Van Essen and co-workers (personal communication), the overrepresentation of the central visual field in the macaque would be less than indicated by Tusa et al. (1978): 80% of V1 devoted to the central 20° of the visual field.

Similarly in AMLS and ALLS of the cat the representation of the central part of the visual field is much smaller than in the other 4 suprasylvian areas (Palmer et al., 1978).

An important question concerns the input-output relationship between the different cortical visual representations. This question is far from being resolved, but it seems clear that both *serial and parallel* processing occurs between the different areas. In monkeys where only V1 receives geniculate afferents (if one excepts scant afferents from interlaminar zones of the LGN to prestriate cortex, Benevento and Yoshida, 1981; Bullier and Kennedy, 1983) all the other areas can be considered secondary areas, i.e. their principal visual input is relayed through area 17. Distinction of different higher levels can be based on different criteria. Van Essen (1979) has argued that in the macaque one can distinguish between second, third and fourth level areas depending on whether they receive input exclusively from V1 (second level: V2), partially from V1 and other areas (third level: V3 and MT) or little or no input from V1 (fourth level: V4 and V3A). Recent anatomical data (Van Essen, personal communication) clearly suggest that not only areas at the same level (as V4 and V3A) but also areas at different levels (as V4 and MT) could operate in parallel. Allman and Kaas have used similar criteria to distinguish levels of processing in the owl monkey. In the cat the situation is less clear. I will argue in the next chapter that while areas 17, 18, and 19 represent a first level, the lateral suprasylvian areas represent a second level, areas 20 and 21 representing possibly a third level and the anterior ectosylvian area a fourth level.

1.1.5 Pulvinar

In all three species (cat, owl monkey and rhesus monkey) there is in addition to the dLGN, *another part of the thalamus* that is visual and includes parts or the whole of the pulvinar and (at least in the cat) parts of the nucleus lateralis posterior. This second visual part of the thalamus, abbreviated here to visual pulvinar complex, occupies a similar position in the visual system of all 3 species. On the one hand it is a link between the superior colliculus (SC) and the visual cortex, providing a second route from the retina to the cerebral cortex, and on the other hand it is a link between visual cortical areas, chiefly between area 17 and more anteriorly located visual areas, supplementing the intracortical connections between visual areas.

In the *macaque* (Fig. 1/13) the two main visual parts of the pulvinar are the inferior pulvinar (IP) and the ventral lateral pulvinar (LPα). Both project to area 17 (Rezak and Benevento, 1979) and receive input from occipital cortex (cortico-recipient) (Ogren and Hendrickson, 1976; Benevento and Davis, 1977). IP in addition receives input from SC (tecto-recipient) (Bene-

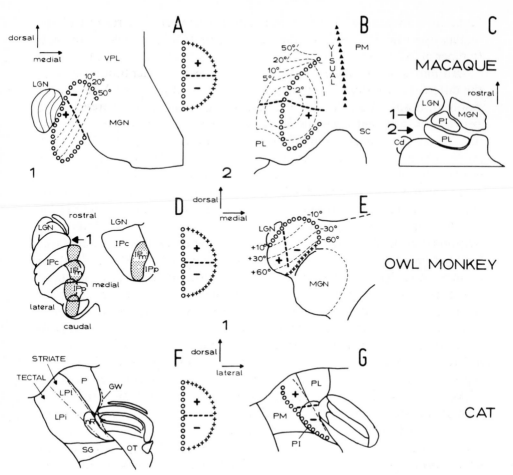

Fig. 1/13. Subdivision of the pulvinar complex of the 3 species. The visual field symbols on the perimeter chart are superimposed on the pulvinar sections to illustrate the visual field representation in the different parts: open circles denote the VM representation, crosses and minuses indicate the periphery of the visual field and the HM representation respectively. In A, B and C illustration of the two visual field representations described by Bender (1981) in the pulvinar of the macaque. The level of the frontal sections 1 and 2 is indicated in the diagram in C (PI inferior pulvinar, PL lateral pulvinar). The inferior map is present in A and B, the lateral map only in B. In D can be seen the division of the inferior pulvinar complex of the owl monkey according to Lin and Kaas (1979) on frontal sections and a dorsal view. IPc central nucleus of inferior pulvinar (IP); IPm, medial nucleus of inferior pulvinar; IPp posterior nucleus of inferior pulvinar. E shows retinotopic organization of IP proposed by Allman et al. (1972) which corresponds according to Lin and Kaas (1979) to a map within IPc (at the level indicated by 1 in D). In F: the 4 divisions of the pulvinar - lateralis posterior complex in the cat: the geniculate wing (Gw), the pulvinar (P), the lateral lateralis posterior (LPl) including the nucleus of Rioch (NR) and the intermediate lateralis posterior (LPi). (SG: suprageniculate nucleus, OT optic tract). The LPl receives striate input, while tectal fibers project to the LPi. In G the visual field representation within LPl is illustrated. In this figure the alternative nomenclature of Niimi and Kuwahara (1973) is indicated: PL = lateral pulvinar (equivalent to Pulvinar in F), PM: medial pulvinar corresponding to lateralis posterior in F and PI: inferior pulvinar corresponding to the nucleus of Rioch. Modified with permission from Bender (1981), Lin and Kaas (1979) and Mason (1978).

vento and Fallon, 1975). These two anatomically defined regions of the pulvinar correspond, although not perfectly, to two visual field representations (Bender, 1981). The map in IP (and the medial part of LPα) is a first order transformation while the map in LPα is a second order transformation, the border between both maps being a representation of the VM. This is another example of a pair of representations sharing the VM representation as border where the second order transformation wraps around the first order transformation. It is possible that other parts of the lateral pulvinar (LPβ and LPγ) which do not project to area 17, are visual since they project to parietal cortex (area 7) and inferotemporal cortex respectively.

In the *owl monkey* Lin and Kaas (1979) have subdivided the inferior pulvinar complex into 3 nuclei (Fig. 1/13) on the basis of cyto- and myeloarchitectonic characteristics and patterns of afferent connections: central IP, medial IP, and posterior IP nuclei. Medial and central IP are cortico-recipient (from areas V1, V2, DM, M, PP and MT) while posterior and central IP are tecto-recipient. The projections from MT are much heavier to medial than to central IP and the projections from SC are much denser to posterior than to central IP. These authors also suggest that each of these subdivisions contain a separate map of the contralateral hemifield. These nuclei all project back to the visual cortex, and although details are not yet worked out each seems to have its own separate cortical termination region e.g. medial IP projects to MT (Lin et al., 1974).

While in monkeys the visual pulvinar complex only includes parts of the pulvinar nucleus which is a large nuclear mass, the visual pulvinar complex of the *cat* includes, in addition to the much smaller pulvinar, parts of the lateralis posterior (LP). This complex has been divided by Graybiel and Berson (1980) mediolaterally into 4 parallel strips (Fig. 1/13) receiving different inputs: (1) the lateral fringe of the pulvinar which receives retinal afferents (retino-recipient zone) and is considered by some authors as part of the dLGN complex (geniculate wing of Guillery et al. 1980) (2) the pulvinar which receives input from the pretectum and projects mainly to area 19 (3) the lateral LP (including the nucleus posterior nucleus of Rioch) receiving occipital afferents (cortico-recipient) and projecting back to area 17, 18 and 19 and (4) the intermediate LP receiving SC afferents (tecto-recipient zone) and projecting chiefly to lateral suprasylvian areas (see Chapter 3).

1.1.6 Callosal Connections

In all three species callosal inputs terminate predominantly in cortical regions *where the vertical meridian is represented* (Shatz, 1977 c; Newsome and Allman, 1980, Zeki, 1970). This property has been used extensively by Van Essen and Zeki (1978) and Van Essen et al. (1982) to trace borders

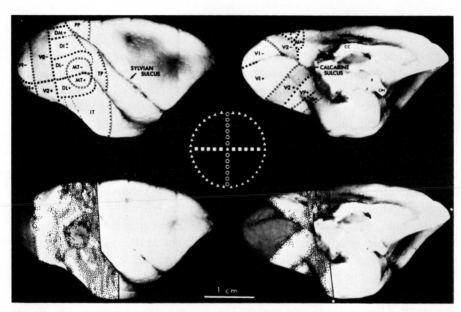

Fig. 1/14. Two dorsolateral and ventromedial views of the hemisphere of an owl monkey. Top
views illustrate the topographic organization of the visual cortex, see Fig. 1/12. The bottom
figures show the pattern of callosal degeneration over the expanse of the cortex for which the
retinotopic organization is shown in the top views. The striated area at the occipital pole is the
striate cortex (V1), the shaded area on the lateral surface in extrastriate cortex is MT. The large
dots signify heavy and moderate degeneration, and the small dots denote light degeneration. The
solid block lines show the anterior extent of the reconstruction. Note the discrete band of
degeneration at the V1–V2 border and at the VA–VP border as well as the thickening of
degeneration at the MT border (Allman, personal communication).

between different visual maps within areas 18 and 19 of the macaque. In all
three species the correspondence between callosal input and vertical meridian
representation is closest at the level of the V1–V2 border and becomes
weaker as one moves in an anterior direction on the cortical surface. Indeed
in the more rostral regions the callosal input is more and more widespread
although still centered on the VM representation. In the owl monkey
Newsome and Allman (1980) have shown that callosal inputs correspond
closely to the V1–V2 border and to the VA–VP border and to a lesser extent
to the DL-MT border, while all three correspond to VM representations
(Fig. 1/14). Similarly in the macaque, callosal inputs correspond closely to
the V1–V2 border and also surround area V3A and separate V3A from V4
(Van Essen and Zeki, 1978). Finally in the cat, callosal input corresponds to
the V1–V2 border and to the lateral border of V3 both of which represent
the VM. In the suprasylvian areas of the cat callosal inputs are much more
widespread and link regions up to 15–20° from the VM (Keller and
Innocenti, 1981).

1.2 Quantitative Aspects of the Retino-Geniculo-Cortical Projections

1.2.1 The Overall Numbers of Cells in the Visual Pathway

For the macaque we have a fairly good estimation of the number of cells at the different levels of the retino-cortical pathway. They are indicated in Table 1/1, an adaptation of Fig. 7 of Barlow (1981). The number of receptors is larger than the number of ganglion cells. The number of geniculate cells is of about the same order of magnitude as that of the ganglion cells. On the contrary *the number of cells in layer IV of area 17* (where the geniculo-striate afferents end) *largely exceeds* (by a factor of about 40) *the number of geniculate cells*. The number of cells in the rest of the primary visual cortex is of the same order of magnitude as the number of area 17 layer IV cells. Thus, a great increase in processing capacity takes place at the entrance of message into the visual cortex. It comes then at this level, as no surprise that Barlow (1981) puts the spatial interpolation process at this level, which allows a fine grain reconstruction of the visual image.

One can define the *global divergence* or *convergence* factor of a neuronal connection by taking the ratio of cell numbers in the two connected struc-

Table 1/1. Number of cells in the retino-geniculo-cortical pathway of the macaque (Adapted from Barlow, 1981)

A. All eccentricities pooled

Retina			dLGN	Visual Cortex			Non-Visual Cortex
Receptors Rods Cones		Ganglion cells		Layer IV area 17	Other layers area 17	Other visual cortical areas	
100*	2.6[0]	1.1[0]	1.1[1]	50[1]	90[1]	–	–
			2.3[2]	84[3]	151[3]	518[3]	481[3]
				72[4]	89[4]		

B. Comparison central (0–10°) and peripheral (>10°) visual field

Retina			dLGN	Area 17	
Eccentricity	Cones	Ganglion cells		Layer IV	Other layers
0–10°	0.27[0]	0.32[0]	0.98[2]	43[4]	53[4]
>10°	2.33[0]	0.78[0]	1.32[2]	29[4]	36[4]

* Numbers are millions of cells.
[0] Rolls and Cowey (1970).
[1] Original figures of Chow et al. (1950) (estimates surface of area 17: 640 mm²).
[2] Estimated from Malpeli and Baker (1975) (77 mm³ for LGN volume) and from Chow et al. (1950) for cell density.
[3] Estimated from the surface of area 17 (17% of neocortex) (1090 mm²), of visual cortex outside area 17 (43% of neocortex) and of non-visual cortex (40% of neocortex) given by Van Essen and Maunsell (1980) and from the cell density given by Chow et al. (1950).
[4] Figures of O'Kusky and Colonnier (1982).

tures. For example the cone-ganglion cell connection has a global convergence factor of 2.5, the ganglion cell-geniculate connection has a global divergence factor of 1 or 2, while the geniculo-cortical connection has a global divergence factor of 40. It should be realized that these global factors are the sum of local operations at the level of single cells. We define the *local divergence* factor as the number of higher-order cells, to which one lower-order cell projects, and the *local convergence* factor as the number of lower order cells from which a single higher order cell receives input. The global divergence factor is thus the ratio of the average local divergence and convergence factors and the global convergence factor is the ratio of the average local convergence and divergence factors. The important point is that a given global factor can be realized by a whole series of combinations of local factors (Fig. 1/15): e.g. the global divergence factor at the geniculo-cortical level of 40 could as well result from an average local convergence factor of 1 and an average local divergence factor of 40, as from a mean local convergence factor of 5 combined with a mean local divergence factor of 200 and so on.

Given the overrepresentation of the central portion of the visual field in the retino-geniculo-cortical pathway of the macaque it is interesting to examine separately the global divergence and convergence for the parts of the pathway subserving central and peripheral vision (see Table 1/1B). It is clear that the convergence between cones and ganglion cells is larger for peripheral parts than for the central part of the retina. For the central retina the global convergence factor in the cone-ganglion cell connection is 1 and human data (Missotten, 1974) suggest that for this connection the local factor is also 1.

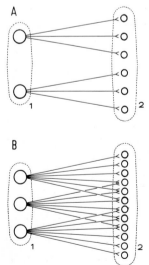

Fig. 1/15. Independence of global and local con- and divergence factors. The global divergence factor in the connection between nuclei 1 and 2 equals 3 both in A and B, yet the local divergence factor is 3 in A and 6 in B. The increase in local divergence factor is compensated by an increase in local convergence factor from 1 to 2.

On the other hand the global divergence factor between retinal ganglion cells and cortex is much larger for parts subserving central vision than for those subserving peripheral vision. One way of achieving this would be to have a constant local divergence factor at every eccentricity while the local convergence factor would increase with eccentricity.

For the other species (cat and owl monkey) the data available do not permit computation of a table similar to Table 1/1. However it is clear that there is also an initial step of global convergence between receptors and ganglion cells (see below) and a second step of divergence between geniculate cells and cortical cells. In particular for the cat the ganglion cells seem to be responsible for *a strong reduction in information transmission capability* since their number has been estimated to be only 100,000 to 200,000 (see Stone, 1978 for review). The number of neurons in area 17 of the cat has been estimated to be about 23 million by Colonnier and O'Kusky (1981). If layer IV occupies about 1/3 of the thickness of the cortex, then there are about 7.7 million layer IV neurons receiving LGN afferents. Hence the global retino-cortical divergence could be quite similar in cat and macaque.

1.2.2 Distribution of Retinal Cell Populations

The distributions of *receptor* cells have been evaluated for all three species and are summarized in Fig. 1/4. In the diurnal macaque there is a sharp peak in the cone distribution at the fovea. This steep decrease in cone density with eccentricity is partially compensated by an increase in rod density. Consequently in the macaque the rod/cone ratio increases with eccentricity (Table 1/2). In the nocturnal owl monkey the number of rods is large and the rod/cone ratio is similar (50/1) over the whole retina. The density of both types of receptors increases weakly with decreasing eccentricity. Finally, the cat which has both a diurnal and nocturnal life has a large number of rods but the distribution of the rods has a minimum at the area centralis (Fig. 1/4). While in the cat the cone density increases from periphery to center of the visual field by a factor of 5 (Fig. 1/4), it increases by a factor of 1.5 in the owl monkey and a factor of 15 in the macaque (factor of 30 in humans).

The *distribution of ganglion* cells has also been estimated in all three species (Fig. 1/5). The measure of density is number of cells/mm^2. It should be noted that 1 visual degree does not measure the same distance of the retinae of the different species due to difference in eyeball diameter. For the macaque 1 visual degree equals .246 mm (Rolls and Cowey, 1970), for the cat $1° = 0.226$ mm (Bishop et al., 1962), and for the owl monkey $1° = 0.15$ mm (Webb and Kaas, 1976). For cat and owl monkey species the distribution is similar in the sense that density is maximum at the area centralis. For the macaque there is a minimum at the fovea since inner retinal layers have been

Table 1/2. Ratio of different cells in central and peripheral retina.

		0° eccentricity	30° eccentricity
A) Rod/cone ratio	cat[1]	10	100
	owl monkey[2]	50	50
	macaque[3]	0	25
B) Cone/ganglion cell ratio	cat[1]	5	19
	owl monkey	0.7	1.7
	macaque[4]	1	2
C) Rod/ganglion cell ratio	cat[1]	50	1500
	owl monkey[2]	32	70
	macaque[3]	0	50

[1] Data from Steinberg et al. (1973) and Stone (1965)
[2] Data from Ogden (1975) and Webb and Kaas (1976)
[3] Extrapolated from human data (Østerberg, 1935)
[4] Data from Rolls and Cowey (1970)

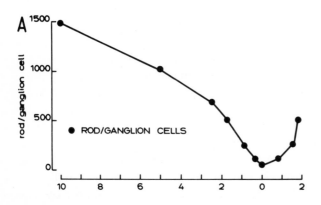

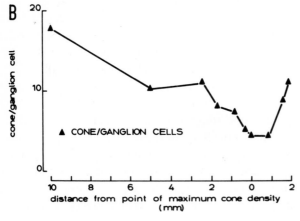

Fig. 1/16. The receptor-ganglion cell ratios in the cat plotted as a function of distance from the area centralis. Adapted with permission from Steinberg et al. (1973).

pushed aside to form the foveal pit. For that region the density of ganglion cells is estimated from the cone density by assuming a 1 to 1 projection. The degree of global convergence between rods and cones on one hand and ganglion cells on the other hand changes with eccentricity [11]. As is illustrated for the cat in Fig. 1/16, convergence in the receptor-ganglion cell connection increases with eccentricity and much more so for rods than for cones. For the rhesus monkey the global cone-ganglion cell convergence remains relatively small at all eccentricities. Rod-ganglion cell convergence is large at large eccentricities (Table 1/2).

1.2.3 Magnification Factors

The receptor densities represent peripheral innervation densities (number of receptors per surface unit). By extension one can still consider the ganglion cell densities as peripheral innervation densities. Both show a strong decrease with increasing eccentricity. On the other hand the central visual structures have a large overrepresentation of the central visual field. The question then arises whether this overrepresentation is just a passive reflection of the peripheral innervation density (retinal factor) or whether this density is modified by adaptation in the central structures.

The most general definition of *magnification* has been given by Myerson et al. (1978) as the "proportion of a structure that is devoted to the representation of a particular visual field zone divided by the proportion of the visual field represented"; this *global normalized cellular magnification factor* (NCMF) is defined as

$$M(\varphi_1, \varphi_2) = \frac{N(\varphi_1, \varphi_2) : N_{Tot}}{A(\varphi_1, \varphi_2) : A_{Tot}}, \text{ where } M(\varphi_1, \varphi_2) \text{ is the magnification}$$

factor for the representation of the zone of the visual field between iso eccentricity contours of radii 1 and 2 centered on the center of gaze, $N(\varphi_1, \varphi_2)$ is the number of cells in the representation of that zone in a given structure, N_{Tot} is the total number of cells in that structure and $A(\varphi_1, \varphi_2)$ and A_{Tot} are the area of that zone and the total area of the visual field respectively. If the cell density in a structure is invariant with respect to eccentricity (e.g. in the LGN), volume measurements in the numerator will yield equivalent values for magnification, and if in addition thickness is also invariant (as e.g. in the cortex), surface measurements in the numerator will give equivalent values of magnification. The factor is normalized since it uses proportions, is cellular since it uses number of cells, and global since it is only a function of eccentricity and not of the visual field radius (e.g. horizontal meridian)

---

[11] It should be noted that physiological studies suggest that ganglion cells receive input from both cones and rods.

along which measurements were made. Thus for the cortex one measures the proportion of cortical surface devoted to a portion of the visual field. For the retina, where density (number of cells/mm^2) changes with eccentricity, one can calculate the normalized cellular magnification from surfaces below the distribution of ganglion cells density as a function of eccentricity measured along different radii (upper and lower vertical meridian and nasal and temporal horizontal meridians). The results of these measurements for the retina and V1 of the owl monkey are shown in Fig. 1/17B. It is clear in both structures that magnification decreases monotonically with eccentricity but much more so in V1 than in the retina. The cortex is even more specialized than the retina for processing of information concerning the center of the visual field. The overrepresentation of the central portion in the visual field in the cortex of the owl monkey is not just a reflection of peripheral innervation density but there is an additional cortical adaptation. It should be noted that Webb and Kaas (1976), using a local linear version of the normalized magnification factor measured along the horizontal meridian, reached the opposite conclusion.

While the normalized cellular magnification factor of Myerson et al. (1977) is the most general definition, it is not the most commonly used nor the one which was first introduced. Daniel and Whitteridge (1961) initially defined *magnification factor* for a cortical surface as the distance in mm corresponding to the projection of 1 visual degree. This is a *local linear non-normalized factor*. Using this factor Daniel and Whitteridge (1961) were able to show that in the old world monkey (mainly the baboon) cortical magnification decreased monotonically with eccentricity. Direct comparison of this linear factor with retinal density of ganglion cells is not possible since the latter measure is an areal measurement. In fact there is a long standing dispute in the literature regarding whether M (the linear magnification) is proportional to D (retinal density) or $\sqrt{D}$ (see Hughes, 1977 and Rovamo and Virsu, 1979 for discussion). The source of error is the confusion between local and linear. Retinal density is evaluated along a given radius (mostly temporal and nasal halves of HM and upper and lower halves of VM) and is a local measure. However what is counted is the number of cells in small squares or rectangles placed along those radii. Since this surface has fixed dimensions in both directions, changes in magnification in both directions (i.e. parallel and orthogonal to the radius along which the squares are spaced) come into play, and density is a true areal measure. Therefore $M^2 = kD$. For this reason an areal magnification factor has been introduced for measurement of cortical magnification by Tusa et al. (1978). They measured the cortical surface (mm^2) devoted to blocks of $10° \times 10°$ and expressed this factor in mm^2/deg^2. This is a *non-normalized, local but areal* magnification factor. Similar to this measure is the magnification factor used by Malpeli and Baker (1975) for the macaque LGN. They used mm^3/steradian, a mea-

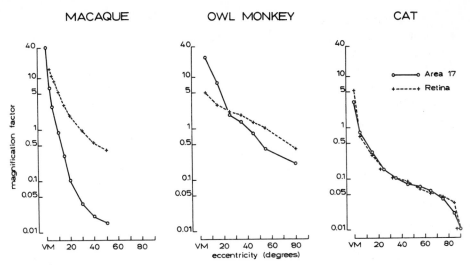

Fig. 1/17. The cortical magnification factor (open circles) and retinal density (crosses) compared in the 3 species. For the macaque, the cortical magnification estimates are from Daniel and Whitteridge (1961) and the retinal ganglion cell density from Rolls and Cowey (1970). They have been normalized so that the density and magnification were normalized at 0° eccentricity (Bishop, 1983). For the owl monkey, magnification factor in striate cortex and retinal ganglion cell layer are compared directly (Myerson et al., 1977). For the cat, cortical magnification factor (Tusa et al., 1978) and ganglion cell density (Stone, 1965) are compared: these data have been normalized 5 degrees out along the HM. Note that in both primates cortical magnification falls off more steeply than the retinal density. Note the high cortical magnification in the owl monkey. This may explain why this animal has a rather good acuity 10 c/deg (Jacobs, 1977 b) despite its small density of ganglion cells (see Fig. 1/5). For comparison (see Fig. 1/18) acuity of the monkey is 40–50 c/deg (De Valois et al., 1974 b) and that of the cat 2–8 c/deg (Vandenbussche and Orban, 1983; Elberger, 1982). Adapted with permission from Bishop (1983), Myerson et al. (1977) and Tusa et al. (1978).

sure directly proportional to an areal magnification factor of a nucleus expressed in mm^3/deg^2. The results of the comparison of non-normalized areal magnification factors for retina, LGN, and V1 of the macaque are shown in Fig. 1/17 A. The cortical areal magnification is obtained by squaring the linear factor of Daniel and Whitteridge (1961). The geniculate factor by converting Malpeli and Baker data to mm^3/deg^2 and the retinal factor by converting Rolls and Cowey's (1970) data into ganglion cells/deg^2. As in the owl monkey, the cortical overrepresentation of the central portion of the visual field in the macaque is not just the expression of peripheral innervation density but also the result of central adaptation. And here we have the additional information that the adapation occurs in two steps, one at retinogeniculate level and one at the geniculocortical level.

While in *both new and old world monkeys the differential cortical magnification is more than just the reflection of peripheral scaling, it seems that in the cat the differential magnification just reflects the differential peripheral innervation density*. Tusa et al. (1978) using a local areal magnification factor

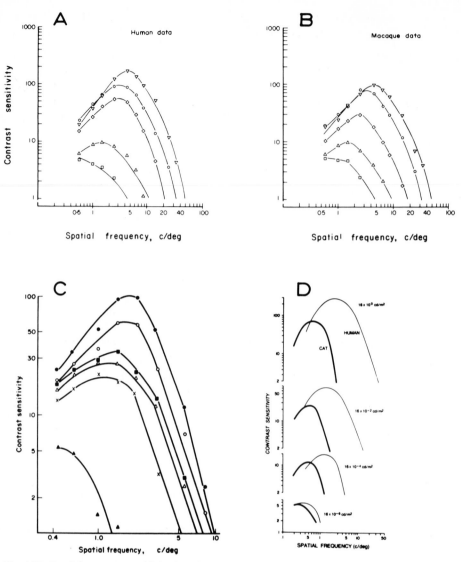

Fig. 1/18. Spatial contrast sensitivity functions measured at different luminance levels in all three species and in humans: A human observers, B macaque, (both from De Valois et al., 1974 b), C owl monkey (Jacobs, 1977b), D cat and humans (Pasternak and Merigan, 1981). In each of the panels the highest sensitivity corresponds to the highest mean luminance level (17 cd/m² in A and B, 11.4 cd/m² in C and 16 cd/m² in D). The other curves are for successive logarithmic attenuations below the highest level (1 log unit step in A, B and C and 2 log unit steps in D). Note that with a 5 log unit attenuation of luminance the contrast sensitivity of the owl monkey peaks above 15, while that of the macaque and human only reaches 6. The procedure was a 4 alternative forced choice technique with the threshold set at 50% correct responses, in A and B, a 3 alternative forced choice with the threshold set at 66% correct responses in C, and a 2 alternative forced choice in which the threshold set at 75% correct responses in D. Most estimates of grating acuity of the cat are higher (usually 4–8 c/deg) than those reported by Pasternak and Merigan (1981). Adapted with permission from De Valois et al. (1974 b), Jacobs (1977) and Pasternak and Merigan (1981).

showed that the change in magnification exactly paralleled the change in density of ganglion cells measured by Stone (1965) (Fig. 1/17 C). The measurements of Albus (1975 a) who used a linear cortical magnification factor, confirm this observation. The data of Sanderson (1971 b) who measured the linear magnification in the cat LGN are also in agreement with this view. Although his calculations were only approximative[12], Sanderson (1971 b) concluded from the comparison of geniculate magnification and retinal density, that differential geniculate magnification is simply a reflection of changes in retinal ganglion cell density. In conclusion then the global divergence in the retinocortical connection is invariant with respect to eccentricity in the cat, but increases with decreasing eccentricity in monkeys, a conclusion also apparent from the data in Table 1/1 B. However, as mentioned earlier, these changes of global divergence do not allow us to draw any conclusion about changes of local convergence or divergence with eccentricity.

1.3 Conclusion

The visual systems of cats and primates share a similar basic layout. Major differences between cat and old world monkeys involve (1) the number of cone types, (2) the number of retinal receptors and ganglion cells, (3) the projection of the visual field on the SC, (4) the layering in the dLGN and (5) the connection between dLGN and cortex. In the three species studied the retino-cortical pathway is topographically organized with emphasis on the representation of the central visual field and is strongly divergent.

---

[12] To evaluate the neural magnification in the LGN along the horizontal meridian (supposedly a local, areal factor) Sanderson (1971b) assumed that the iso-elevation lines were parallel. This could be true in first approximation for small changes in azimuth but cannot hold for large changes in azimuth, since this would imply that magnification is constant along the VM. This probably explains that his calculated LGN to retinal magnification ratio slightly increased with eccentricity.

Chapter 2. The Visual Cortical Areas of the Cat

In the first part of this chapter I will describe the multiple representations of the visual field on the cortical surface in the cat. While it is established that there are multiple visual cortical maps in the cat, the exact number of visual field representations and the organization of some of them is still an open question. It is clear that areas 17, 18, and 19 each contain a single representation of the visual field. However the exact nature of the visual field representation at the 18–19 border is still in debate. As one goes further out to the lateral suprasylvian areas, and to areas 20 and 21, problems grow as the question of the number of representations in these areas is not fully resolved. The existence of multiple cortical maps raises an important question concerning the relationships between them: are these maps serially connected or do they operate in parallel? In the second part of this chapter I will argue that there may be at least four levels of visual processing in the cat cortex of which the first level is represented by areas 17, 18, and 19. Since the rest of this study is devoted mainly to areas 17, 18, and 19, some aspects of their retinotopic organization will be treated in more detail: the variability in the maps, the scatter superimposed on the retinotopy, and the borders between the areas.

2.1 Description of the Visual Cortical Areas

2.1.1 Area 17: The Prototype of Visual Cortical Areas

Area 17[1] is the *largest* of all visual cortical areas (310–380 mm²) and is located medioposteriorly on the cerebral hemispheres of the cat (Fig. 2/1). It is surrounded anteriorly and laterally by area 18, medially by the area prostriata (in the depth of the splenial sulcus) and posteriorly by area 20 (Fig. 2/1). Area 17 is uniquely defined by its cyto- and myeloarchitectonic properties (Fig. 2/2). Area 17 has a thicker layer IV than the neighbouring area 18 (O'Leary, 1941). Area 18 has two characteristic fiber bands (seen on myelin stains) running in layer IV and V and a coarse myelination of radial

---

[1] Area 17 of the cat is also called striate cortex by analogy to area 17 of the monkey, in which the striation (stria of Gennari) is much clearer.

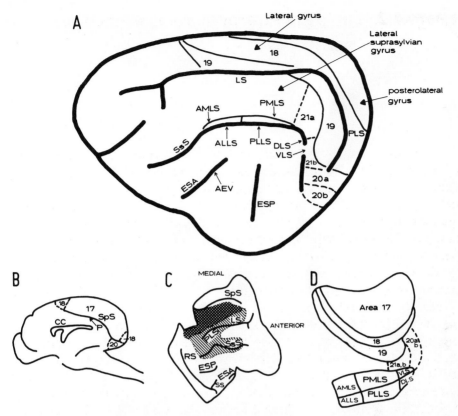

Fig. 2/1. The visual cortical areas of the cat: A) positions of the visual areas on the exposed dorsal and lateral surfaces of the left hemisphere; B) positions of the visual areas on the medial surface of the right hemisphere. The different sulci are indicated: LS: lateral sulcus; PLS: posterolateral sulcus; SsS: suprasylvian sulcus; ESA: anterior ectosylvian sulcus; ESP: posterior ectosylvian sulcus; SpS: splenial sulcus. CC indicates the corpus callosum. While areas 17, 18, 19, 20, and 21 lie chiefly on the exposed surface, the suprasylvian areas: the anteromedial and antero-lateral lateral suprasylvian areas (AMLS, ALLS), the posteromedial and posterolateral lateral suprasylvian areas (PMLS, PLLS) and the ventral and dorsal lateral suprasylvian areas (VLS, DLS), the anterior ectosylvian visual area (AEV) and the area prostriate (P) are buried in sulci. C) surface of the primary visual area (area 17) (heavy hatching) and of the other visual cortical areas (light hatching) on a twodimensional representation of the cat hemisphere according to Van Essen and Maunsell (1980). RS: rhinal sulcus, other abbreviations as in A and B. The striate cortex of the cat represents 12% of the neocortex and the whole of the visual cortical areas 31% of the neocortex. D) A schematic unfolded map of cat visual cortical areas showing the topographical relationships among areas and also their relative surface areas. Adapted with permission from Van Essen and Maunsell (1980) and Van Essen (1979).

fibers (Hubel and Wiesel, 1965; Tusa et al., 1978). By its heavier myelination area 18 can be distinguished from area 17. The area prostriata in the spenial sulcus and area 20 have a poor myelination compared to area 17 (Tusa et al., 1978).

Electrophysiological mapping techniques allow the investigation of the retinotopic organization of visual areas. Each visual neuron has a *receptive*

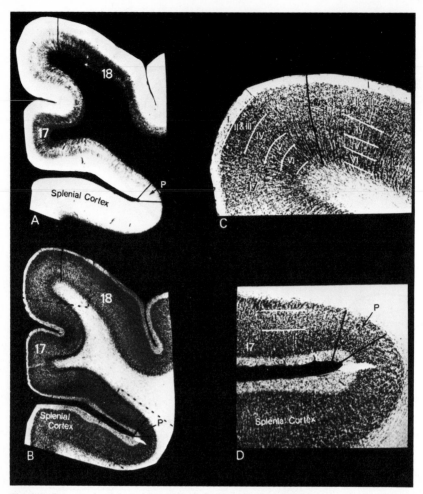

Fig. 2/2. Cyto- and myeloarchitectonic definition of area 17. A) Extent of area 17 within a fiber stained coronal section. B) Section adjacent to that in A, showing the extent of area 17 within a cellular stained section. C) Enlarged photograph of the 17/18 border. D) Enlarged photograph of the 17/prostriata (P) border. Adapted with permission from Tusa et al. (1978).

field (RF) i.e. a small region of the retina (or equivalently of the visual space) from which it can be influenced, i.e. excited or inhibited. For mapping experiments one uses mainly the excitatory RF since this can be plotted with hand-held stimuli moved through or flashed into the RF, while listening to the discharges of the cell over a loudspeaker to detect increases in discharge rate elicited by the stimuli. By recording from single cells (or small clusters of cells) in many different positions of an area and mapping their RF, one can reconstruct the relationships between the position on the cortical surface and position in the visual field (Fig. 2/3). This electrophysiological mapping technique was developed by Hubel and Wiesel (1962) who described the

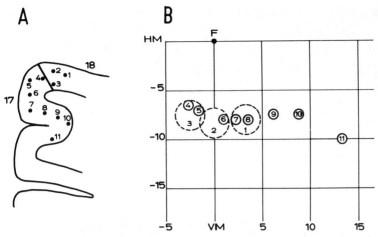

Fig. 2/3. Principle of the electrophysiological visual field mapping technique. A: location of recording sites on a coronal section (Anterior 3.6), oblique line: 17–18 border; B: receptive field plots from single cells (or small clusters of cells) recorded at the sites indicated in A. The full circles represent RFs recorded from cells in area 17 and dotted circles RFs recorded from cells in area 18. F: fixation point; HM: horizontal meridian; VM: vertical meridian. Note (1) the increase in azimuth of the RFs as one moves away from the 17–18 border in either area and (2) the location of RFs 3, 4, and 5 in the ipsilateral visual field. Adapted with permission from Tusa et al. (1978).

retinotopical organization of area 17 representing the central portion of the visual field. These experiments were extended by Tusa et al. (1978) who showed that area 17, as anatomically defined structure, contains *a single, complete and straightforward (i.e., first order, point-to-point) representation of the contralateral hemifield*. This representation, called V1 [2], includes, in addition to the contralateral visual hemifield, a narrow strip of the ipsilateral hemifield (Fig. 2/3), adjoining the vertical meridian (VM). Since in paralyzed animals it is difficult to reach a precision better than 1° or 2° in ascertaining the position of receptive fields with respect to the visual axis and since the strip is narrow (2°), this strip is not represented in most drawings of visual field maps (Fig. 2/4). The full contralateral visual hemifield is represented in area 17: 60° down, 60° up, and 90° laterally (Fig. 2/8). The lower quadrant is represented anteriorly, the upper quadrant posteriorly, and the extreme lateral field medially. The border between areas 17 and 18 represents the vertical meridian (Fig. 2/4).

In area 17 the *central part of the visual field is overrepresented: 50% of the cortical area is devoted to the central 10° of the visual field* (Tusa et al., 1978). Consequently cortical magnification decreases with eccentricity

---

[2] V refers to a visual map defined physiologically, maps may or may not be equivalent to cytoarchitectonic areas.

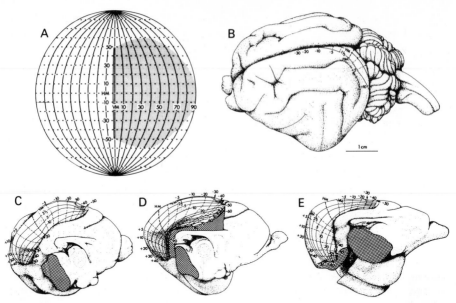

Fig. 2/4. Summary diagram of the representation of the visual field in area 17 of the cat. A) A perimeter chart showing the extent of the visual field represented in area 17. The perimeter chart is based on a world coordinate scheme in which the azimuths are represented as solid lines and the elevations are represented as dashed lines. The location of the visual field in area 17 is illustrated in the four sketches of cat brain (B to E). B) A dorsolateral view; C) A posteromedial view; D) A medial view with the cingulate gyrus removed to expose the superior bank of the anterior and middle portions of the splenial sulcus; E) A ventromedial view with the hippocampal fusiform gyrus removed to expose the superior bank of the posterior portion of the splenial sulcus. Adapted with permission from Tusa et al. (1978).

(Fig. 2/9). For uniformity reasons I use in this chapter the areal magnification factor introduced by Tusa et al. (1978) (see Chapter 1). The comparison between the changes in cortical (area 17) magnification factor along the horizontal meridian (HM) and the density of ganglion cells along the horizointal meridian (Stone, 1965) shows that the changes in cortical magnification directly reflect the changes in retinal ganglion cell density (Fig. 1/17). The magnification factor stresses the cortical projection of the central visual field. However one should remember that in the cat about half of area 17 (i.e. approximatively 170 mm^2) is devoted to the peripheral visual field ($>10°$ eccentricity). In the old world monkey (macaque) proportionally less striate cortical surface is devoted to the peripheral visual field (10% or more for eccentricities $>10°$). Since area 17 is so large in the monkey, even in this species a substantial part of the cortical surface (at least 110 mm^2) is devoted to the periphery of the visual field. This observation cast doubts on older theories about cortical and collicular visual systems in which the forebrain channel was concerned with central or focal vision and the midbrain channel with peripheral or ambient vision (Trevarthen, 1968).

Area 17 is an heuristic example of a visual cortical area since both histological criteria (cyto- and myeloarchitecture) or electrophysiological mapping criteria can be used to define the area and both definitions fit each other.
Therefore the terms area 17 (or striate cortex) and V1 can be used interchangeably. Since area 17 is the prototype of visual cortical areas, other
characteristics distinguishing area 17 from its neighbouring areas can be used
to derive additional strategies and criteria to define new functional visual
areas. Area 17 has input and output connections different from neighbouring
areas (see Chapters 3 and 10), and differences in connections have been used
to validate definitions of new visual areas (e.g. Tusa and Palmer, 1980). Area
17 is separated from area 18 by a narrow band of callosal projections (see
Chapter 3), and the projection bands of the corpus callosum have been used
to delineate different extrastriate areas (Zeki, 1970; Van Essen et al., 1982,
Newsome and Allman, 1980). Area 17 receives a topographically organized
projection from the dLGN (see Chapter 3). Topographically organized projections from a structure of known retinotopic organization have been used
to study less wellknown visual areas or structures (Albus and Meyer, 1981;
Montero, 1981). Finally area 17 neurons have properties distinct from those
of neighbouring areas (see Chapters 7, 8, 9). Differences in response properties have been used to validate distinctions between visual areas (e.g. Baker
et al., 1981).

2.1.2 Areas 18 and 19

Areas 18 and 19 are two smaller areas (each about 1/6 of the surface of
area 17) wrapping laterally around area 17 (Fig. 2/1). As with area 17, they
can be defined on the grounds of their cyto- and myeloarchitectonic characteristics (Otsuka and Hassler, 1962; Hubel and Wiesel, 1965; Tusa et al.,
1979). Compared to areas 17 and 19, area 18 has a thicker lamina III which
contains large pyramidal cells. Area 18 can also be distinguished from its two
neighbouring areas by its heavy myelination. Only the lateral border of area
19 can be dificult to define histologically (Albus and Beckmann, 1980). Each
of the anatomical entities contains *a single visual field representation* and in
the cat, areas 18 and 19 are used synonymously with V2 and V3 respectively.

There is however a dispute with respect to the *extent of visual field*
represented in the two areas as well as with the exact organization of the
retinotopy at the 18–19 border. All authors (Hubel and Wiesel, 1965; Donaldson and Whitteridge, 1977; Tusa et al., 1979; Albus and Beckmann, 1980)
agree that the lower field is represented anteriorly and the upper field posteriorly in both areas and that the VM is represented both at the 17–18 border
and at the lateral edge of area 19. However the different authors disagree on
the part of the visual field represented at the 18–19 border (compare

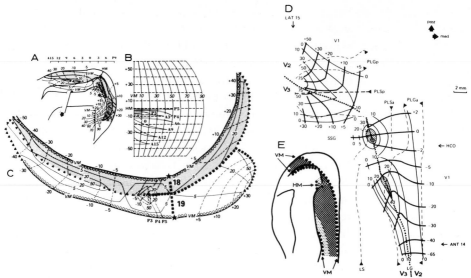

Fig. 2/5. Representation of the visual field in areas 18 (V2) and 19 (V3) of the cat: A, B, C according to Tusa et al. (1979); D and E, according to Albus and Beckmann (1980). A) A dorsolateral surface view of cat cortex with the lateral and posterior lateral sulci opened to expose the banks of these two sulci. The topographic representation of the visual hemifield found in areas 18 (shaded) and 19 are shown on this drawing. B) A perimeter chart showing the progression of receptive field centers in areas 18 and 19 along nine coronal planes spaced every 3 mm and at P4.0 and P5.0. For each coronal plane the progression of receptive field centers within area 18 is at the bottom and that of area 19 is on the top. C) A schematic representation of the visual hemifield in areas 18 and 19 on the unfolded cat cortex. The part of the representation found along coronal planes P3.0, P4.0, and P5.0 are dotted on the flat map. The remaining coronal planes similarly cross the diagram systematically throughout the map. D) Basis retinotopic map of V2 and V3 in the cat. The map has been prepared from two animals, and is projected upon the extended surface of a right hemisphere. HCO, Interaural plane of the Horsley Clarke coordinate system; ANT 14, frontal plane 14 mm anterior to the interaural plane HCO; LAT 15, parasagittal plane 15 mm lateral from the midline of the brain. The first visual area (V1) is located medial and posterior from V2. Most of the representation of the upper hemifield in V2 and in V3 is hidden in the posterior portion of the postlateral sulcus as can be seen from the surface view in E. E) A part of the representation of the vertical meridian in V3 is visible on the lateral gyrus and on the medial and the posterior edge of the suprasylvian gyrus. Filled circles in E: representation of the vertical meridian in V1/V2 and in V3. Open circles in E: representation of the horizontal meridian in V2 and V3. Striped area: V2; dotted area: V3; Abbreviations in D: PLGp, a: posterior respectively anterior part of posterolateral gyrus, PLSp, a: posterior respectively anterior part of the posterolateral sulcus; LS: lateral sulcus. SSG: suprasylvian gyrus. Dotted line: V2–V3 border. Hatched areas: 18–19 border islands. Adapted with permission from Tusa et al. (1979) and from Albus and Beckmann (1980).

Fig. 2/5A and B). Initially Hubel and Wiesel (1965) suggested that the far lateral fields were represented at the 18–19 border. However subsequent reports suggested that it could be lateral fields of variable azimuth (Donaldson and Whitteridge, 1977) the horizontal meridian (Bilge et al., 1967; Tusa et al., 1979) or an imaginary line parallel to the horizontal meridian (Albus and Beckmann, 1980). In fact it seems that there may be a difference between the

18–19 border in the upper and lower visual field quadrant. The disagreement between Albus and Beckmann (1980) (see Fig. 2/5A) and Tusa et al. (1979) (see Fig. 2/5B) may be due to the difference in sampling strategy: (every 200–300 μ for Albus and Beckmann, 1980 compared to every 1000 μ for Tusa et al., 1979). Initially it was thought that the representation of the visual field in areas 18 and 19 was incomplete (Whitteridge, 1973; Tusa et al., 1979; Woolsey, 1971). Taking into account the large size of the receptive fields in the parts of area 18 subserving peripheral fields, the visual field can be considered to be completely represented in area 18 (compare the plots of Tusa et al., 1979 and Albus and Beckmann, 1980 in Fig. 2/8) and almost completely in area 19, the far lateral fields lacking in the lower quadrant (Fig. 2/8).

As in area 17, *the central visual field is overrepresented in areas 18 and 19* (see Fig. 2/9). Since areas 18 and 19 are smaller areas than area 17, magnification is smaller in areas 18 and 19 than in area 17. This difference may be more pronounced for the peripheral field than for the central field. Indeed the changes in magnification along the horizontal meridian (Fig. 2/10) are steeper in areas 18 and 19 than in area 17. The difference in magnification along the horizontal meridian between areas 18 and 19 is probably due to the fact that, as a closer inspection of Fig. 2/9B shows, in area 18 the vertical

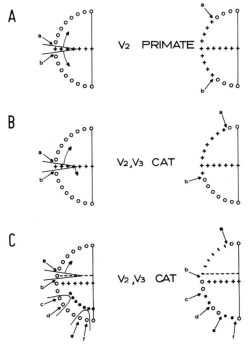

Fig. 2/6. Mapping of a visual hemifield onto a half circular target, illustrating second order transformations. The vertical line represents the VM, crosses the HM, open circles the far periphery, minuses a line above the HM and dots less peripheral fields in the lower quadrant. A) In a simple second order transformation as in V2 of primates, the HM representation is split in such a way that adjacent points on opposite sides of the HM (a and b) are represented at widely separated sites on the map. B) According to Tusa et al. (1979) the second order transformations in V2 and V3 are similar to those of V2 of primates except that the HM represents more of the border of the upper quadrant than of the lower quadrant. C) According to Albus and Beckmann (1980) the second order transformation is more complex. There is a split of the visual field along a horizontal line 5° to 10° above the HM. In addition there are splits (e.g., between c and d) in the far periphery of the lower quadrant so that less peripheral parts of the lower quadrant are represented at the border. The more peripheral parts are grouped into islands. While in the transformations of A and B there is only one field discontinuity (between a and b), there are several in this transformation: between a and b, c and d, and between e and f.

meridian is overrepresented compared to the horizontal meridian. The transformation of the visual field is more complicated in areas 18 and 19 than in area 17. Both areas contain *a second order representation of the visual field.* This is to say that adjacent points in the visual field are not always represented in adjacent points in the cortical map (i.e. field discontinuity in the terminology of Van Essen et al., 1981). The map of V2 of the primate is a classical example of such a discontinuity (Fig. 2/6A). The visual field is split at the level of the horizontal meridian and both upper and lower field are compressed in their lateral parts so that most of the border of the map represents the HM (crosses) and only a small part the extreme periphery (circles). The representation of V2 and V3 in the cat seems to differ from that in V2 of the primates in that only the periphery of the upper field is compressed. In addition, the level of the split is different according to the authors: the horizontal meridian (Fig. 2/6B) according to Tusa et al. (1979) and an horizontal line 8–10° above the HM (Fig. 2/6C) according to Albus and Beckmann (1980). According to the latter authors there is an additional complication in that the lateral periphery of the lower field is not represented continuously at the border of the maps but only at the level of the *islands.* The presence of these islands is another reason why the maps are second order representations of the visual field.

2.1.3 The Lateral Suprasylvian Areas

Visual responses in the region of the middle suprasylvian gyrus were first described by Marshall et al. (1943), Clare and Bishop (1954), and Hubel and Wiesel (1969). The extensive mapping study of Palmer et al. (1978), showed that the visually responsive region extends along both banks of the middle and posterior suprasylvian sulci. Since this region corresponds grossly to the anatomically described lateral suprasylvian area (Heath and Jones, 1971), Palmer et al. (1978) retained that nomenclature in the designations of the *six retinotopic subdivisions* of that region: anteromedial and anterolateral, posteromedial and posterolateral, and dorsal and ventral lateral suprasylvian areas (abbreviations AMLS, ALLS, PMLS, PLLS, DLS and VLS respectively) (Fig. 2/7D). In the anterior and posterior areas the lower fields are represented in the depth of the suprasylvian sulcus and the upper fields in the upper parts of the bank of the sulcus. The separation between the anterior and the posterior areas is the vertical meridian. In the ventral and dorsal areas there is no systematic representation of elevations, only the azimuths are represented. The area centralis is represented on the outer border of the maps and any radial path directed inwards corresponds to movement into the periphery along the horizontal meridian. This parcellation of the lateral suprasylvian area into 6 maps is further supported by anatomical data. In the

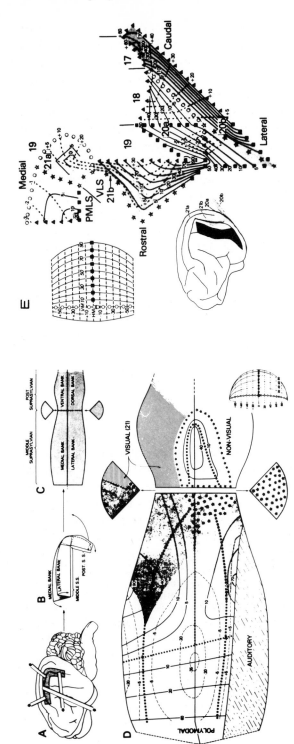

Fig. 2/7. Visual field representation in the lateral suprasylvian areas (A, B, C and D) and in areas 20 and 21 (E). D) A composite flat map of all six lateral suprasylvian areas on the middle and posterior suprasylvian sulci. The sulcus was first straightened (B), then fully opened (C, D). In order to do this, small sectors of cortex had to be cut free at the junction of the middle and posterior suprasylvian sulci. In B and C, the continuity of the medial bank of the middle suprasylvian sulcus with the ventral bank of the posterior suprasylvian sulcus can be seen. Similarly for the lateral and dorsal banks of the middle and posterior suprasylvian sulci, respectively. The insert shows the perimeter charts with the principal visual field landmarks. E) A schematic diagram of the representation of the visual field found in areas 20a, 20b, 21a, and 21b on the unfolded cortex. Inserts: perimeter chart and location of areas 20a, 20b, 21a and 21b on the lateral view of the cat hemisphere with the posterior ectosylvian gyrus removed (the portions of areas 20a and 20b on the medial surface have been swung out). In both schemes (D and E) azimuths are illustrated as full lines and elevations as dashed lines. Adapted with permission from Palmer et al. (1978) and Tusa and Palmer (1980).

cytoarchitectonic study of Sanides and Hoffmann (1969) the suprasylvian sulcal cortex was divided into 5 areas of which 3 correspond to AMLS, PMLS, and VLS while the 2 other correspond to the polymodal cortex in front of AMLS and to area 21. Study of the anatomical connections of the lateral suprasylvian area also supports the parcellation: the thalamic afferents to PMLS and PLLS are different (Palmer et al., 1978), the projections from AMLS, ALLS, PMLS and PLLS to the LP-pulvinar complex are different (Updyke, 1981), while area 17 projects to PMLS and AMLS, it does not to PLLS and ALLS (Kawamura and Naito, 1980) and the callosal connections of all 6 areas are different (Segraves and Rosenquist, 1982b). The only conflicting report is from Albus and Meyer (1981) who conclude that the whole of the lateral suprasylvian areas and areas 20 and 21 only contain 4 visual field representations.

The representations of the visual field in the lateral suprasylvian areas are *incomplete* (Fig. 2/8). In the anterior areas mainly the lower field is represented, in the posterior areas the lower field and the horizontal meridian, and in the dorsal and ventral areas the horizontal meridian. Except for the 2 anterior areas, central vision is overrepresented in the lateral suprasylvian areas (Fig. 2/9). If one considers the magnification factor along the horizontal meridian (Fig. 2/10), the magnification is lower in the posterior and dorsal and ventral areas than in area 17 but the relative changes as a function of eccentricity are similar. On the contrary in the anterior areas the changes along the horizontal meridian are quite small. While the anterior areas contain a first order transformation of the visual field, the transformation in the dorsal and ventral areas is more complicated (Table 2/1). In fact a point in visual space is represented by a line rather than by a point in the map. Palmer et al. (1978) call this a point-to-line representation. The representation in the posterior areas is even more complicated (mixed transformation) since they contain both a point-to-point transformation in their rostral parts and a point-to-line transformation in their caudal parts (Palmer et al., 1978).

Table 2/1. Types of visual field representation

Area 17 = V1	First order point-to-point transformation
18 = V2	second order point-to-point transformation
19 = V3	second order point-to-point transformation
AMLS & ALLS	first order point-to-point transformation
VLS & DLS	point-to-line transformation
PMLS & PLLS	mixed (first order point-to-point and point-to-line) transformation
20a	first order point-to-point transformation
20b	mixed (second order point-to-point and point-to-line) transformation
21a	mixed transformation (map discontinuity)
21b	mixed (first order point-to-point and point-to-line) transformation
AEV	?
splenial visual area (P)	?

Note: point-to-line transformation always concerns the area centralis and sometimes more lateral points of HM.

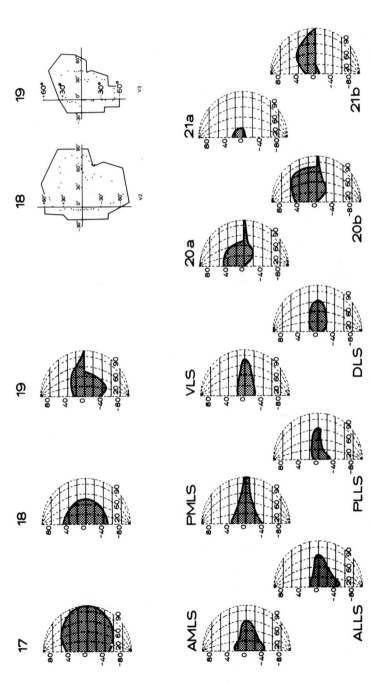

Fig. 2/8. Extent of the visual field represented in the visual cortical areas of the cat. The perimeter charts show the extent of the representations (using only RF centers) according to Palmer et al. (1978); Tusa et al. (1978, 1979) and Tusa and Palmer (1980). The diagrams in the upper right corner indicate the area of the visual field represented in areas 18 and 19 according to Albus and Beckmann (1980). The most peripheral fields are presented by their outer borders (continuous lines) and by their centers (points). Adapted with permission from Palmer et al. (1978), Tusa et al. (1978, 1979), Tusa and Palmer (1980) and Albus and Beckmann (1980).

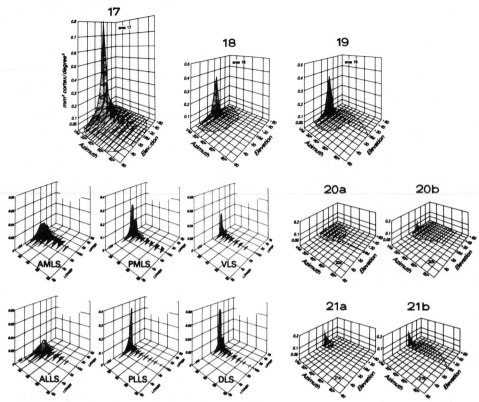

Fig. 2/9. Three-dimensional plots showing the magnification factor as a function of position in the visual field for each of the visual cortical areas. Azimuth and elevation form the base of each cube and the areal magnification factor (in square multimeter per square degree) is given as distance above the plane. Adapted with permission from Palmer et al. (1978), Tusa et al. (1978, 1979) and Tusa and Palmer (1980).

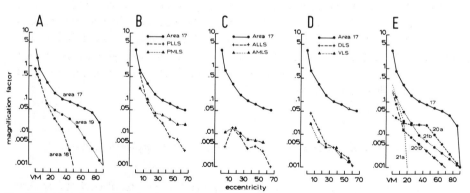

Fig. 2/10. (Areal) magnification factors plotted as a function of eccentricity along the horizontal meridian for each of the visual cortical areas. In each of the panels the curve of area 17 is repeated for comparison purposes. Adapted with permission from Palmer et al. (1978), Tusa et al. (1978, 1979), Tusa and Palmer (1980). Note that in areas 18 and 19 the magnification is twice as large along the VM as along the HM (Albus and Beckmann, 1980).

2.1.4 Areas 20 and 21

According to Tusa and Palmer (1980) areas 20 and 21 each contain 2 maps. All 4 maps mainly represent the upper visual field. In areas 20a and 20b and 21a the lower visual field is represented rostrally and the upper field caudally. Area 21b contains only a representation of the upper visual field. In all 4 areas magnification is at least one order of magnitude lower than in area 17 (Fig. 2/9). However changes along the horizontal meridian are even steeper than in area 17 (Fig. 2/10). Except for area 20a, which contains a first order transformation of the visual field, all 3 other areas contain a mixed transformation of the visual field, since the area centralis is represented in all 3 by a line. The point-to-point transformation in these areas is different: first order in area 21b, second order in area 20b (split representation of the HM) and even more complex in area 21a. The latter representation could be described as a map discontinuity (Van Essen et al., 1981) where the whole of the periphery of the upper field has been compressed.

2.1.5 Additional Visual Areas?

Kalia and Whitteridge (1973) have described a small visual area in the depth of the splenial sulcus: the splenial visual area corresponding to the cyto-architectonically defined area prostriata (Sanides and Hoffmann, 1969). However Tusa et al. (1978) using NO_2 anesthesia rather than chloralose anesthesia were unable to elicit visual responses from this area. A similar area has been described in the macaque by Van Essen et al. (1982), at the anterior tip of the calcarine sulcus. Both in the cat and the macaque the area prostriata is interposed between striate cortex and allocortex. According to Kalia and Whitteridge the splenial visual area is topographically organized. Recently Mucke et al. (1982) and Olson and Graybiel (1981) have described an additional visual area in the ventral bank of the anterior ectosylvian sulcus. Mucke et al. (1982) called this area the anterior ectosylvian visual area (AEV). Retinotopy in this area is either unclear (Mucke et al., 1982) or complex (Olson and Graybiel, 1981).

2.2 The Levels of Processing in the Visual Cortical System of the Cat

An important issue for the understanding of the visual cortex concerns the way in which information flows through the different cortical areas, in other words whether the cortical areas operate serially or in parallel. Initially Hubel and Wiesel (1962, 1965, 1967) considered a purely serial hypothesis illustrated in Fig. 2/11A. In such a scheme each area represents a hierarchi-

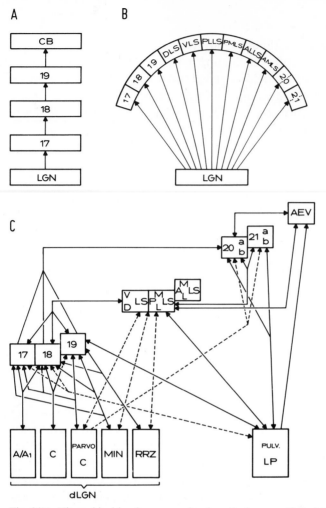

Fig. 2/11. Hierarchical levels among visual cortical areas. A) Serial hypothesis: each area is at a hierarchically higher level. CB: Clare Bishop or lateral suprasylvian area. B) Parallel hypothesis: all areas are at the same (primary) level. C) Serio-parallel hypothesis: areas 17, 18 and 19 represent a primary visual complex (see text). A/A1: dorsal layers of dLGN; C and parvo C: magnocellular C lamina and parvocellular C laminae of LGN respectively; MIN: medial interlaminar nucleus of dLGN; RRZ retino-recipient zone of pulvinar or geniculate wing; pulv-LP: pulvinar-lateralis posterior complex. The dashed and full lines have only be used for the sake of clarity.

cally higher level and processes further the information provided by the lower level. All connections in the serial hypothesis are *"feeding" connections* which provide input for the processing in the next area (Fig. 2/12). However the dLGN of the cat projects not only to area 17 but also to area 18 (see Chapter 3). This raises the possibility that both areas 17 and 18 are primary visual areas (i.e. receiving input from the specific thalamic relay nucleus) and thus

A Types of connections

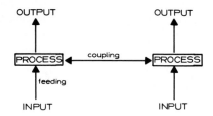

B Strength of connections

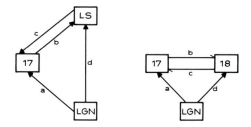

Fig. 2/12. Intracortical associative connections. A) Two functional types of connections. B) Strength of connections can differentiate between areas at different or the same hierarchical levels. LS: lateral suprasylvian area.

operate in parallel. This suggests that in the cat the connections between areas 17 and 18, which in fact are reciprocal (Wilson, 1968), are of a nature other than "feeding" connections and I call them *"coupling" connections*. This type of connection does not provide input for the processing in a cortical area but rather allows one process to modulate the other. While "feeding" connections are essential to the normal operation of an area, "coupling" connections are not and they could only control the gain of processes operating in an area or in some of its parts.

In fact it seems that in the cat the parvocellular C_{1-3} laminae of the LGN project to all or most known visual cortical areas (Raczkowski and Rosenquist, 1980). Therefore, one could hold another extreme view that all visual cortical areas (except maybe AEV) are primary areas and all operate in parallel (Fig. 2/11B). This extreme view has little chance of being verified since the projections of the main laminae of the LGN are more restricted and since the projections of the parvocellular laminae of the LGN to the different cortical areas are not equally strong. In fact, for many areas outside areas 17 and 18, the LP-pulvinar complex, rather than the LGN, is the dominant thalamic afferent structure. It seems therefore likely that *both serial and parallel processing*[3] occur among the different visual cortical areas which

---

[3] This parallel processing can be twofold: there may be different systems at the retinal level (e.g., X, Y, or W) which project to different areas, i.e., the different areas receive a different retinal message, or there may be branching (eventually, but not necessarily due to branching axons) within one afferent system whereby the different areas receive the same message.

then *operate on different hierarchical levels.* The question then becomes which criteria can be used to distinguish areas operating in parallel from areas operating serially. I will review different types of data, both physiological and anatomical, which in the opinion of the author (see Van Essen, 1979 for a different view) suggest that there are at least four hierarchical levels of processing in the visual cortical system of the cat: the level of the primary complex (areas 17, 18, and 19), the level of the suprasylvian areas, the levels of areas 20 and 21, and the level of AEV (Fig. 2/11C).

Among the *anatomical criteria* the absence of connections between 2 areas with the same input or a unidirectional connection seems to be good evidence for parallel and serial operation respectively. However most if not all cortical areas are reciprocally connected and one has to look for asymmetries in the connections to distinguish "feeding" from "coupling" connections. Such an asymmetry could be indicated by the lamination of the connections. Initially it was thought that corticocortical connections only originate in the superficial (supragranular) layers (II and III), in opposition with the cortico-subcortical projections which originate in the deep (infragranular) layers (V and VI) (Gilbert and Kelly, 1975). In fact recent studies in the squirrel monkey (Tigges et al., 1981), in the owl monkey (Lin et al., 1982), and in the macaque (Rockland and Pandya, 1979; Van Essen et al., 1981; Lund et al., 1981) have shown that the origin of corticocortical connections is supra-granular for forward connections (i.e. away from area 17) but is (mainly) infragranular for connections in the reverse directions (towards area 17). In fact the asymmetry between forward and reverse connections is even greater if one also considers the layers of termination: forward connections end in layer IV, reverse connections outside layer IV (Tigges et al., 1981; Rockland and Pandya, 1979; Lund et al., 1981). Thus these connections are reciprocal but highly *asymmetrical in their lamination.* Since this type of connection occurs between V1, which in the monkey is the primary area, and V2 which is not, and since this connection pattern resembles that of the LGN-V1 connection, this asymmetric lamination could be considered as typical for "feeding" connections, the forward projection to layer IV representing the feedforward[4] and the reverse projection from the deep layers representing the feedback[5]. This systematic feedback to hierarchically lower areas may be very important for noise suppression in the input. While it is clear that the described asymmetry in lamination could be characteristic of "feeding" connections, it is less clear what lamination pattern "coupling" connections

---

[4] This view is strongly dependent on our ideas of information processing within area 17, in which the geniculate afferents end in layer IV, from where cells project either to the supra- or infragranular layers (see Figs. 14/3 and 14/4).

[5] The recent results of Sandell and Schiller (1982) suggest that the intracortical feedback from area 18 to area 17 in the squirrel monkey, projects mainly to the infragranular layers and hence could modulate the subcortical projections from these layers.

should have. [6] Indeed, for the only pair of cortical areas for which there is good evidence (see below) that they operate in parallel, i.e. for areas 17 and 18 of the cat (Tretter et al., 1975), the lamination pattern of the connections is not wellknown. However, one could consider that the lamination pattern should be much more symmetrical linking similar layers e.g. linking only the superficial layers or all layers. Another characteristic of the connections which may help to distinguish "feeding" and "coupling" connections between structures with a common input is the *relative strength of the connections*. If an area (LS in Fig. 2/12) is serially connected to another cortical area (17 in Fig. 2/12) and both receive a common input (LGN in Fig. 2/12), one has to suppose that the direct input from LGN to LS (d) is much weaker than the corticocortical connection (b) or than the LGN input to area 17 (a). On the contrary if two areas (17 and 18 in Fig. 2/12) operate in parallel on a similar input, then the 2 inputs from the lower order structure (a and d) should be about equally strong and both stronger than the corticocortical connections (b, c). Unfortunately most studies on cortical connectivity in the cat do not mention the strength of connections or only use qualitative statements (strong, scant). Another criterion which could be used to distinguish hierarchical levels among the cortical areas of the cat is the comparison between the strength and the layer of termination of the two thalamic inputs to the visual cortical areas, dLGN and LP-pulvinar complex, or if this information lacks the relative strength of the descending connections between cortical areas and dLGN or LP-pulvinar. If a cortical area has stronger connections with the dLGN than with the LP-pulvinar, this could be seen as evidence that it is operating at a lower level than an area for which the reverse is true [7].

Different *physiological* criteria can be used to distinguish between areas operating serially or in parallel. Electrical stimulation can be used to detect the input from a given structure. This does not distinguish between coupling and feeding connections but can help to decide whether or not an area gets input from the LGN and is primary or not. The effect of *cooling or ablation* of one area on the properties of another area is a major functional test for the distinction between feeding and coupling links. Finally similarity in response properties between areas can be seen as an argument that areas perform a similar operation, eventually on different inputs, and thus operate in parallel. In particular simple cell-like RF organization is typical of primary visual cortices (Hubel and Wiesel, 1962; Tretter et al., 1975; Orban and

---

[6] Up to now most corticocortical connections studied either in the cat or monkeys seem to be of the feeding type (Ungerleider, personal communication, Bullier and Kennedy, personal communication); the connection between MT and V4 could be of the coupling type.

[7] This need not imply that the LP-pulvinar operates at a higher level than the LGN, but that the information originating from the LP-pulvinar is only mixed with the direct retino-cortical pathway at later stages of processing.

Callens, 1977 a; Orban and Kennedy, 1981; Schiller et al., 1976; Kennedy et al., 1980).

Most data bearing on the question of parallel versus serial processing in the cat concern the relationship between areas 17 and 18 and the hierarchical position of the lateral suprasylvian (LS) areas. These data clearly suggest that *17 and 18 operate in parallel* while the *LS areas represent a further level of processing* (Fig. 2/11C). The anatomical data clearly show that both areas 17 and 18 have a similar reciprocal connection with the main laminae of the dLGN (A, A1 and C) (Garey et al., 1968; Holländer and Vanegas, 1977; LeVay and Gilbert, 1976). Physiologically, this is confirmed by the fact that the proportion of cells with monosynaptic input from the LGN (Tretter et al., 1975) and the proportion of cells with simple-like RF organization, are equally large in both areas (Tretter et al., 1975; Harvey, 1980 a; Orban and Callens, 1977 a; Orban and Kennedy, 1981). That area 18 operates in parallel with area 17 is also indicated by the little influence of ablation or cooling of area 17 on the properties of area 18 neurons (Dreher and Cottee, 1975; Sherk, 1978). The lateral suprasylvian areas receive no input from the main LGN laminae but from the parvocellular laminae and MIN. However in addition to LGN input, the LS areas receive a strong input from the LP-pulvinar complex which terminates in layer IV (Rosenquist et al., 1974). Reciprocal connections to the LGN are very weak compared to those to the LP-pulvinar complex (Updyke, 1981). This suggests that the major thalamic input to LS areas is the LP-pulvinar complex rather than the dLGN. In addition LS (at least PMLS, which corresponds grossly to the Clare-Bishop area (Hubel and Wiesel, 1968) in the older terminology, has a reciprocal connection with 17 and 18 of the feeding type: areas 17 and 18 projection to PMLS originates in layer III and the return projection in layers V, VI (Gilbert and Kelly, 1975). The recent fluorescent tracer studies of Bullier and Kennedy (personal communication) show that the return projection originates both in infra- and supragranular layers. Physiologically the response properties of PMLS neurons are clearly different from those of 17 and 18 (Spear and Baumann, 1975) and their properties depend on the integrity of area 17 input (Spear and Baumann, 1979), although the latter result has been disputed (Guedes et al., 1983).

The position of area 19 is less clear, but there are a number of arguments that allow us to consider it *as part of the primary visual complex of the cat* (Orban et al., 1982 c). The anatomical data give conflicting information. The reciprocal connections between 17 and 19 seem to be asymmetrical in layering: the forward projection originates in layer III of area 17 and the reverse projection in layer VI of area 19 (Gilbert and Kelly, 1975). However, according to Bullier and Kennedy (personal communication) the reverse projection arises in similar numbers from the infra- and supragranular layers. Area 19 has a weak input from the main laminae of the LGN, most of its geniculate afferents originating in MIN and the parvocellular C laminae, as for LS. However in opposition to LS, the LGN input to area 19 is as strong as the LP-pulvinar input (Holländer and Vanegas, 1977; Bullier and Kennedy, personal communication). In addition the reciprocal connection from area 19 to the parvocellular C laminae and MIN is strong (Updyke, 1977). Therefore, the main thalamic afferent area 19 seems to be the LGN. Physiologically there are many cells (> 50%) driven monosynaptically by LGN stimulation (Kimura et al., 1980; Dreher et al., 1980). In addition about 25% of cells have a simple-like receptive field organization (compared to 65% in 17 and 18) (Duysens et al., 1982 b). Finally cooling of area 17 has been reported by at least one group (Kimura et al., 1980) to have little effect on the properties of area 19 neurons. Therefore, as others (Stone et al., 1979), we consider area 19 to be the third member of the primary visual complex of the cat, although area 19 may occupy a special place in this complex.

There is hardly any information concerning the relationships between the different LS areas. The absence of LGN input to AMLS and ALLS (Raczkowski and Rosenquist, 1980) may suggest that these areas occupy a slightly different level from that of the other suprasylvian areas. The 4 visual areas 20 a, b and 21 a, b are considered to be a third level. As the LS areas, they receive weak LGN input (Raczkowski and Rosenquist, 1980) and a strong LP-pulvinar input (Tusa and Palmer, 1980) and input from the primary complex level (areas 17, 18, and 19) (Symonds and Rosenquist, 1979). The return projection from area 20 to area 17 seems only to arise from the infragranular layers (Bullier and Kennedy, personal communication). In addition areas 20 and 21 receive input from LS areas (Tusa and Palmer, 1980; Symonds and Rosenquist, 1979). Since area 20 provides input to area 21 it may be that thus 2 areas are not exactly on the same hierarchical level. Finally AEV has been put on a still higher level (Fig. 2/11C) since it has been reported to be connected reciprocally with LS areas and area 20 and to receive input from the LP-pulvinar complex but not from the primary complex nor the dLGN (Olson and Graybiel, 1981; Mucke et al., 1982).

2.3 Additional Observations on the Retinotopic Organization in the Primary Complex

2.3.1 Variability of the 3 Cortical Maps

There are 2 main sources of variability in the retinotopic maps of areas 17, 18, and 19. The first source of variability concerns *the position of visual field landmarks* in stereotaxic (Horsley-Clarke) coordinates.[8] The principal

---

[8] The zero of these brain coordinates are the interaural plane (in the anteroposterior direction) and the midline (in the mediolateral direction).

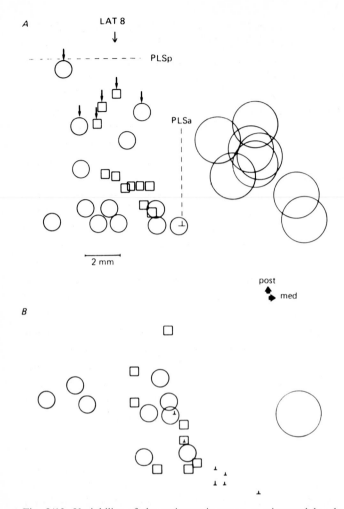

Fig. 2/13. Variability of the retinotopic maps as witnessed by the cortical locations of the representations of the area centralis and the periphery of the horizontal meridian in V2 and V3. The area centralis at the V1–V2 border is indicated by large diameter circles, that in V3 by small diameter circles. The horizontal meridian periphery at the V2–V3 border is given by open squares. A) Representations arranged with respect to the anterior beginning of the postlateral sulcus. Representations marked by an arrow are located on the anterior bank of the postlateral sulcus (posterior portion). B) Two of the representations (area centralis in V3 and horizontal meridian at the V2–V3 border) are arranged with respect to the cortical location of the third (area centralis at the V1–V2 border). For seven animals the location of the anterior beginning of the postlateral sulcus is given by ⊥. Adapted with permission from Albus and Beckmann (1980).

landmark is the projection of the area centralis (AC). According to Albus and Beckmann (1980) the AC representations at the V1–V2 border are found over an area measuring 8 × 8 mm centered on (posterior) P5 and (lateral) L2. According to the same authors the AC representation in V3 occupies an area measuring 10 × 7 mm (Fig. 2/13). Similarly Tusa et al. (1979) mention that in

3 out of 20 cats, the AC representation in area 17 was located 4 mm more posteriorly than the usual stereotaxic coordinates (P4). Another landmark is the representation of the periphery of the horizontal meridian which clusters around two main positions approximatively 5 mm apart, either on the lateral bank or the anterior bank of the posterolateral sulcus according to Albus and Beckmann (1980). These findings indicate that the 3 maps (V1, V2, and V3) as a whole can be shifted over the cortical surface in anteroposterior or mediolateral directions.[9] Therefore, published maps always represent V1, V2, and V3 of a cat and not of the cat. One should therefore be extremely cautious when using the "average" maps to guide penetrations into one area by stereotaxic coordinates alone. Such an approach must be limited to experiments where one is aiming at parts far distant from the borders, as for example at area 17 on the medial bank of the lateral gyrus at P3. However when one is aiming at regions close to the borders (i.e. any part of area 18 and 19 since both are relatively narrow) and especially to the AC representation in V1, control procedures are necessary to ascertain that one is recording in the area intended. Since on Nissl-stained sections the V1–V2 border is fuzzy (Fisken et al., 1975; Hubel and Wiesel, 1965), the control procedure should either include a myelin stain or physiological procedures of which velocity sensitivity seems to be the most reliable (Orban et al., 1980). This casts some doubt on the earlier work on area 17 done without such controls.

The second source of variability is *the number of islands* (Donaldson and Whitteridge, 1977) in the representation of the visual periphery at the V2–V3 border and their position in the lower visual quadrant (Fig. 2/5D). The most common arrangement seems to include 2 islands: one on the HM, or just below, and a second one between elevations $-10°$ and $-20°$. Sometimes both islands are further down in the visual field. The number of islands is also variable from 0 to 3. In 3 animals out of 20, Tusa et al. (1979) found no islands but a continuous representation of the far periphery at the V2–V3 border in the lower visual field. Such interindividual variations have also been seen in the arrangement of extrastriate areas of the owl monkey (Allman and Kaas, 1975). These authors suggested that such abnormalities may be more common in domesticated animals that are no longer subjected to the rigors of natural selection.

2.3.2 RF Scatter

In their initial microelectrode study of area 17, Hubel and Wiesel (1962) made the observation that at the "microscopic" level the retinotopic representation breaks down. They observed that there was a random staggering of

---

[9] A similar variability has been reported for the auditory cortical areas of the cat (Imig and Morel, 1983).

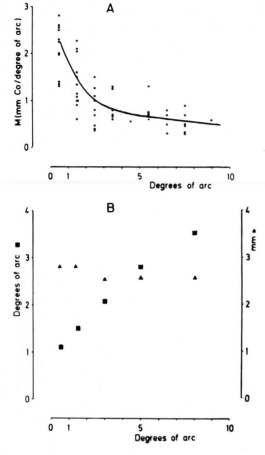

Fig. 2/14. Quantification of the retinocortical projection. A) (Linear) magnification factor (ordinate) as a function of
distance from the area centralis projection (abscissa). The factor is calculated
for 9 eccentricity classes. RF centers distant from the area centralis: $0-0.9°$;
$1.0-1.9°$, etc... $9.0-10.0°$. The continuous line is drawn by hand. B) Squares:
Total radial scatter of RFs. Each value is
calculated from $12-19$ individual values
in each eccentricity class. The values are
corrected by 10% because the netshift of
RF positions within 200 m cortical distance was found to contribute to the
scatter measurements in that order of
magnitude. Triangles: Width of spatial
subunits in area 17 as calculated for 5
eccentricity classes. Adapted with permission from Albus (1975 a).

field position superimposed on changes in mean value which corresponded
to the topographic arrangement. This RF scatter has been examined in detail
by Albus (1975 a) for the projection on area 17 of the central 10° of the visual
field. He observed that the scatter increased with eccentricity as did the size
of the RFs and the inverse of the magnification (Fig. 2/14). Due to the scatter
one has to move about 2.5 mm over the cortical surface before reaching a new
population within which the RFs are completely separated from the first one.
Therefore, Albus has concluded that a *spatial subunit* spans about 2.5 mm on
the cortical surface and that the width of a subunit was constant for different
eccentricities between 0 and 10°. The conclusions of Albus (1975 a) agree with
those of Hubel and Wiesel (1974 b), who from their study of the monkey
cortex concluded that each retinal ganglion cell is connected to the same
number of cortical cells irrespective of its position in the retina. From this
constant degree of retinocortical local *divergence* observed over a restricted
range of eccentricities (0–10°) Albus concludes that the whole striate cortex

is structurally uniform, although he notes that this seems to be inconsistent with some of the physiological non-uniformities he observed (changes in proportions of RF types and in binocularity with eccentricity). In fact our own work (Orban and Kennedy, 1981; Orban et al., 1981 a, b) has shown that functional properties change dramatically with eccentricity (see Chapters 4, 6, 7, 8). Indeed a point seemingly missed by Albus and Hubel and Wiesel is that the degree of local *convergence* in the retinocortical projection may be much more determinant for functional properties than the degree of local divergence. There is now evidence that this degree of local convergence changes with eccentricity (see Chapter 12). In the monkey a change in local convergence in the retinocortical projection does not need to imply a change in local retinocortical divergence as the global divergence of retinocortical connection changes with eccentricity (see Chapter 1). However in the cat changes in local convergence imply parallel changes in local divergence since the global divergence in the retinocortical projection is constant over the whole visual field (Chapter 1).

   That there is scatter superimposed on the retinotopic arrangement is a *direct consequence* of the local divergence and convergence in the retinocortical projection. Local divergence and convergence are themselves the structural basis of information processing within a topographically organized structure. Therefore one can understand that scatter in the maps increases as one moves from the receptor to higher levels of processing (Tusa and Palmer, 1980). A possible important function of scatter has been pointed out by Bishop (1979). According to Bishop the scatter of RF positions in both eyes is the mechanism by which the variation in binocular disparity is produced. Indeed disparity increases with eccentricity (Blakemore, 1970; Nikara et al., 1968) exactly as does the RF scatter.

2.3.3 The 17–18 Border and the Question of the Naso-Temporal Overlap

   The V1–V2 border is an important border since it includes *the representation of the AC* and the overwhelming majority of cortical studies are directed toward this representation. As pointed out earlier, the variability in the position of the maps on the cortical surface calls for proper control procedures. In addition to histological criteria (Nissl stain for layering and myelin stain), physiological criteria can be used. One obvious criterion is the movement of the RFs as the recording electrode advances through the border. Unfortunately at least where the lower visual quadrant is concerned, this movement of the fields is small given the high magnification (Fig. 2/15) and can actually be zero over a strip approximatively 1 mm wide (Dreher and Cottee, 1975; Hubel and Wiesel, 1965; Orban et al., 1980). There is a strip of high magnification at the 17–18 border and, as pointed out by Orban et al.

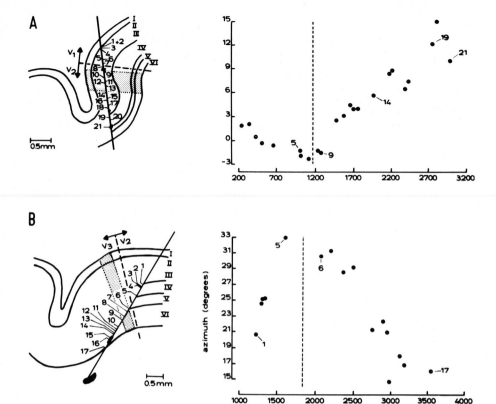

Fig. 2/15. Changes in RF azimuth in penetrations crossing the 17–18 (A) and the 18–19 (B) borders. Left-hand side, histological reconstruction of the penetrations. Hatched areas indicate histological transition zones, dashed lines physiological borders. Right-hand side, azimuth-distance curves. The azimuths were corrected by assuming that the mean disparities of the binocular cells in each animal were zero. Vertical stippled lines indicate physiological border. Cells 7 and 8 in the penetration through the 18–19 border responded tonically to changes in whole field illumination (see Chapter 6).

(1980), the magnification in this strip is higher than the values reported for the magnification in the AC representation of area 17 or 18. This can easily be explained by the finer sampling in our experiments compared to classical mapping studies. Because of this high magnification, azimuth-distance curves are of little use for the precise location of the V1–V2 border. RF width is not a useful indicator of the 17–18 border since either it does not change until 1500 µ past the border (Fig. 2/16). However *other physiological changes* occur at the level of the 17–18 border (Orban et al., 1980). This is illustrated in Fig. 2/16 which averages data from 5 different penetrations through the 17–18 border, both in superficial and deep layers, and in 5 different animals (all RFs within 10° from the fixation point). Velocity characteristics (half height upper

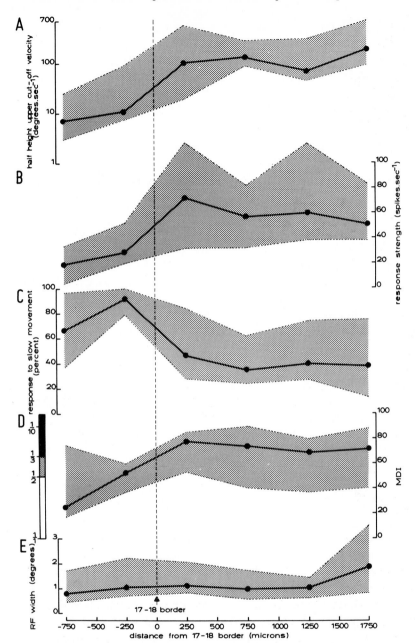

Fig. 2/16. Physiological changes across the 17–18 border: half height upper cut-off velocity (A), response strength (B), response to slow movement (C), mean direction index (D) and RF width (E). For definitions see Chapters 8 and 4. Data from 5 penetrations pooled. Each penetration was subdivided in segments 500 μ long, referred to the physiologically defined 17–18 border point. For each segment (2 before and 4 after the border) the medians and first and third quartiles are indicated at the middle of the segment. While changes in velocity characteristics and in direction selectivity occur at the 17–18 border (within 500 μ), the RF width changes only once the electrode has moved 1500 μ into area 18.

cut-off velocity and response to slow movement (see Chapter 8 for definition), response strength, and direction selectivity (mean direction index –
MDI see Chapter 8 for definition) change clearly at the border as one expects
from the regional differences described by Orban et al. (1981 a, b). Using
these physiological indications, it is generally possible in individual penetrations to trace the 17–18 border between 2 successively recorded cells (see
Fig. 3 in Orban et al., 1980).

In their initial description of the retinotopy of area 17, Hubel and Wiesel
(1962) mention that almost all RFs were confined to the contralateral visual
field and that some RFs stopped abruptly at the level of the VM. They further
noted that the spillover of RFs into the ipsilateral visual field was only 2–3°,
i.e., of the order of magnitude of possible errors in determining the AC
location. In their map of area 17, Tusa et al. (1978) indicate a representation
of an ipsilateral visual field strip adjoining the vertical meridian of 1.5 to 2°
(Fig. 2/3). They also note that this is approximatively the range of error when
one infers the position of the AC from the blind spot plots. Given the
importance of the *naso-temporal overlap* (i.e., the projection from a central
vertical strip of retina to both hemispheres) for stereoscopic depth perception
at the fixation point, several authors have tried to ascertain that there is a
representation of the ipsilateral visual field in areas 17 and 18. By sealing the
eyes to rings so as to avoid eye movements, and by plotting the position of
the RFs at the 17–18 border in both hemispheres, Blakemore (1970) was able
to show that there is a 1.5°-wide strip representing the ipsilateral field adjoining the vertical meridian. The estimation of AC position can be improved by
taking into account the mean disparity of the binocular cells which should be
zero (Nikara et al., 1968; Cooper and Pettigrew, 1979 a) to correct the mean
distance between the blind spot and AC, measured by Bishop et al. (1962).
Using this method Kato et al. (1978) and Orban et al. (1980) have found that
the visual field representation in area 17 extended up to 2° into the ipsilateral
hemifield. Finally Berman et al. (1982) have estimated the position of the AC
from the geometric center of the area devoid of blood vessels. With this
method, Berman et al. (1982) also found an ipsilateral representation 2° wide.
Therefore, it seems now to be established that in area 17 there is a representation of the ipsilateral visual field with a naso-temporal overlap of 1.5 to 2°,
if one considers the RF centers, or 3 to 4° considering the RF borders.
According to Albus and Beckmann (1980) the representation of the ipsilateral field in area 18 is 5° wide if one considers RF centers and 10 or 20° if
one considers RF borders. We have observed RF centers up to 3° into the
ipsilateral field in area 18. At the lateral border of 19 a representation of the
ipsilateral visual field has also been found (Albus and Beckmann, 1980).

The degree of naso-temporal overlap measured in areas 17 and 18 by
electrophysiological mapping fits with the naso-temporal overlap measured
anatomically (Fig. 2/17) in the retina by retrograde transport after several

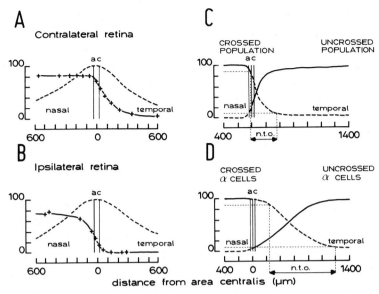

Fig. 2/17. The naso-temporal division of crossed and uncrossed projecting ganglion cells along a horizontal band through the central area. A) Contralateral retina; the stippled line indicates the total ganglion cell density, which peaks in the central area. The 2 vertical lines are 100 μm distant and show the possible error in assessing the peak of the central area. Crosses and the left ordinate show the percentage of labelled cells. B) Equivalent analysis of the ipsilateral retina. C) The crossed/uncrossed separation of the ganglion cell population projecting to the thalamus; crossed and uncrossed populations are balanced 70 μm temporal from the area centralis. D) As in C but for α cells only. ac: area centralis (peak of the maximum of total ganglion cell density – indicated by stippled lines); nto: naso-temporal overlap defined as the region between lines where the crossed population falls from 90 to 10%. Note the asymmetric location of the nasotemporal overlap with respect to the area centralis: the projection of points at the same distance in front and beyond the fixation point is more compressed on the nasal retina (in front) than on the temporal retina (beyond). Adapted with permission from Illing and Wässle (1981).

injections of HRP into the dLGN of one side (Cooper and Pettigrew, 1979 b; Illing and Wässle, 1981). At the level of the area centralis, the naso-temporal overlap is about 200 μ wide according to Cooper and Pettigrew (1979 b) and 400 μ wide according to Illing and Wässle (1981). Given the diameter of the cat's eye 400 μ corresponds to 2° in the visual field. According to both reports, the naso-temporal overlap is larger for α-cells than for the whole population projecting to the thalamus (Fig. 2/17). The width of the naso-temporal overlap (in visual degrees) increases both above and below the area centralis. The increase is inversely proportional to the square root of ganglion cell density so that in fact the naso-temporal decussation is about 25 ganglion cells wide at all levels. Since the cortical magnification (in area 17) follows ganglion cell density, the anatomical width (mm of retina) of the naso-temporal overlap is equal in the representation of the central and the peripheral visual field, but of course in visual field terms (visual degrees), the degree of overlap increases with distance from the fixation point.

2.3.4 The 18–19 Border and the Question of the Visual Field Islands

At the V2–V3 border magnification is small and the border can be reconstructed in oblique penetrations from the *azimuth-distance curves* (Fig. 2/15). In our own data on areas 18 and 19 representing the lower field, we have seen penetrations in which the most lateral RF at the V2–V3 border had its center as much as 35° from the fixation point or as little as 15°. This supports the idea (Donaldson and Whitteridge, 1977) that the periphery of the lower visual field is not represented continuously but by patches or islands (Fig. 2/5D). At the border the RFs are very large and some fields right on the border are difficult to outline and seem to extend throughout most of the visual field. Such fields responded to changes in diffuse illumination (see Chapter 6). We observed these large RFs at the V2–V3 border, both at the level of islands or between them. Albus (personal communication) has also found them throughout the border, contrary to the initial claim (Sanides and Albus, 1980) that they may be restricted to the parts of V2–V3 border between islands. These bridges between islands correspond to the patches of callosal projections extending from the 17–18 border into lateral area 18 (Sanides and Albus, 1980; Keller and Innocenti, 1981). This suggests a possible *function of the islands:* it is a means by which a representation of the whole visual field in area 18 is conserved (by large RFs in and around the islands) whilst allowing a vertical strip of the visual field surrounding the VM to be magnified. The latter representation is linked to a similar representation in area 18 of the other hemisphere by callosal connections. Although the large RFs make the topographic map less precise, there is no doubt that there is a single although distorted and non-topological (i.e. second order) representation of the visual field in area 18.

2.4 Conclusion

Areas 17, 18, and 19 of the cat, each contain a complete, or almost complete representation of the contralateral visual hemifield (V1, V2, and V3 respectively). In all three areas there is an overrepresentation of the central part of the visual field. While the retinotopic projection in area 17 is a first order point-to-point transformation of the retinal map, the transformations in areas 18 and 19 are more complex. Areas 17, 18, and 19 represent in all likelyhood, the first step of cortical processing in the cat visual system (primary cortical complex). Since the retinotopic maps are to a certain degree variable, adequate procedures have to be taken to ensure that recordings are made in the cortical area intended.

Chapter 3. Afferent Projections to Areas 17, 18, 19 of the Cat: Evidence for Parallel Input

The three major sources of afferents to the visual cortical areas are the visual thalamus, the visual claustrum, and other cortical areas. The visual thalamus includes the dorsal lateral geniculate nucleus, the relay on the direct retinocortical route, and the pulvinar lateralis posterior complex.

3.1 The Relay of Retinal Afferents: The Dorsal Lateral Geniculate Nuclear Complex

In the cat the direct route from the retina to the visual cortical areas goes through a *thalamic relay:* the dorsal lateral geniculate nuclear complex (Fig. 1/3). This complex includes the laminated part of the dorsal lateral geniculate nucleus (dLGN) the medial interlaminar nucleus (MIN) of the dLGN and the retino-recipient zone (RRZ) of the pulvinar-lateralis posterior (LP) complex, also called the geniculate wing (Guillery et al., 1980). The latter relay site can be considered as belonging to the pulvinar (Berman and Jones, 1977) or to the dLGN nuclear complex (Guillery et al., 1980). The ventral part of the LGN (vLGN) although receiving retinal afferents, does not project to the cortex.

The laminated dLGN contains several *laminae* (Figs. 3/1 and 3/2). In Nissl stains three layers are readily apparent: the dorsal A lamina, the middle A1 lamina and a lower lamina B located above the optic tract. While lamina A receives input from the contralateral eye and A1 from the ipsilateral one, the input to lamina B is more complex. Based on projections from the two eyes studied by degeneration or autoradiographic techniques, Guillery (1970) and Hickey and Guillery (1974) have further divided the B lamina into lamina C which receives input from the contralateral eye, lamina C_1 which receives input from the ipsilateral eye, lamina C_2 which has again input from the contralateral eye and lamina C_3, which has no detectable retinal input but receives a projection from the superior colliculus (SC) (Torrealba et al., 1981) (Fig. 3/1). The laminae C_1 to C_3 contain very small cells while the C lamina contains large cells in its dorsal part and smaller cells in its ventral part (Hickey and Guillery, 1974). There is a clear separation between laminae A, A1 and B by relatively cell-free interlaminar plexi, but there is no obvious

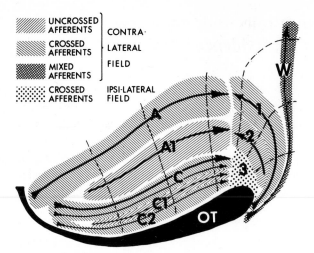

Fig. 3/1. Schematic representation of the pattern of retinal representation in the main laminae of the dorsal lateral geniculate nucleus (A, A1, C, C1, C2), in the medial interlaminar nucleus (1, 2, 3), and in the geniculate wing (W), as these would appear in a horizontal section through the dorsal half of the geniculate complex. Note that in the ventral regions, the relationship would be similar, except that the lamina 1 would lie next to lamina C, not next to lamina A. In the most dorsal tip of the nucleus, lamina 3 would lie between layers A and 1. Each arrow shows a single hemiretinal representation, and the point of each arrow is toward the vertical meridian, the tail toward the peripheral retina of each representation. Thick arrows show the coarsefibered components, thin ones show the fine components. The thin, interrupted lines indicate the approximate position of the lines of projection for each group of retinal representations (projection columns, see Chapter 1). Note the two components within lamina C. Adapted with permission from Guillery et al. (1980).

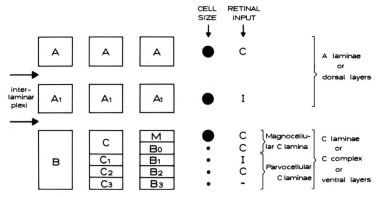

Fig. 3/2. Comparison of the different schemes of lamination for the laminated part of dLGN. C contralateral and I ipsilateral.

separation between C_1, C_2 and C_3 and the separation between C and C_1 is hard to see (Hickey and Guillery, 1974). The whole of laminae C, C_{1-3} is called the C complex or C laminae or ventral layers. By contrast the A laminae are labelled dorsal layers. Since laminae C_{1-3} characteristically contain only very small cells they are often labelled parvocellular C laminae, and lamina C is then referred to as magnocellular C lamina, although only its dorsal part contains large cells. Based on functional properties Rodieck (1979), in following Famigletti (1975), proposed to divide lamina C into a dorsal part with large cells (lamina M) and a ventral part which contains small cells (lamina B_0). In this scheme the parvocellular C_{1-3} laminae are called B_{1-3}. The M lamina corresponds then to the central interlaminar nucleus (CIN) of Thuma (1928). Although this scheme is very attractive most anatomical work has been done with the A, A1, C, C_{1-3} scheme and this has to be followed here, although it seems highly desirable that anatomists pay more attention to the subdivisions of lamina C in the future.

Although no lamination is apparent in Nissl-stained sections of MIN, autoradiographic techniques indicate that MIN has a hidden lamination (Fig. 3/1). The MIN contains at least two laminae, one for each eye. The region which receives input from the ipsilateral eye is a small central region, surrounded dorsally, medially and ventrally by a larger crescent shaped region that receives input from the contralateral eye (Kratz et al., 1978). Recently Guillery et al. (1980) have described a third lamina in the MIN corresponding to an ipsilateral field representation in the contralateral eye. It is noteworthy that MIN seems to be a thalamic nucleus which is found only in carnivores (Rodieck, 1979). The geniculate wing contains very small cells, of a size similar to that of the parvocellular C laminae (Leventhal et al., 1980) and receives input from both eyes (Guillery et al., 1980).

Both the MIN and the laminated part of dLGN are strictly *retinotopically* organized (Sanderson, 1971 a) while the geniculate wing has only a coarsely

Table 3/1. Different morphological classes of LGN cells

Class	Size	Description (Guillery, 1966)		Location	Function	
		Dendritic tree appendages	Dendritic tree location		LeVay and Ferster (1977)	Friedlander et al. (1981) Stanford et al. (1981)
1	large ($\varnothing$ 20–40 μm)	no	does not respect laminar borders	A, magno-cellular C, MIN	relay: Y	relay: Y
2	medium ($\varnothing$15–25 μm)	grape-like appendages	does not cross laminar borders	A, magno-cellular C, MIN	relay: X	relay: Y, X
3	small ($\varnothing$10–25 μm)	clusters of stalked appendages	—	A, magno-cellular C, MIN	inter-neuron	relay: X
4	intermediate	free	dendrites parallel to the laminae	parvo-cellular C_{1-3}	—	relay: W

retinotopic organization. MIN and possibly the ventral C laminae not only contain a full retinotopic projection of the contralateral hemifield, as do the A laminae, but they also have a representation of the ipsilateral hemifield, arising from ganglion cells in the temporal retina of the contralateral eye. While in the laminated part of the dLGN there is a proportionally larger representation of the central visual field this is less true for MIN (Sanderson, 1971 a). Following Guillery's (1966) original classification, cells in the dLGN are classified *morphologically* into 4 types using chiefly cell size and dendritic tree characteristics (Table 3/1). Classes 1, 2, and 3 occur in the A laminae, the magnocellular C lamina and MIN, while class 4 occurs in the parvocellular C_{1-3} laminae.

3.2 The Geniculocortical Projection

To provide retinotopic cortical maps, a topographically organized projection from the dLGN onto the visual cortices is required. This has indeed been shown (Rosenquist et al., 1974). The *different parts of the dLGN complex have different cortical targets* (Fig. 3/3). In view of the many changes in properties of cortical neurons with eccentricity in the visual field, it would be interesting to know whether projections from the different parts of the LGN to the cortical areas change with eccentricity. Unfortunately little data (e.g. Meyer and Albus, 1981 b) are at present available on this point.

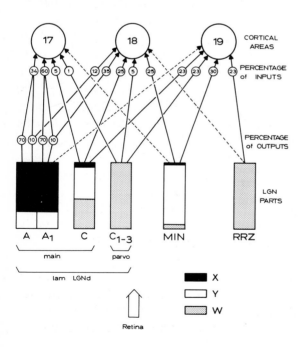

Fig. 3/3. Anatomically established projections from the different parts of the dLGN nuclear complex to areas 17, 18, 19. Within each part, the approximate proportion of physiological LGN types are indicated. Numbers in upper row indicate proportions of afferents from different parts to a given cortical area. Numbers in lower row indicate proportions of a given LGN part projecting to different areas.

Laminae A and A1 project only to areas 17 and 18 with the exclusion of other visual areas (Fig. 3/3). While area 17 receives a heavy input from A and A1, area 18 receives a weaker input from both laminae and the input from lamina A is more variable than from lamina A1 (Geisert, 1980; Holländer and Vanegas, 1977). While laminae A and A1 account for 94% of the thalamic input into area 17, they account for only 47% of the input to area 18 (Holländer and Vanegas, 1977). Only one report (Holländer and Vanegas, 1977) out of 5 (Geisert, 1980; Gilbert and Kelly, 1975; Holländer and Vanegas, 1977; Maciewicz, 1975; Niimi et al., 1981) found a very small projection from the A laminae to area 19.

Geisert (1980) with double labelling experiments has shown that 70% of laminae A and A1 cells project to area 17 only and 10% to areas 17 and 18 while hardly any cell projects to area 18 only. The cells with double projection in these laminae are markedly larger than the mean and probably correspond to class 1 cells of Guillery (1966). From these double labelling experiments Geisert (1980) estimated the proportion of interneurons in the LGN to be approximately 20%, which is between previous estimates by LeVay and Ferster (1977) (25%) and Lin et al. (1977) (10%). From their intracellular staining experiments Friedlander et al. (1981) recently reached the conclusion that the proportion of interneurons must be very small.

Lamina C projects to areas 17, 18, and 19 (Geisert, 1980; Holländer and Vanegas, 1977; Leventhal et al., 1980; Maciewicz, 1975). While lamina C provides only 4% of the input to area 17, it provides about 20% of the input to areas 18 and 19 (Holländer and Vanegas, 1977). From the data of Holländer and Vanegas (1977) it appears that the lamina C cells projecting to area 18 are markedly larger than those projecting to areas 17 and 19, although Holländer and Vanegas (1977) injected only one animal in area 19. It is thus likely that the class 1 cells of lamina C project to area 18. Given the possible physiological correlation, it would be interesting to know whether the input from lamina C to area 19 arises only from the smallest, more ventrally located, cells. The data of Leventhal et al. (1980) suggest that the vast majority of lamina C cells projecting to 19 are small cells, of the same size as those in the parvocellular C lamina, but the data of Geisert (1980), Holländer and Vanegas (1977) and Leventhal et al. (1980) suggest that some of the large cells of lamina C also project to area 19.

The *parvocellular C laminae* (C_{1-3}) project to areas 17, 18 and 19. However, they account for less than 5% of the inputs to areas 17 and 18, while they are a substantial input to area 19 (20%) according to Holländer and Vanegas (1977). Recently Raczkowski and Rosenquist (1980) have shown that these projections of the C_{1-3} laminae to areas 17, 18 and 19 are part of a wide projection to almost all visual cortical areas with the exception of ALLS and AMLS (Palmer et al., 1978). In his labelling experiments Geisert (1980) could not distinguish between the magnocellular C lamina and parvocellular C_{1-3} laminae. However in the C laminae as a whole there were 50% of the cells projecting to both 17 and 18. In opposition to the A laminae, the size of those cells was not larger than the mean, and seemed to be bimodally distributed including very large cells (probably the class 1 cells of top lamina C) and smaller cells (probably from the parvocellular layers). With separate injections into each of the 3 areas 17, 18, and 19, Geisert (1980) observed HRP labelling in about 65 to 70% of the cells in each case. Even with a small proportion of interneurons this indicates that a number of C laminae cells must send a triple branching axon to the three areas.

The *projection from the MIN* to area 17 is very scant: it was observed by Ferster and LeVay (1978), Geisert (1980), Gilbert and Kelly (1975), Leventhal (1979) and Niimi et al. (1981) but not by Holländer and Vanegas (1977) nor by Kennedy and Baleydier (1977). MIN projects to areas 18 and 19. According to Holländer and Vanegas (1977) it accounts for 25% of the input to area 18 and 40% of the input to area 19. It is clear from Table 1 in Holländer and Vanegas (1977) that more rostral portions of area 18 receive a heavier input from MIN (40%) than more caudal parts (10%). A similar result has explicitly been reported by Leventhal et al. (1980). After injections of horseradish peroxydase (HRP) into regions of area 18 subserving peripheral vision ($>20°$ ecc) 60% of MIN cells were labelled, while less than 20% of MIN cells were labelled after injection in area 18 representing the central 5° of the visual field. This indicates that the proportion of input from MIN increases with elevation or with eccentricity. Holländer and Vanegas (1977) injected only 1 animal in area 19 at rostral levels; the difference in strength of MIN input to areas 18 and 19 they observed may simply be a reflection of this eccentric location of the injection site in area 19. Geisert (1980) also observed double labelled cells in MIN after injection of areas 17 and 18. Their size was not larger than those of the average MIN population.

The *geniculate wing* projects only to area 19 (Leventhal et al., 1980; Holländer and Vanegas, 1977) and accounts for 20% of the input to area 19 (Holländer and Vanegas, 1977). However after massive HRP injection into the 17–18 border Hughes (1981) observed a small projection from the region corresponding to RRZ onto the 17–18 border.

3.3 Functional Streams in the Retino-Geniculocortical Projection

It now seems well established that there are at least *three functional streams* arising from the retina, relaying separately in the different parts of the dLGN complex and projecting differently to the visual cortical areas. At the retinal level three functional types have been described. The identity of two of these types: X or brisk sustained and Y or brisk transient cells is now well established (Enroth-Cugell and Robson, 1966; Cleland et al., 1971). Y cells have fast-conducting axons and X cells more slowly conducting axons. The third group has been described only recently although it constitutes about half of all ganglion cells (Stone and Hoffmann, 1972). It is a looser collection of sluggish and "rarely encountered" types (Cleland and Levick, 1974 a, b) which have been grouped under the label W (Stone and Fukuda, 1974). Stone and Fukuda (1974) advocated the use of a single label (W) for these cells because of their similarity in conduction velocity (which is very slow), retinal distribution and central projections. For our purpose it is convenient to consider them as a functional entity since they mainly relay through the parvocellular C laminae, but they may well be a collection of types as stressed by Rodieck (1979) in his review. In view of the widespread projection of the parvocellular C laminae to at least 8 or 9 different visual cortical areas, it could well be that the different subtypes of the W system have different cortical targets.

3.3.1 Functional Properties of Retinal and Geniculate X, Y, W Cells (Table 3/2).

The *same tests* can be used to distinguish between the 3 functional types of retinal and of LGN cells. These tests have been reviewed recently (Stone et al., 1979; Rodieck, 1979 and Lennie, 1980). It will suffice to note that tests of linearity or derived tests such as the second harmonic analysis (So and Shapley, 1981) are useful to distinguish between X and Y geniculate cells but do not allow a positive identification, unless one is sure that one can only sample from X or Y cells (e.g., because of the position of the electrode in the dorsal laminae). Indeed recently Levick and Thibos (1980) and Sur et al. (1981) have reported linear and non-linear sluggish cells in the cat retina. *The tests which seem now to be most generally used for classification of LGN cells are RF diameter and its correlate grating acuity, conduction velocity, and sensitivity to fast movements* especially those of the contrast which cause response from the surround (Bullier and Norton, 1979 a, b; Lehmkuhle et al., 1980). RF diameter increases with eccentricity, but at all eccentricities Y cells have larger diameters than X cells. Y and W cells have approximately equal RF diameters (Wilson et al., 1976; Dreher and Sefton, 1979). Particularly interesting are the properties distinguishing between X, Y and W cells which can be applied to cortical cells, in order to identify the type of afferents to a cortical cell: these include conduction velocity, linearity of summation, spatial distribution of responses to ON-OFF flashed stimuli [response planes (Stevens and Gerstein, 1976) or spatio-temporal maps (Bullier and Norton, 1979 a, b)] and velocity sensitivity (Dreher and Sanderson, 1973; Orban et al., 1981 c). These properties will be discussed in Chapter 11.

Table 3/2. Properties of X, Y, W cells (modified from Stone et al., 1979)

	Y-cells	X-cells	W-cells
Functional properties			
Receptive field layout	ON-center/OFF-surround or OFF-center/ON-surround	As for Y-cells	Some have layout as Y and X cells; others have ON-OFF centers, some have purely inhibitory centers, some are directionally selective or color-coded
Receptive field center size	Large (0.5°−2.5°)	Small (0.2°−1°)	Large (0.4−2.5°)
Velocity sensitivity	Respond well to rapid stimulus motion	Relatively poor response to rapid stimulus motion	Relatively poor response to rapid stimulus motion
Linearity of center-surround summation	Non-linear	Linear	Linear or non-linear
Response to standing contrast	Phasic or transient in most cells; some are tonic or sustained, especially near area centralis; all are tonic when dark adapted	Most give tonic responses in mesopic conditions, many are transient when ligth adapted	Either tonic of phasic
Periphery effect	Present	Usually absent	Absent
Axonal velocity	Fast, 30−40 m/sec	Slow, 15−23 m/sec	Very slow, 2−18 m/sec
Retinal distribution			
Proportion of population	5%	Approximately 40−55%	Approximately 40−55%
Distribution in different parts of the retina	Concentrated near area centralis	Concentrated at area centralis	Concentrated at area centralis and in streak
Naso-temporal division (Fig. 3/4)	Nasal cells project contralaterally, most temporal cells ipsilaterally; strip of intermingling centered slightly temporal to area centralis	Nasal cells project contralaterally, temporal cells project ipsilaterally, narrow strip of intermingling centers on area centralis	Nasal cells project contralaterally, most temporal cells also project contralaterally; about 40% of temporal cells project ipsilaterally
Morphological correlation in retina	α cells	β cells	γ and other cells
dLGN distribution (Fig. 3/3)	Some in A laminae Many in magnocellular C & MIN	Many in A laminae Few in magnocellular C	Parvocellular C laminae, geniculate wing, MIN
Morphological correlation in dLGN	Class 1−2	Class 2−3	Class 4

3.3.2 Correlation with Retinal Morphology

The 3 *functional* types of ganglion cells have been correlated with the 3 *morphological* types described by Boycott and Wässle (1974): α, β and γ cells. α cells have large somata and wide dendritic trees and β cells have medium size somata and small dendritic trees, while γ cells have large dendritic trees but very small somata. Boycott and Wässle (1974) briefly described a 4th type (δ cells) and recently other types have been reported (ε cells by Leventhal et al., 1980). The correspondence between α and Y cells has been established by the experiments of Cleland et al. (1975) and Wässle et al. (1975). The correlation between β and X cells seems established (see Rodieck, 1979 for review) although the quantitative comparison between dendritic trees of β with RF center of X cells is discouraging (Lennie, 1980). The correlation between W cells and γ cells is very loose, given the many other morpohological types that are candidates for correlation with W cells. The correlation between morphological and functional types is important since the proportions, retinal distribution and even central projections can be more easily established for the morphological types (Fig. 3/4) (Wässle and Illing, 1980;

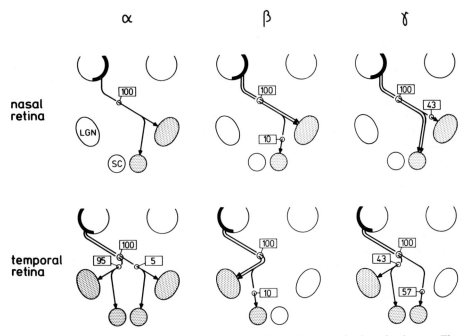

Fig. 3/4. Comparison of the retinotectal and the retinothalamic projections in the cat. The numbers give percentages within each of the three ganglion cell classes. The left column shows the α cell projections from the nasal and from the temporal retinae. The middle column summarized the β cell projections and the right column the γ cell projections. The whole ganglion cell population is made up from 4.5% α cells, 56% β cells, and 40% γ cells. From Illing and Wässle (1981) with permission.

Illing and Wässle, 1981). α or Y cells constitute about 5% of the ganglion cells – although physiological recording yields a proportion of 25% Y cells due to sample bias of electrodes (Stone, 1973) – and their density peaks at the area centralis (Illing and Wässle, 1981). According to Wässle et al. (1981 a) each retinal point is covered by 2 α cells (1 ON center and 1 OFF center). The axon of almost every α cell branches (Fig. 3/4) and sends a branch to the superior colliculus (SC), lam dLGN and MIN and the nucleus of the optic tract (NOT) (Bowling and Michael, 1981). Branching of axons may be an important property of the retino-geniculo-cortical Y system, as class 1 LGN cells, identified as Y cells, also send branching axons to the areas 17 and 18. Therefore the proportion of cortical cells receiving Y afferents may be much larger than the proportion of Y ganglion cells (5%) suggests. The β cells (and thus probably the X cells also) form 55% of the ganglion cells (Illing and Wässle, 1981) and are concentrated in the area centralis. According to Wässle et al. (1981 b) each retinal point is covered by 6 β cells (3 ON center and 3 OFF center). β cells project mainly if not exclusively to the dLGN (Fig. 3/4). The γ cells make up 40% of all ganglion cells (Illing and Wässle, 1981) and are concentrated in the area centralis and possibly also in the visual streak (Rowe and Stone, 1976, but Hughes, 1980). γ cells project both to the dLGN and the midbrain (Fig. 3/4). About 40% of γ cells have branching axons.

3.3.3 Separation of Functional Streams at LGN Level

The vast majority of geniculate cells projecting to the cortex have RF properties similar to those of ganglion cells (Cleland et al. 1971, 1976; Wilson et al., 1976; Hoffmann et al., 1972). This suggests that there is *little or no mixing* of excitatory signals at this level in the visual pathway. The separate projections through the LGN of the 3 functional streams is further demonstrated by the simultaneous recording of geniculate cells and their retinal afferents (Cleland et al., 1971). Only 5–10% of cells in the A, A1, and C lamina have properties intermediate between X and Y (mixed X/Y cells in Wilson et al.'s (1976) terminology or IM cells in Bullier and Norton's (1979 a) terminology). According to Bullier and Norton (1979 a) these cells are in fact X cells with large RFs and should be considered as X cells.

3.3.4 Correlation with LGN Morphological Types (Table 3/1)

LeVay and Ferster (1977), following Wilson et al. (1976), have proposed an attractive correlation between functional and morphological types of LGN cells. They suggested that class 1 and 2 cells of Guillery (1966) correspond to Y and X cells respectively while class 3 of Guillery (1966) would be interneurons. In the same vein Wilson et al. (1976) have suggested that W cells of the parvocellular layer would correspond to class 4 cells of Guillery (1966). According to LeVay and Ferster (1977) X cells would be further characterized by the presence of a "laminar body" in the neuron. Kalil and Worden (1978), Schmidt and Hirsch (1980) and Geisert (1980) however showed that the proportion of cells with laminated bodies is much too small compared to the proportion of X cells in the A laminae. While the correlation between W cells and class 4 neurons has been confirmed by intracellular staining techniques (Stanford et al., 1981), the correlation between class 1 and 2 and X and Y cells has not been confirmed by the intracellular injection experiments of Friedlander et al. (1981). *Indeed while all class 1 are Y cells, class 2 cells can be both X or Y cells and class 3 cells are X cells.* These findings imply that many class 3 cells are relay cells rather than interneurons. This is confirmed by the anatomical study of Meyer and Albus (1981 b) who showed that class 3 cells project to areas 17 and 18.

The correlation of functional types with morphological types is important because cortical projections of the morphological types can be established with retrograde transport techniques. Both LeVay and Ferster (1977) and Meyer and Albus (1981 b) found that class 2 cells project mainly to area 17. It then follows that the smaller Y cells (group 2) project only to area 17 while the large Y cells (group 1) project to both areas 17 and 18. This is in keeping with the observation that the proportion of cells projecting to both areas 17 and 18 in A and A1 laminae is smaller than the proportion of Y cells in those laminae (10% compared to 22% Geisert, 1980). Meyer and Albus (1981 b) also reported that the change in relative numbers of class 1 and class 2 LGN cells projecting to areas 17 and 18 is very significant but occurs gradually across the 17/18 border and is not strictly related to that border as defined by cytoarchitectonic or physiological criteria. This may be in keeping with our observation that contrary to velocity sensitivity, RF width does not change at the 17–18 border but only 1500 µ past the border (see Fig. 2/16). Indeed the type of geniculate afferents (X or Y and hence class 2 and 1) may be more strongly correlated with RF width than with velocity characteristics of the cortical cells (see Chapter 11).

3.3.5 Distribution of Functional Streams in dLGN Nuclear Complex (Table 3/3)

The *proportion of functional types are very different in the different* parts of the *dLGN nuclear complex.* In the A laminae X cells outnumber Y cells and W cells are almost absent. It has been constantly found that the proportion of Y cells is 1.6 times (range 1.4 to 1.9) larger in lamina A1 than in lamina A. This is in keeping with the fact that lamina A1 provides input from the

Table 3/3. Distribution of functional types in the different parts of dLGN

	% X cells	% Y cells	X/Y ratio	% W cells
A laminae				
Wilson et al., 1976 [+]	67	23	3/1	0
Cleland et al., 1976 [+]	62	28	2/1	5
Bullier and Norton, 1979 a [*+]	50	40	1/1	–
Sireteanu and Hoffmann, 1979 [*]	50	50	1/1	–
Friedlander et al., 1981	65	35	2/1 – 1/1	–
Magnocellular C lamina				
Wilson et al., 1976 [+]	12	40	1/3	43
Cleland et al., 1976	5	43	1/9	52
Parvocellular C laminae				
Wilson et al., 1976	0	0	–	100
Cleland et al., 1976	0	0	–	100
MIN				
Kratz et al., 1978 [*]	0	100	–	–
Dreher and Sefton, 1979 [+]	4.5	84	1/19	7.5

[*] Varnished metal electrodes, may bias recording towards larger cell somata
[+] Sum of percentages smaller than 100 because of intermediate cells

ipsilateral eye to both areas 17 and 18, while A and C provide the input from the contralateral eye to areas 17 and 18 respectively. The proportion of Y cells in the A laminae has been reported to increase with eccentricity (Hoffmann et al., 1972; see also Dreher and Sefton, 1979). In lamina C there is a relative absence of X cells and a high proportion of Y and W cells. According to Wilson et al. (1976) and Mitzdorf and Singer (1977) there is a clearcut separation between Y (and X cells) recorded dorsally in lamina C and W cells recorded in the ventral part of lamina C. The parvocellular C laminae contain only W cells. In MIN all or almost all cells belong to the Y type.

It seems therefore that *functionally the dLGN complex contains 3 parts:* the A laminae characterized by a large X/Y ratio (2/1); the interlaminar nuclei: the medial nucleus (MIN) and central nucleus (CIN) or top part of lamina C which have a large Y/X ratio (9/1) and the small cell part (bottom of lamina C, the parvocellular C laminae and RRZ) which contains almost exclusively W cells. The A laminae project to area 17 and to a lesser extent to area 18, the interlaminar nuclei to area 18 and less to area 19 and the small cell part to area 19 and weakly to areas 17 and 18.

3.3.6 Input to Different Areas of Primary Visual Complex

In conclusion (Fig. 3/5A) the X cells almost exclusively reach area 17 since the cells projecting to area 18 from laminae A are probably all Y cells except

A   anatomy

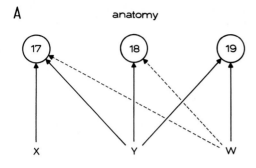

B   physiology

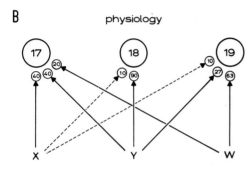

Fig. 3/5. Comparison of the anatomical (A) and physiological (B) identifications of inputs to the 3 cortical areas. The anatomical estimation is derived from Figure 3/3. Recently Meyer and Albus (1981b) have provided some anatomical evidence for X input to area 18 (not indicated). The physiological estimations are the data from Table 3/5.

a small strip along the 17/18 border (Meyer and Albus, 1981 b). A small proportion of X cells could reach area 18 or 19 through lamina C. Y cells project more widely to areas 17, 18 and 19, exactly as at the lower level they project to SC, lam dLGN and MIN. The Y input reaches area 19 mainly through MIN which possibly has a larger projection to cortical regions subserving peripheral vision than to regions subserving central vision. Thus area 19 subserving central vision may have only a scant Y input. The W cells project mainly to area 19, although they also provide a weak input to areas 17 and 18. On anatomical grounds, Meyer and Albus (1981 b) have suggested that the strength of the W projection to area 18 increases with eccentricity. *Thus it seems that although Y and W cells project to more than 1 area, areas 17, 18 and 19 are the main targets of X, Y and W systems respectively* (Stone et al., 1979). Any understanding of the functional role of these systems calls then for a comparison of properties of these cortical areas. The difficulties encountered by Lennie (1980) when attempting to find a role for Y cells may then be imputed to his failure to consider cortical areas other than area 17. Also the separation between geniculostriate system and extrastriate areas followed in many handbooks may be more appropriate for the monkey than for the cat.

3.4 Physiological Identification of the Functional Type of Afferents to Areas 17, 18 and 19

Since *conduction velocities* can be measured quite easily in electrical stimulation experiments, the differences in conduction velocity of the different functional types (see Table 3/2), have been used to identify the afferents to the different cortical areas. It is well established that the different functional types of LGN cells have conduction velocities matched to those of their afferents (Cleland et al., 1971, 1976; Dreher and Sefton, 1979; Hoffmann and Stone, 1971; Hoffmann et al., 1972; Wilson et al., 1976). Hence both conduction velocity of LGN afferents to the cortex (comparing latencies to optic radiation stimulation in 2 positions (S2 and S4 in Fig. 3/6A) or conduction velocity of the retinal afferents to the LGN (comparing latencies to optic chiasm and optic radiation just above the LGN, S1 and S2 in Fig. 3/6A) could be used to identify the functional type of the afferents to the cortex. Comparison of both types of measurements shows that the conduction veloc-

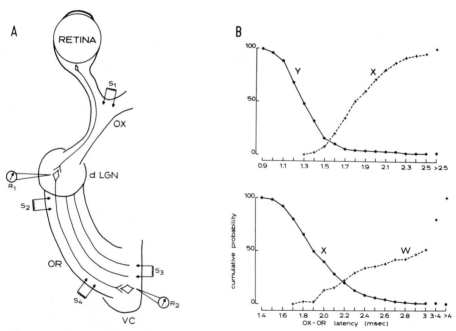

Fig. 3/6. How well do OX–OR latency differences separate the different functional input types? A. Experimental set-up to measure orthodromic conduction velocities of retinal afferents of LGN cells (stimulating at S_1 and recording at R_1), antidromic conduction velocities of LGN cells (stimulation at S_3 and recording at R_1) and conduction velocity of afferents to cortical cells (comparing stimulation at S_1 and S_3 at recording site R_2 or comparing stimulation at S_2 and S_4 at recording site R_2). B. Cumulative probabilities of OX–OR latency differences for Y- and X-recipient (above) cortical cells and for X- and W- recipient (below) cortical cells. Based on OX latencies of LGN cells in three studies (Dreher and Sefton, 1979; Hoffmann et al., 1972 and Wilson et al., 1976).

Table 3/4. Conduction velocities of functional types

	Y (msec)	X (msec)	W (msec)
Conduction velocity of LGN afferents measured by antidromic latency of LGN cells to VC stimulation			
Cleland et al., 1971	0.5–1.1	0.9–4	–
Hoffmann et al., 1972	0.4–1.4	0.9–2	–
Stone and Dreher, 1973	0.4–1.5	0.6–5.5	–
Cleland et al., 1976	0.2–1.8	0.9–4	1.6–10
Wilson et al., 1976	0.5–1.4	0.9–4	1.8–11.8
Dreher and Sefton, 1979	0.4–1.2	0.9–4	–
Conduction velocity of retinal afferents measured by orthodromic latency of LGN cells to OX stimulation			
Hoffman et al., 1972	0.9 –1.6	1.4–3	–
Wilson et al., 1976	0.8 –1.5	1.4–2.4	1.8–8
Dreher and Sefton, 1979	0.85–1.6	1.3–2.85	2 –7.5

ity of retinal afferents allows a more reliable identification of the functional input types (Table 3/4).

The conduction velocity of LGN cells can be evaluated by measuring the latency of antidromic activation from the visual cortex (VC) (see Fig. 3/6A). Y LGN fibers have the fastest conduction velocity as witnessed by a short antidromic latency to VC stimulation. X LGN axons have a medium conduction velocity as indicated by a somewhat larger antidromic latency to VC stimulation. W fibers have the slowest conduction velocity as shown by their long antidromic latency to VC stimulation. While all these studies agree that on average Y LGN fibers have faster conduction than X LGN fibers and that those in turn are faster than W LGN fibers, there is considerable overlap (Table 3/4). Considering only the two largest studies Cleland et al. (1976) and Wilson et al. (1976), there is about 25% chance of error in classifying LGN fibers as X or Y only by their antidromic latency (the best separation is around 0.9 or 1 msec). Similarly the distinction between X and W fibers based only on antidromic latency will induce 20 to 25% misclassifications, the best separation being around 2.5 msec.

The cortical latency to optic radiation (OR) stimulation means very little. Indeed a long latency response of a cortical cell to LGN stimulation or to stimulation of the optic radiation (OR) just above the LGN, can be due either to monosynaptic activation by slow afferents or polysynaptic activation by fast afferents. Therefore *most studies compare response latencies of cortical cells to stimulation of two sites on the retino-geniculo-cortical pathway.* Since the conduction velocity of LGN afferents is not very reliable, the two sites usually chosen are the optic chiasm (OX) and the optic radiation just above the LGN (OR). The implication is that the difference in latency to stimulation of these sites should be compared to the orthodromic latency of LGN cells to optic chiasm (OX) stimulation in order to determine the type of afferents. Indeed both measurements reflect the conduction velocity of the retinal afferents. There is however an additional factor intervening in the cortical measurements namely the variability of the transmission time at the cortex which, to some extent, blurs the distribution. Hence identification of afferents is more valid for first order cortical neurons than for subsequent ones because of the lower variability introduced by a smaller number of cortical synapses. It should also be noted that the use of OX−OR latency differences[1] depends critically on the assumption that there is only one synapse at the LGN level and that recurrent collaterals of corticofugal fibers do not contribute to OR responses of cortical cells. According to Dreher et al. (1980) comparison of ON[2]-OX and OX-OR latency differences suggest that recurrent collaterals are not a problem.

The available data show that there is *on the average a clear separation between the OX latencies of the 3 functional types of LGN cells:* the distributions overlapping to some extent, but less than those of antidromic VC latency (Table 3/4). Since the identification of the type of afferents to cortical cells depends critically on the distribution of OX latencies of LGN types, I have prepared the cumulative probabilities of these latency distributions using data of Dreher and Sefton (1979), Hoffmann et al. (1972) and Wilson et al. (1976) (Fig. 3/6B). The comparison between latencies of X and Y cells show that the best separation is at 1.55 msec: cortical cells with OX−OR latency differences of 1.5 msec or less should be considered as receiving Y afferents (8% error), and those with OX−OR latency differences of 1.6 msec or more as receiving X afferents (10% error). The data of Eysel et al. (1979) fully confirm this decision criterion. Indeed, Singer et al. (1975), Tretter et al. (1975) and Dreher et al. (1980) all consider 1.5 msec or less to be characteristic of Y afferents. Henry et al. (1979) based on their own recordings of LGN afferents in the cortex (only 17 fibers) place the limit at 1.65 msec. Bullier and Henry (1979 b) consider cells with latency differences <1.4 msec as Y and those with latency differences >1.7 msec as X cells. This reduces the errors (to 2 and 5% respectively) and takes into account the variability introduced by the cortical synapses but leaves some cells unclassified. The separation between X and W afferents is less clear (see also Dreher et al., 1980). The best separation is at 2.15 msec: cortical cells with latency differences of 2.1 or less can be considered as receiving X afferents (16% error) while those with latency differences of 2.2 msec or more as receiving W afferents (20% error). Indeed Dreher et al. (1980) use the criterion 2.2 msec and larger to define W afferents.

The above reviewed criteria for distinguishing between cells with Y, X and W afferents have been applied to the distribution of OX−OR latency differences for cortical cells in different areas (Bullier and Henry, 1979 a, b;

---

[1] Difference in latency of cortical cell response to optic chiasm and optic radiation stimulation.
[2] Optic nerve.

Table 3/5. Proportion of cells receiving X, Y, W afferents in the three cortical areas estimated from OX–OR latency differences

Area 17				Area 18				Area 19			
	X	X	W		Y	X	W		Y	X	W
Stone and Dreher (1973)* (n = 43)	30%	70%		Stone and Dreher (1973)* (n = 34)	94%	6%		Dreher et al. (1980) (n = 50)	28%	9%	63%
Singer et al. (1975) (n = 130)	40%	33%	27%	Tretter et al. (1975) (n = 61)	93%	7%	–	Kimura et al. (1980)** (n = 56)	32%		68%
Henry et al. (1979) (n = 56)	34%	50%	16%	Harvey (1980) (n = 152)	95%	5%	–				
Bullier and Henry (1979 b)** (n = 93)	46%	50%	4%	Dreher et al. (1980) (n = 55)	84%	16%	–				
Dreher et al. (1980) (n = 78)	47%	31%	22%								
median	43%	41%	18%	median	93%	7%	–				

Number between brackets indicates the number of cells studied.
* Relying primarily on OR latencies although for most cells OX latencies were available
(Y afferents OX–OR latencies 0.9 to 1.7 msec)
(X afferents OX–OR latencies > 1.5 msec)
** Relying on conduction velocity estimated between LGN and OR.

Dreher et al., 1980; Harvey, 1980 a; Henry et al., 1979; Singer et al., 1975; Tretter et al., 1975) and the results are listed in Table 3/5. In addition estimates of Y afferents to areas 17 and 18 by Stone and Dreher (1973) and of W afferents to area 19 by Kimura et al. (1980) are also indicated in Table 3/5. It should be noted that Singer et al. (1975) did not interpret their longest OX–OR latency differences as indicative of W afferents since at that time there was no evidence that W cells relayed through the dLGN. Bullier and Henry (1979b) discard the 4% cells with possible W afferents using the argument that the cells were recorded outside the layers of termination of W afferents (see later), while Henry et al. (1979) seem to accept the possibility of very slowly conducting input (W cells) into area 17.

The different studies agree quite well and *reveal marked differences between afferents to areas 17, 18, and 19* (Table 3/5). Area 17 receives a mixture of afferents dominated by X and Y afferents in about equal proportions and somewhat less than 20% of W afferents. Area 18 on the contrary receives almost exclusively Y afferents. Area 19 receives mainly W afferents (over 60%) and a substantial proportion of Y cells (25–30%). According to Dreher et al. (1980) these Y axons reach area 19 indirectly, while Kimura et al. (1980) suggest that they reach area 19 directly (probably through MIN). While X cells represent 30 to 50% of the afferents to area 17, less than 10–15% of the afferents to area 18 or 19 are X cells. The latter cells could also be either Y cells or W cells. While the W cells project mainly to area 19 and hardly to area 18, they contribute 4–27% of the afferents to area 17. Given the less distinct separation between X and W, this may be either an over- or underestimation. Y cells project to all three areas and seem to diverge at the geniculocortical level at least as much as at the retinogeniculate level (Friedlander et al., 1981).

Finally there is good agreement between the physiological and morphological identification of afferents to the 3 cortical areas (Fig. 3/5). The major discrepancies are possible X afferents to areas 18 and 19 suggested by the physiology which may actually relay through lamina C, and the difference in strength of W input to areas 17 and 18 revealed by stimulation experiments and unexpected by from anatomical studies.

3.5. The Termination of Geniculate Afferents in the Visual Cortex

Two issues have been addressed with respect to the termination of geniculate afferents in the visual cortical areas: the *laminar distribution of afferents* and the *spatial distribution of input from the two eyes*. Laminar differences in functional properties of cells have been reported by several authors (Gilbert, 1977; Leventhal and Hirsch, 1978; Kato et al., 1978; Henry et al., 1979). Recently there has been a tendency to explain the laminar

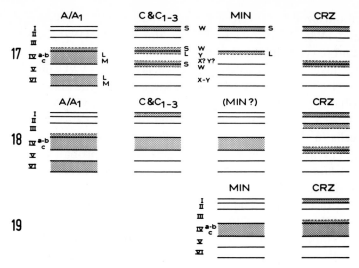

Fig. 3/7. Laminar distribution in areas 17, 18, and 19 of the termination of afferents from different parts of dLGN nuclear complex and the cortico-recipient zone (CRZ) of the pulvinar LP complex. S, M, L refers to afferents from small, medium and large LGN cells respectively. For area 17 the possible layering of three functional afferents (X, Y, W) termination is indicated.

differences in functional properties in terms of the differences in afferents terminating in the different layers (Gilbert, 1977; Leventhal, 1979). The correlation between laminar position of cells and types of afferents however is *not necessarily as tight* as between laminar position and destination of efferents. A cell situated in one layer may contact afferents in other layers by sending dendrites to these layers and in view of the wide distribution of dendritic trees of some cortical cells, especially pyramidal cells, this is a distinct possibility. Indeed recent evidence from intracellular staining experiments in area 17, suggests that many of the stellate or pyramidal cells receiving monosynaptic input lie outside layers IV and VI (Martin and Whitteridge, 1981). Therefore great caution is required in establishing correlations between laminar position of cells, especially pyramidal cells, and termination of afferents which supposedly provide input to those cells.

Laminar distribution of afferents has been mostly studied in area 17 (Fig. 3/7). The A laminae project heavily to layer IV and deep layer III and to a lesser extent to layer VI (LeVay and Gilbert, 1976; Rosenquist et al., 1974). Ferster and LeVay (1978) have shown that large afferents, presumably from class 1 geniculate cells, terminate in IV a, b while thinner afferents, presumably from class 2, cells terminate in IV c. This has been confirmed by Leventhal (1979), showing that large LGN cells in the A laminae terminate in IV a, b and medium-sized cells in IV c. The conclusion of both authors that X cells terminate in IV c and Y in IV a, b rests on the assumption that class 1 are Y cells and class 2, X cells, but this is not the case (Friedlander et al.,

1981). If some medium sized LGN cells are Y cells then Y cells could project both to IV a, b and IV c. According to LeVay and Gilbert (1976) the C laminae (magno- and parvocellular parts) project to layer I, the lower half of layer III, the top of layer IV, and to the border of layers IV – V. Using the report of Leventhal (1979), one can infer that the large cells of the magnocellular C lamina probably account for the projection to upper layer IV, while the projections to layer I, lower half of layer III and the layers IV – V border arise from small cells in the parvocellular C laminae. In keeping with this Ferster and LeVay (1978) observed very thin axons, arising probably from the parvocellular C laminae, terminating in layer I. Finally according to Leventhal (1979) small cells of the MIN project to layer I and larger cells of MIN to the top part of layer IV. The termination of the different afferents have been interpreted (Leventhal, 1979) as evidence that the different afferent systems to area 17 terminate in different layers: Y cells in upper layer IV, X cells in lower layer IV, and W cells in layer I, lower III, and the border between IV and V. In considering the different terminations of afferents one should keep in mind that afferents from the A laminae make up more than 90% of the total LGN projection to area 17 and that these fibers end predominantly in layer IV.

Less information is available on the termination of afferents in areas 18 and 19 (Fig. 3/7). According to LeVay and Gilbert (1976) and Miller et al. (1980) the A laminae (lamina A1 more than lamina A cf. supra) project to layer IV and deep layer III of area 18 and also provide a weak input to layer VI of area 18. The C laminae terminate in layers I and IV. One may speculate that the layer I projection is from small cells from the parvocellular layers, while the layer IV projection arises from lamina C which provides substantial input to area 18. According to Rosenquist et al. (1974) MIN project also to layer IV of area 18. The data of these authors also suggest that MIN projects to layer IV in area 19. According to Benevento and Miller (personal communication) all thalamic afferents to area 19 (geniculate wing, C laminae, and MIN) have the same laminar pattern of termination, projecting to layer IV and weakly to layer I.

LeVay and Gilbert (1976) observed that the projections to layer IV and also to layer VI traced by anterograde transport after injection of a single A or A1 lamina were *patchy*. The patches were more clear after injection of lamina A1 than of lamina A. In keeping with this, Shatz et al. (1977) observed clear ocular projection bands in layer IV of the ipsilateral cortex after injection of H^3-proline into one eye and more continuous labelling (although with some patches) in layer IV of the contralateral cortex. The ocular projection bands were about 0.5 mm wide in area 17 and thus similar in size to the physiologically defined ocular dominance columns of which they probably form the morphological substrate (see Chapter 9). In area 18 the bands were about double in size. It should be stressed that the ocular projection bands, as well as the ocular dominance columns, are less clearly organized in layer IV of the cat than in layer IV c of the monkey (Shatz et al., 1977), which agrees with the larger proportion of binocular cells in layer IV of the cat compared to layer IV c of the monkey.

3.6 Other Subcortical Afferents: Pulvinar-Lateralis Posterior Complex, Intralaminar Nuclei, Claustrum, and Brainstem

The *pulvinar-lateralis posterior (LP) complex* relays information from the pretectum and colliculus superior (SC) to the visual cortical areas and therefore represents a *secondary route from the retina to these cortical areas* (Fig. 1/3). However this route projects almost exclusively outside areas 17 and 18. In addition, the pulvinar-LP complex is involved in *corticocortical loops*. The pulvinar-LP complex includes the pulvinar, or lateral pulvinar, the lateralis posterior (LP) or medial pulvinar (MP) (Niimi and Kuwahara, 1973) and the nucleus posterior of Rioch or inferior pulvinar (Niimi and Kuwahara, 1973). *This complex can be divided medio-laterally (Fig. 1/13) in 4 parts* (excluding the lateral fringe of the pulvinar or geniculate wing): (1) the pulvinar which is the most lateral part and receives afferents from area 19 (Updyke, 1977) and corresponds to the pretecto-recipient zone of Graybiel and Berson (1980), (2) the lateral part of LP (LPl) (Updyke, 1977) which includes the nucleus posterior and receives projections from areas 17, 18, and 19 in topographic register (Updyke, 1977) and corresponds to the cortico-recipient zone of Graybiel and Berson (1980), (3) the intermediate part of LP (LPi) which receives afferents from the colliculus superior (tecto-recipient zone of Graybiel and Berson, 1980) and most medially (4) the medial part of LP (LPm) of which no visual connections are known. It is worth mentioning that Raczkowski and Rosenquist (1981) have described 3 retinotopic maps in the pulvinar LP complex corresponding to the first 3 parts.

While the LPl has a widespread projection to the cortex (Fig. 3/8) including at least areas 17, 18, 19, and PMLS and PLLS (Graybiel and Berson, 1980; Hughes, 1981; Miller et al., 1980) the pulvinar projects only to area 19 (Graybiel and Berson, 1980) and the LPi only outside areas 17, 18 and 19, notably to PMLS and PLLS (Graybiel and Berson, 1980, Hughes, 1981). Miller et al. (1980) have compared the termination of LPl afferents (CRZ in Fig. 3/8) in areas 17, 18 and 19. While LPl afferents terminate in layer I and the layer IV–V border of area 17, they project in addition to upper layer III in area 18. There seems to be a partial overlap between parvocellular C laminae and LPl projections. In area 19 LPl projected densely to layer IV and more lightly to layer I and lower layer III.

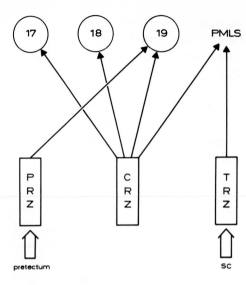

Fig. 3/8. Projections from the different parts of pulvinar LP complex to the different cortical areas (PMLS is one of the 6 suprasylvian areas, see Chapter 2). PRZ, CRZ and TRZ: pretecto-recipient zone, cortico-recipient zone and tecto-recipient zone respectively.

The *intralaminar nuclei of the thalamus* (the central lateral nucleus and to a lesser extent, the paracentral nucleus and the central medial nucleus) have been shown anatomically to project to areas 18 and 19 (in addition to PMLS and PLLS) (Kennedy and Baleydier, 1977; Hughes, 1981). It has been argued that this may convey signals related to ocular motility or to visual attention. It is also possible that the central lateral nucleus, which has a widespread projection to the cortex, exerts a more global influence over the level of arousal of the telencephalon.

There is a bilateral projection from the dorsal part of the *claustrum* upon areas 17, 18 and 19 (Riche and Lanoir, 1978; Hughes, 1981; LeVay and Sherk, 1981). The ipsilateral projections are stronger than the contralateral ones (Hughes, 1981).

The claustrum is reciprocally connected with areas 17, 18 and 19, receiving cortical projections from layer VI and projecting back to layer IV.

Hughes (1981) observed labelled cells in the *brainstem* after HRP injection into the 17–18 border. Labelled cells were found mainly in the locus coeruleus and subcoeruleus, and the dorsal tegmental nucleus. Ipsilateral brainstem projections to the visual cortex were denser than contralateral ones. Albus (1981) has reported a bilateral input from the basal forebrain and the lateral hypothalamus to areas 17, 18 and 19.

3.7 The Ipsilateral Corticocortical Connections

The importance of the corticocortical connections between 17, 18 and 19 for the question of parallel versus serial processing has been discussed in the previous chapter. Here it suffices to recall that there are reciprocal connections between areas 17 and 18, 17 and 19 and 18 and 19 (Garey et al., 1968; Kawamura, 1973; Wilson, 1968; Heath and Jones, 1970; Squatrito et al., 1981 a, b). The laminar origin of these projections has been studied in some detail (see Chapters 2 and 10). Relatively little is known about the termination of the corticocortical afferents, although Fisken et al. (1975) report that the projection from area 18 to area 17 terminated in the middle cortical layers while Lund et al. (1979) report termination of afferents from area 19 in layer I of area 17.

3.8 The Connections Through the Corpus Callosum

At the level of areas 17, 18 and 19 the callosal connections principally connect the *projections of the vertical meridian* and adjacent parts of the visual field: i.e. the 17–18 border and the lateral edge of area 19 (Sanides, 1978; Shatz, 1977 a, b, c). At the level of the suprasylvian areas the callosal connections cover much larger parts of the visual field (Keller and Innocenti, 1981) which is in keeping with the importance of the suprasylvian areas in interhemispheric transfer of visual discriminations (Berlucchi and Sprague, 1980).

The 17–18 border projects to the contralateral 17–18 border (homotopic projections), the lateral border of area 19 (Willson, 1968), and some of the suprasylvian areas (heterotopic projections) (Keller and Innocenti, 1981; Segraves and Rosenquist, 1982 b). The lateral border of area 19 projects to the contralateral area 19 border (homologic projection) and most other visual cortical areas (heterotopic projection) (see Table 3/6). By combined injection of HRP (transported retrogradely) and H^3 leucine (transported orthogradely) into identified visual cortical sites (i.e. the part of the visual field represented at the injection site was determined by electrophysiological mapping), Segraves and Rosenquist (1982 b) established that callosal connections link cortical parts representing identical parts of the visual field.

The same authors (Segraves and Rosenquist, 1982 a) showed that *callosal projection* cells are located mainly in layers II, III, and IV of areas 17, 18 and 19 (see also Shoumura, 1974 and Shatz, 1977 c) and a small number also in layers V and VI of area 19. These cells are medium to large pyramidal cells with, in addition, a few layer IV stellate cells. They occupy the visual cortex representing the visual field near the vertical meridian (VM): up to 5° from VM in area 17 up to 5–10° from VM in area 18 and up to 20° from VM in area 19.

Callosal afferents terminate mainly in layer II, III, and IV (Garey et al., 1968; Fisken et al., 1975; Shoumura, 1974; Segraves and Rosenquist, 1982 b). The callosal afferents to the 17–18 border extend very little into area 17 at least in layer IV (Fisken et al., 1975; but Sanides, 1978) and more widely into

Table 3/6. Origins and destinations of visual callosal axons.*
(modified from Segraves and Rosenquist 1982b)

	17	18	19	AMLS	PMLS	VLS	ALLS	PLLS	DLS	20a	20b	21a	21b
17	×	×	×	×	×							×	
18	×	×	×	×	×	×						×	
19	×	×	×	×	×	×	×	×	×	×	×	×	
AMLS	×	×	×	×	×		×	×	×				
PMLS	×	×	×	×	×			×	×	×		×	
VLS						×		×	×				×
ALLS							×	×					
PLLS				×		×		×	×				
DLS						×		×	×				
20a				×				×	×	×	×		
20b		×		×							×		×
21a		×	×	×				×	×			×	
21b										×	×		

* A column indicates the afferents to an area
A line lists the efferents of an area
Homotopic projections are on the diagonal (left up – right down)

area 18 (Fisken et al., 1975; Sanides, 1978). Therefore in terms of visual field the callosal afferents spread to a wider region in area 18 than in area 17. This may be only marginally true because of the high magnification strip in area 18, surrounding the VM representation (Orban et al., 1980). Moreover callosal afferents form patches which extend from the 17–18 border further into area 18. According to Sanides and Albus (1980) these patches correspond to regions between the islands i.e., to representation of parts of visual field close to the VM (see also Segraves and Rosenquist, 1982 b). In area 19 the spread of callosal afferents is of the same width as in areas 17 or 18 according to Sanides (1978), but given the lower magnification in area 19, this corresponds to a larger part of the visual field.

3.9 Conclusion

Most afferents to the visual cortical areas originate in other visual structures. The retina projects to the visual cortex directly through the LGN complex or indirectly via the pulvinar-LP complex. In the retino-geniculo-cortical pathway 3 separate functional systems funnel information into the visual cortex. The targets of these systems seem to be different in terms of areas and layers. In addition to projections ascending from the retina, there are many corticocortical loops involving either intracortical and callosal connections, connections over the pulvinar-LP complex or connections through the claustrum.

Chapter 4. Receptive Field Organization in Areas 17, 18 and 19 of the Cat

As pointed out in Chapter 2, each visual neuron, and thus also each visual cortical neuron has a *receptive field* i.e. a small retinal region, or its counterpart from the visual field, from which it can be influenced. Receptive field organization refers to the layout of the different parts (or subregions) within the receptive field (RF). When tested with different visual stimuli, cortical cells display a wide variety of response patterns. Exactly as zoologists and botanists exploring new continents a few centuries ago, neurophysiologists studying new cortical areas need a *taxonomy* to describe this variety. This allows them to compare the results of different experiments during each of which they can only observe a limited number of cortical cells. It also makes possible exchanges of information between experimenters. In principle, each functional property of cortical cells, as orientation selectivity, binocularity, direction selectivity, velocity sensitivity etc. can be used to derive a taxonomy. And indeed many of the results which will be presented in the subsequent chapters are just examples of such taxonomies. However, in as much as these different properties are independent, one would need a large set of such taxonomies and thus of experimental tests, in order to categorize the cells. Therefore, one has to look for a more fundamental taxonomy which in a way could contain or imply all the others. The properties of a cortical cell result from the inputs to the cell (i.e. different afferents converging onto the cell) and the intrinsic (i.e. membrane) properties of the cell. One of the important contributions of Hubel and Wiesel (1959, 1962, 1965) to cortical physiology has been to use the *receptive field organization*, which to a certain extent reflects the *input pattern*, to derive a taxonomy for the visual cortical cells.

The concept of receptive field organization was discovered by Hartline (1938) in the limulus eye and introduced into studies of the cat retina by Kuffler (1953). Kuffler showed that in the light adapted state the retinal ganglion cell had a RF organized in 2 concentric mutually antagonistic parts: the center and surround. To a first approximation the center represents a direct input from the receptors and the surround an indirect input from the receptors through the horizontal cells. Furthermore the center surround antagonism explains why ganglion cells respond better to a small, approximately circular, stimulus than to a diffuse one. Hence Kuffler's work had shown that receptive field organization is a reflection of the inputs to the cell and can explain the other properties of the cell.

Hubel and Wiesel applied this principle to the cortex. They were able to do so since they discovered that in order to study cortical RF organization one has to use a near optimal stimulus and that an elongated light bar of optimal orientation is such a stimulus. From their experiments Hubel and Wiesel derived a three-member taxonomy for the cat visual cortex: the simple, complex and hypercomplex scheme. This scheme has been used in a more or less orthodox way for twenty years, and has proven to have correlations with cortical layering and hence with input-output relationships, with functional properties and with the ontogenesis of the cortex. This validates Hubel and Wiesel's initial assumption that RF organizations represent a fundamental taxonomy. However these twenty years of use have also shown the shortcomings of the scheme, which in recent years may have discouraged some of the experimenters. These shortcomings call for better and more refined criteria to classify the different types of RF organization.

4.1 Twenty Years with the Simple-Complex-Hypercomplex Scheme

In their initial study of area 17 of the cat Hubel and Wiesel (1962) made the discovery that not all cortical cells are alike but fall into categories of which they recognized two: cells with 'simple' and 'complex' fields (Fig. 4/1). Hubel and Wiesel used *hand-held light stimuli which they flashed ON and OFF* to categorize receptive fields. *Simple fields* were defined as follows (Hubel and Wiesel, 1962, p. 110) (1) they were subdivided into distinct "excitatory" and "inhibitory" regions;[1] (2) there was summation within the separate "excitatory" and "inhibitory" regions, (3) there was antagonism between the "excitatory" and "inhibitory" regions and (4) it was possible to predict responses to stationary or moving spots of various shapes from a map of the "excitatory" and "inhibitory" regions. A field for which one of these requirements was not fulfilled was classified as *complex* i.e. non-simple, including those which could not be plotted with stationary stimuli and should have been left unclassified. However Hubel and Wiesel (1962) noted that a moving stimulus was a powerful stimulus and that some cells gave no response to stationary stimuli. Hubel and Wiesel (1962) went on to describe the response of simple cells to moving slits as a brief response to crossing a very confined region, in opposition to a sustained response to movement over a much wider region characteristic of a complex cell. Hubel and Wiesel (1962) classified 233 cells out of 303 in area 17 (i.e., 77%) as simple and the remaining as complex. However they admitted that for 116 of the simple cells they had mainly used moving stimuli, which was paradoxical, since among those, the cells which would have given no response to stationary stimuli should have been clas-

---

[1] Hubel and Wiesel meant excitation by light ON and excitation by light OFF when they used excitation and inhibition respectively – quotation marks are from the author.

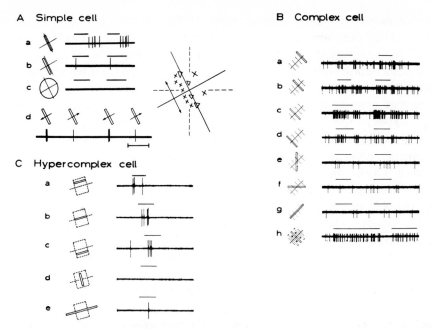

Fig. 4/1. The 3 RF types described by Hubel and Wiesel. A) Cell with simple RF activated from ipsilateral eye only. RF just temporal to area centralis. Field elongated and obliquely oriented. Left excitatory flanking region stronger than right. a. 1° x 10° slit covering central region; b. 1° x 10° slit covering left flanking region; c. 12° spot covering entire RF; d. transverse movement of slit (1° x 10°) oriented parallel to axis of field – note difference in response for the two directions of movement. Background and stimulus intensities – 1.9 and 0.69 log cd/m² respectively. Scale, 10°; time, 1 sec. B) Responses of a cell with a complex field to stimulation of the left (contralateral) eye with a slit 1/8 x 2 1/2° RF was in the area centralis and was about 2° x 3° in size. a–d, 1/8° wide slit oriented parallel to RF axis; e–g, slit oriented at 45 and 90° to RF axis. h, slit oriented as in a–d, is ON throughout the record and is moved rapidly from side to side where indicated by upper beam. Responses from left eye slightly more marked than those from right, ocular dominance (Group 3). Time 1 sec. C) Responses of a hypercomplex cell recorded in area 19, right hemisphere. RF was 10° below and to the left of the center of gaze. Excitatory portion roughly 2° x 2°, represented by interrupted rectangle. a through c, stimulation with an optimally oriented slit, 1/8° x 2°, in various parts of RF in right (ipsilateral) eye. d: same slit, shown at 90° to optimum orientation. e: optimally oriented slit 5 1/2° long, extending beyond excitatory region on both sides. For each record upper line shows when stimulus light was ON. Duration of each sweep, 1 sec. Intensity of slit 1.0 log cd/m²; background 0.0 log cd/m². Adapted with permission from Hubel and Wiesel, 1959, 1962, 1965.

sified as complex. Actually Hubel and Wiesel (1962) admitted that some of the cells they classified as simple with moving stimuli might have revealed complex properties with further study (presumably with stationary stimuli). Thus, from the beginning it was unclear whether or not one should rely exclusively on stationary stimuli and stick exclusively to the 4 conditions mentioned earlier to define a simple cell.

Since *moving stimuli* were apparently more powerful than stationary ones and since Hubel and Wiesel seemed to imply that one could use moving stimuli to classify cells as simple or complex, Pettigrew et al. (1968 a) tried to define classification criteria based on quantitatively measured responses to moving slits. Simple units had (1) a sharply defined response to movement of the stimulus over a small region of the retina (1° or less) (2) a tendency for the response to be of low frequency or poorly sustained (3) absence or weakness of spontaneous activity (4) a preference for slowly moving stimuli (around 2°/sec). Complex cells had the opposite properties: a wider response region (generally more than 3°), a high frequency or sustained response, brisk spontaneous activity in most cases and a preference for a fast oscillatory motion of the stimulus.

Most investigators refer to these two references when they classify their units as simple or complex, *without being specific* on how they mix the two groups of criteria. Those studies of area 17 subserving central vision broadly fall into two categories: those with a high proportion of simple cells (> 60%) (Ikeda and Wright, 1975 a; Kato et al., 1978; Berman et al., 1982; Rose, 1977; Sherman et al., 1976; Singer et al., 1975; Palmer and Davis, 1981 a) and those with low proportions of simple cells (< 30%) which all come from the laboratory of Hubel and Wiesel: Kelly and Van Essen (1974), Gilbert (1977), Ferster (1981). It is noteworthy that while the first group of studies reliably describe differences in functional properties of simple and complex cells (e.g. in orientation tuning or binocularity) the second group denies these differences. As pointed out by Kato et al. (1978) disagreement is mainly due to different decisions with respect to (1) cells which do not respond to stationary stimuli on the plotting table[2] (2) cells which have only one subregion, either ON or OFF, in their field.

In their study of areas 18 and 19 Hubel and Wiesel (1965) classified all cells of these areas as either complex or hypercomplex (Fig. 4/1). *Hypercomplex cells had fields* similar to those of complex cells except that these cells responded less to a long stimulus than to a short one. Hypercomplex cells formed 5–10% of the cells in area 18 and about half of the cells in area 19. Hubel and Wiesel (1965) believed that areas 18 and 19 were "higher centers in which images from area 17 were further elaborated". They saw the absence of simple cells outside area 17, and the absence of hypercomplex cells in area 17 as evidence for a hierarchical connection between areas 17, 18 and 19. Indeed they suggested a serial connection between geniculate, simple, complex, and hypercomplex cells, each cell type representing a step further in the hierarchy of visual processing.

Since then hypercomplex cells have been described *in area 17 as well* (Gilbert, 1977; Henry et al., 1978 a; Kato et al., 1978) and it has become clear that *some of them resemble simple cells and others complex cells* (Dreher, 1972; Gilbert, 1977; Kato et al., 1978). A number of studies have shown that

---

[2] That is when testing with hand-held stimuli.

hypercomplexity is not an all or nothing phenomenon but that the degree of end-stopping can vary from 0 to 100% (Gilbert, 1977; Henry et al., 1978 a; Kato et al., 1978; Rose, 1977; Wilson and Sherman, 1976). All subsequent studies of area 18 cells have shown that in this area, as in area 17, two groups can be distinguished which are similar to the simple and complex types described in area 17 (Dreher and Cottee, 1975; Ferster, 1981; Hammond and Andrews, 1978; Harvey, 1980 a; Orban and Callens, 1977 a; Orban and Kennedy, 1981; Orban et al., 1975; Tretter et al., 1975). Ferster from the same laboratory as Hubel and Wiesel has even found a larger proportion of simple cells in area 18 than in area 17 (31% compared to 25%). It thus seems that the evidence on which Hubel and Wiesel based their hierarchical scheme of information flow between areas 17, 18 and 19 (i.e. absence of simple cells and predominance of hypercomplex cells outside area 17) has not been confirmed. The finding that complex cells can be monosynaptically activated from the LGN (Hoffmann and Stone, 1971; Singer et al., 1975) as well as observations that complex cells respond to stimuli to which simple cells do not respond (Duysens et al., 1982 b; Hammond and MacKay, 1977; Movshon, 1975), put the hierarchical scheme between simple and complex cells in considerable doubt.

In subsequent studies of areas 17 and 18, other criteria were introduced which seemed to be useful in distinguishing so called simple and complex cells. *Responses to moving dark and light edges* were introduced by Goodwin and Henry (1975) and used extensively by Kato et al. (1978) and in many of the subsequent studies (Berman et al., 1982; Bullier and Henry, 1979 a, b, c; Harvey, 1980 a, b; Henry et al., 1979; Kulikowski et al., 1981; Orban and Kennedy, 1981). *Inhibitory sidebands* demonstrated by raising the spontaneous activity with a conditioning stimulus and moving a test slit through the RF have been used as characteristics for simple cells (Bishop et al., 1973; Sherman et al., 1976) or simple family cells (Kato et al., 1978). Even with these increased number of tests and criteria it seems that there are cells with properties intermediate between simple and complex cells and these have been referred to as B cells (Harvey, 1980 a; Henry et al., 1978 b, 1979; Orban and Kennedy, 1981; Orban et al., 1980) or A cells (Harvey, 1980 a; Henry, 1977; Orban and Kennedy, 1981).

As a conclusion of this overview of classifying cells one can say that the terms simple and complex should be *dropped* since they imply a hierarchical connection which is not necessarily valid and since they have lost their defining power (see also Henry, 1977). Any new classification scheme should take into account the problems (Bishop, 1983) which have plagued the description of cortical fields: (1) a number of cells do not respond to stationary stimuli when one uses hand-held stimuli, (2) a number of cells show only one subregion (ON or OFF), (3) cells can show varying degrees of end-stopping or hypercomplexity, (4) cells can have intermediate properties between simple and complex cells. In our laboratory we have developed the A, B, C, S scheme (Duysens et al., 1982 b; Orban and Kennedy, 1981) which is very similar to the one in use in Henry's and Bishop's laboratory (Bullier and Henry, 1979 a, b, c; Harvey, 1980 a, b; Henry et al., 1979; Kulikowski and Bishop, 1981 b, 1982; Kulikowski et al., 1981) and which seems to meet those requirements. Before presenting this scheme it is however useful to critically consider the properties used for classification.

4.2. Criteria for Classifying Cortical RFs

One of the originalities of Hubel and Wiesel's work was the use of RF organization as the cornerstone of a taxonomy. They carefully *avoided using functional properties as classifying criteria*. On the contrary Pettigrew et al. (1968 a) and Henry et al. (1979) have introduced, in addition to RF structural criteria, functional criteria such as for example velocity sensitivity. This should be avoided since it may prevent a classification scheme from being transferred from one area to the other. If for example simple cells have to respond only to slow movements as they do in area 17 subserving central vision, then hardly any cell in area 18 and few cells in area 17 subserving the far periphery of the visual field would qualify as simple cells. In their exploration of RF organization Hubel and Wiesel (1962, 1965) used rather simple tests such as movement of a single stimulus through the field and flashing of a single stimulus at different locations in the field. These tests certainly do not reveal the whole RF organization and more complicated tests as the interaction between two stimuli either moving (Bishop et al., 1973) or flashed (Heggelund, 1981 a, b) give further insight. Given the success of the Hubel and Wiesel scheme it seems that the basic tests they used reveal enough of the RF structure to allow a valid taxonomy. In their scheme 6 criteria (Fig. 4/2) were more or less explicitly used: (1) overlap of ON and OFF regions, (2) RF dimensions, (3) end-stopping, (4) spatial summation within subregions, (5) antagonism between subregions and (6) predictions of responses from the RF map.

The last three have been little used since they have proven difficult to handle and/or of little discrimination power. It is obvious that such properties as direction (Emerson and Gerstein, 1977 b) or velocity selectivity (Duysens et al., 1983) cannot be predicted from any RF map produced by a single stationary flashed stimulus and therefore the criterion (6) has hardly been used. The 5th criterion, antagonism, is difficult to use on the plotting table since it supposes the use of two stimuli. Consequently it has been little used. However quantitative techniques as e.g. the interaction test used by Movshon (1978) and Heggelund (1981 a, b) make it easy to test antagonism.

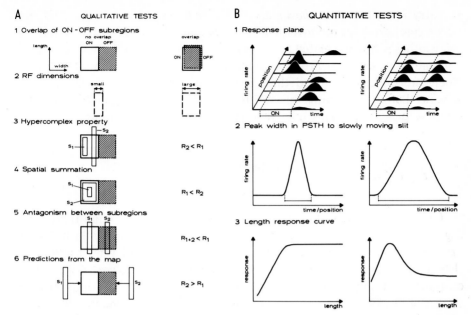

Fig. 4/2. Different tests used to classify RFs. A: qualitative tests (hand-plotting) and B: quantitative tests. S_1, S_2 stimuli, R_1, R_2, R_{1+2} responses to stimuli S_1, S_2, and S_1 and S_2 presented together respectively. In the quantitative tests the response plane (outcome of a position test) distinguishes between overlapping and non-overlapping ON, OFF subregions, the peak width in the PSTH between narrow and wide RFs and the length-response curve between end-free and end-stopped cells.

Movshon (1978 b) and Heggelund (1981 a, b) have shown that both simple and complex cells show antagonism between parts of the RF, the difference between simple and complex cells being that the antagonism occurs within a single region in the complex cells and between subregions in simple cells. And thus criterion (5) is not different from criterion (1). Summation (criterion 4) has also proven difficult to apply (see Henry, 1977 for review). Indeed from Hubel and Wiesel's (1962) description it was never clear whether they meant length or width summation. Both simple and complex cells show length summation and in this respect summation is not discriminative. Width summation is difficult to investigate on the plotting table. With light bars width summation depends on the contrast level in simple cells (Henry et al., 1978 a). With gratings Movshon et al. (1978 a, b) have shown that many simple cells show linear spatial summation while complex cells do not. However linear summation is not an attribute of all simple cells (see Fig. 7/16) and could depend upon the type of geniculate input (X or Y afferents) to the cortical cells. Since X afferents distribute almost exclusively to area 17 linearity of summation may be of little help outside area 17.

This leaves us with the three first criteria, which are relatively easy to handle even on the plotting table, can be applied to areas 17, 18, 19, and seem to carry *information on the inputs to the cell*. Indeed overlap of ON and OFF regions implies a convergence of ON and OFF center LGN afferents, RF width is probably related to the number of afferent LGN rows (see below) and end-stopping most probably indicates an intracortical inhibitory input. Therefore we have retained these criteria in our A, B, C, S classification scheme. Before describing this scheme, the 3 classification criteria and the methodological problems related to them will be further discussed.

4.2.1 The ON-OFF Overlap or the Parcellation of the RF into Subregions

There is now general agreement that with hand-held stimuli there are a number of cortical cells which seem unresponsive to stationary flashed stimuli. This confirms the original observation of Hubel and Wiesel (1962). In area 17, as much as 15 to 30% of the cells respond weakly or not at all to stationary stimuli (Kato et al., 1978; Orban and Kennedy, unpublished; Singer et al., 1975). In area 18 the proportion is slightly smaller: 9 to 15% (Orban and Kennedy, unpublished; Tretter et al., 1975) and this probably explains why Ferster (1981) found a somewhat higher proportion of simple cells in area 18. This apparent inadequacy of stationary stimuli may not

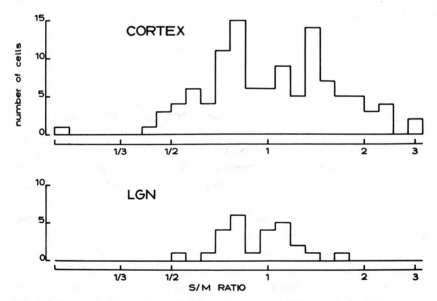

Fig. 4/3. S/M ratios for preferred direction of movement of 111 cortical cells (areas 17, 18 and 19) (A) and of 26 LGN cells (B). The S/M ratio compares the maximum firing rate elicited by an optimal slit (optimal orientation, length, and width) flashed at the optimal position in the RF, with maxium firing rate elicited by the same slit moving at optimal velocity (as determined by a VR curve). All geniculate cells and 83% of the cortical cells had ratios between 1/2 and 2.

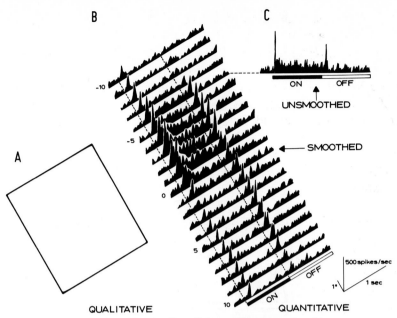

Fig. 4/4. Response plane of C family cell (area 19) apparently without response to stationary flashed slits on the plotting table. Qualitative investigation only revealed a response to a moving slit (discharge region drawn to scale in A). The average responses (PSTHs) to a slit flashed ON and OFF (1 sec each) at different positions (labelled −10 to 10) in the field is shown in B. The presentations at different positions are randomly interleaved (multihistogram method). The response to the stationary flashed slit was mainly a very short phasic ON–OFF response (16 msec duration), see unsmoothed PSTH in C. The center of the RF revealed with stationary flashed slits (see response plane in B) corresponded to the RF discharge region disclosed on the plotting table (drawn in register). The average spontaneous activity of this cell was 28 spikes.sec-^{1}.

reflect the properties of the cells but those of the human ear. Indeed when one compares quantitatively the firing rate elicited by stationary flashed and moving light bars one finds (Duysens and Orban, 1981) that on average the *cortical cells respond as well to a stationary slit flashed at the optimum position as to a slit moving in the preferred direction at optimal speed*, all other parameters being equal and optimal (Fig. 4/3) (see also Emerson and Coleman, 1981). The response which is most easily missed consists of short phasic responses to ON or OFF mixed in a high level of spontaneous activity (Fig. 4/4). This explains the commonly held belief that absence of response to stationary stimuli is typical of complex cells. Thus, if one uses quantitative assessment, both types of stimuli (moving or stationary flashed) are equivalent for the study of RFs.

On the plotting table moving edges reveal systematically more subregions than do stationary flashed ON and OFF (Orban and Kennedy, 1981). Kulikowski et al. (1981) stress that when using quantitative assessment

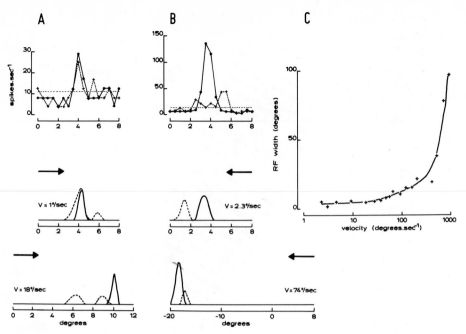

Fig. 4/5. Influence of stimulus velocity on RF characteristics. A and B: influence of velocity on discharge regions of single edges; (A) B cell from area 19: (B) S cell from area 17. Full lines: ON and light edge responses; stippled lines: OFF and dark edge responses. While at low velocities (middle) the spatial disposition of edge discharge regions fits the spatial disposition of ON and OFF regions (top), this is not true at faster velocities (bottom). The horizontal stippled lines in top graphs indicate significiance level. C: apparent RF size plotted as a function of stimulus velocity. Area 18 C cell with unclassified VR curve (half-height upper cut-off at 392°/sec). Note that up to 10°/sec (the working range of velocity low-pass cells) the apparent RF width hardly changes.

moving light and dark bars (or probably moving edges) are more useful to investigate the RF structure than stationary flashed bars. Our own observations (Orban and Duysens, unpublished) show that moving edges are useful for quantitative assessment as long as the cell responds well to slowly moving stimuli. When a cell responds only to fast moving stimuli, then the difference in latency between ON and OFF regions or between responses to light and dark edges, comes into play and influences the apparent position of the response to dark and light edges. In this way discharge regions for edges which are overlapping may become separate or the reverse (Fig. 4/5). This problem which arises from the conversion of the time axis in PSTHs to a position axis, can be offset on the plotting table by moving the edges over short amplitude and by marking where the responses start and stop.

Therefore it is clear that to reveal subregions in the RF, moving edges are superior to stationary stimuli flashed ON and OFF on the plotting table but that with quantitative assessment stationary stimuli are of more general use (i.e. can be used as well in area 18 as in area 17 or 19). It should be stressed that when both responses (to moving edges and to ON/OFF) can be elicited adequately there is an *excellent agreement* between them: ON regions correspond to light edge discharge regions and OFF regions to dark edge discharge regions (Palmer and Davis, 1981 b, see Fig. 4/5 and 4/19). The most notable exception on the plotting table is again linked to the weakness of the human ear: some cells with high spontaneous activity may have a common discharge region for dark and light edges which corresponds to only an ON response. This is due to the fact that in some complex-like cells the OFF response is much more phasic than the ON response and is missed (Fig. 4/14).

4.2.2 Position Test

As a quantitative test for overlap of ON-OFF subregions we currently use a "position test" (Duysens et al., 1982 b) which interleaves in random order presentations of a light bar flashed ON and OFF at different positions in the RF. The outcome of this test is similar to the response planes of Emerson and Gerstein (1977 a) except that we avoid sequence effects by *randomization of stimulus positions* (Fig. 4/4). The stimulus is generally ON or OFF for 1 sec although we sometimes had to use longer durations, when the cell had a sustained ON response and it was difficult to decide whether the firing at light OFF was a true OFF response or the continuation of the sustained ON response. For a few cells we had to use shorter or longer ON durations, since in cells with overlapping subregions the OFF response can be modulated by the preceding ON stimulation. It is possible that the use of conditioning stimuli in conjunction with stationary stimuli (Palmer and Davis, 1981 a) may improve the separation between overlapping and non-overlapping fields. It should also be noted that recent evidence from our laboratory (Duysens, Orban and Cremieux, unpublished) shows that dark adaptation has a strong effect on the response planes, blurring the distinction between overlapping and non-overlapping fields.

4.2.3 RF Dimensions

There is now considerable agreement that the RF sensitivity profile is much sharper in the width than in the length of the RF and that it is therefore preferable *to use only width to evaluate the RF dimension* (Henry et al., 1978 a; Kato et al., 1978; Orban and Kennedy, 1981; Wilson and Sherman, 1976). The length sensitivity profile depends very much on the method used to evaluate it (e.g. differential method with a short stimulus versus integrative method by lengthening the stimulus (Orban et al., 1979 a) (see Chapter 7) or

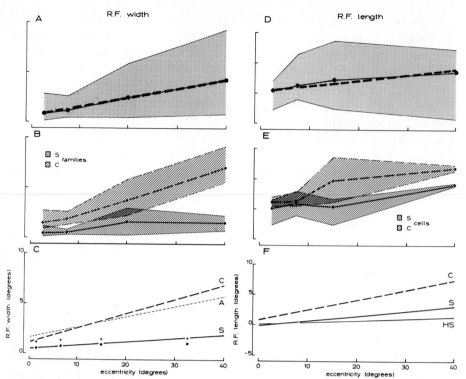

Fig. 4/6. Changes in RF dimension (hand-plotting) as a function of eccentricity. A: mean RF width (full line) and extent of RF width distribution (hatching) plotted for four eccentricity classes of area 17. The regression line for the whole population (stippled line) was nearly coincident with the line connecting means. B: mean RF widths and extent of RF width distributions of S (full line) and of C (stippled line) *family* plotted as a function of eccentricity. C: regression lines of RF width as a function of eccentricity for S, C and A *families*. Crosses and dots indicate mean diameter of Y and X geniculate cells respectively according to the data of Hoffmann et al. (1972). D: mean RF length (full line) and extent of RF length distribution (hatching) plotted for four eccentricity classes in area 17. The regression line (stippled line) is also indicated. E: mean RF lengths and extent of RF length distributions of S (full line) and of C (stippled line) *cells* plotted as a function of eccentricity. F: regression lines of RF length as a function of eccentricity for S, C, and HS cells.

qualitative versus quantitative methods (Kato et al., 1978). In addition the presence of weak end-zones which are not recognized can change the estimation of RF length. It should be noted, however, that on the average both measures (RF width and length) correlate and that for example both the average RF width and RF length increase with eccentricity at a similar rate (Fig. 4/6). As shown in Fig. 4/6 the variability of RF length is much larger and the separation between large and small fields is much poorer with RF length than with RF width. Therefore, only RF width should be used as a measure of RF dimensions and not RF length (Ferster, 1981) nor RF area (Hubel and Wiesel, 1962).

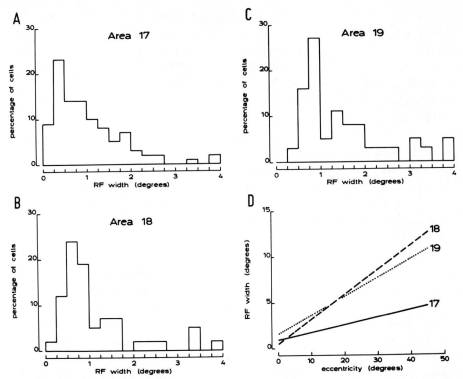

Fig. 4/7. RF width of cortical cells (hand-plotting). A through C: RF width distribution in areas 17, 18 and 19 subserving central vision (0–5°). Number of cells: 88, 42 and 37 respectively. There is a hint of periodicity in the distribution of areas 18 and 19 (fundamental of about 0.75° and 0.8° in areas 18 and 19 respectively). D: regression lines giving the mean increase in RF width with eccentricity in the 3 areas (n = 156, 151 and 118 in areas 17, 18 and 19 respectively). For all 3 areas the correlation was better than 0.5. Note the difference in steepness of the relationship between area 17 on the one hand and areas 18 and 19 on the other.

RF width is not only important because of its correlation with optimal spatial frequency (Maffei and Fiorentini, 1977) but because of *a possible correlation with the number of rows of geniculate afferents*. Indeed all the distributions of RF width of cortical cells in different areas (Fig. 4/7) have a large mode at small width, followed by more or less separated modes at larger widths. This is especially clear in area 19 (Duysens et al., 1982 b) where the different modes are multiples of each other. This suggest that small fields (which by definition belong to the first mode) receive afferents from a single row of geniculate afferents while large fields receive (directly or indirectly) afferents from multiple rows of geniculate afferents (mostly 2 but up to 6 rows). In area 17 which receives X, Y, and W afferents, with X cells having smaller RF diameter than Y or W afferents, the separation of modes is blurred. RF width of large fields increases more steeply with eccentricity than that of small fields (Duysens et al., 1982 b; Orban and Kennedy, 1981; Wilson and Sherman, 1976, see also Fig. 4/6). This is further evidence that large fields receive directly or indirectly afferents from multiple rows of geniculate afferents while small fields receive input from a single row (for elaboration of this argument see Wilson and Sherman, 1976).

While it is intuitively clear that it is preferable to use quantitative techniques for the evaluation of cortical cell properties, quantitative measurements of RF width are difficult to obtain. Again there is no problem when the cell responds well to slowly moving stimuli. Quantitative measurements of RF width, by means of a PSTH, rely on the conversion of time in the PSTH to position and pose a problem when the cell responds only to fast stimuli. Indeed the *apparent RF width increases with velocity* (Orban et al., 1981 a and Fig. 4/5 c). Therefore if RF width has to be estimated from PSTHs corresponding to fast velocities, one will overestimate the field width. This again can be overcome on the plotting table by fast oscillatory motions of small amplitude, which enable one to localize the RF and to outline it. Therefore, up to now we have preferred to use RF width estimated on the plotting table, a procedure which again can be used in all areas. However, for those cells in which both methods (qualitative and quantitative) can be compared there is a good agreement: cells with small or large fields on the plotting table will also have small or large fields respectively when evaluated quantitatively (Duysens et al., 1982 b; Kato et al., 1978). It should be noted however that the qualitative assessment underevaluates the width of the field (Kato et al., 1978).

Quantitative estimation of RF width from the PSTH obtained in response to a slowly moving stimulus (Kato et al., 1978), is difficult when the cell responds only to fast moving stimuli as e.g. the velocity high-pass cells (Orban et al., 1981 a). The RF width cannot be measured from the response planes obtained with stationary stimuli since S family cells have a much narrower response region for moving stimuli than for stationary flashed ones. One has thus to look for other quantitative methods for distinguishing between narrow and wide fields. It is very striking that for optimal velocities small field cells (S and B families) have sharp peaks in their PSTHs whereas large fields (A and C families) have broad rugged peaks (Fig. 4/8). *The sharp width-activity profile of small field cells* is probably due to the presence of inhibitory sidebands (Fig. 4/9). Indeed it has long been known that S family cells have inhibitory sidebands (Bishop et al., 1973; Kato et al., 1978; Sherman et al., 1976; Palmer and Davis, 1981) but also B family cells seem to have sidebands (Bishop, personal communication; Orban and Duysens, unpublished). B family cells probably correspond to the complex cells with sidebands described by Albus and Fries (1980) and the few simple cells (having by their definition inhibitory sidebands) with overlapping edge regions described by Sherman et al. (1976). There is only indirect evidence that A family cells may have no inhibitory sidebands. Indeed among their complex cells,

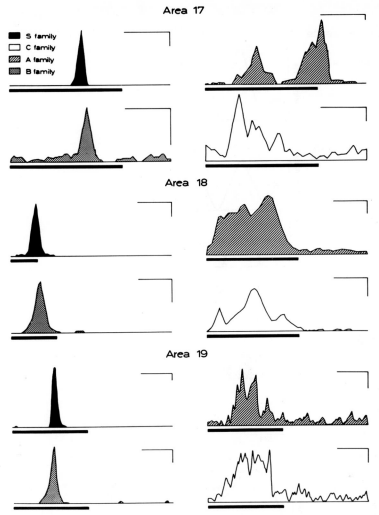

Fig. 4/8. PSTHs representing the average responses to moving slits of the 4 families in each area. Within each area the velocity used was the same for the 4 cells (9°/sec in areas 17 and 19 and 55°/sec in area 18). Calibration marks 250 msec and 25 spikes/sec. Horizontal black bars indicate movement duration. Note that all small field cells (S and B families) have a sharp peak corresponding the feeling of a crisp response on the plotting table while large field cells (A and C families) have wide peaks corresponding to the feeling of a sustained response on the plotting table.

having by definition no sidebands, Sherman et al. (1976) had a small proportion of cells with a single subregion or separate subregions for edges. Also there were no hints of sidebands in the PSTHs of the few A family cells which had a high spontaneous activity in our sample. Therefore the detection of inhibitory sidebands with conditioning stimuli may be the quantitative technique to distinguish between small or large fields, with the additional benefit that

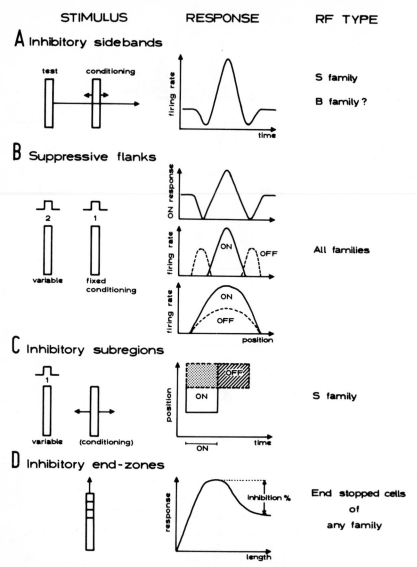

Fig. 4/9. Different inhibitory subregions in the RF. A: inhibitory sidebands (Bishop et al., 1973). B: suppressive flanks (Movshon, 1978 a, b and Heggelund, 1981 a, b). C: inhibitory subregions (Palmer and Davis, 1981). D: inhibitory end-zones (Hubel and Wiesel, 1965). In the left column the stimulus configuration is shown: in most cases 2 stimuli are required to demonstrate the inhibition; in the middle column the outcome of the test is shown; in the right column the RF type in which the inhibitory subregions occur are indicated. While inhibitory sidebands are elicited by 2 moving stimuli, suppressive flanks are demonstrated by using 2 stationary stimuli flashed in phase. The latter regions can either be located on each side of the ON subregion or within the ON subregion. To demonstrate inhibitory subregions (here an inhibitory ON subregion indicated by stippling) one uses a moving conditioning stimulus and a stationary stimulus flashed at different locations (see Fig. 4/19). Inhibitory end-zones can equally well be demonstrated with moving as with stationary flashed stimuli of increasing length (Orban et al., 1979 a).

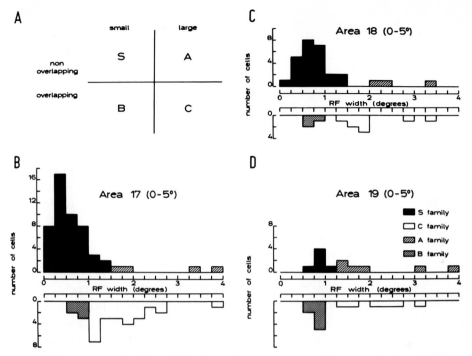

Fig. 4/10. Definition of the 4 families. A: principle of classification using the 2 criteria: RF width and spatial location of discharge subregions. B through D: separation of small and large RFs among cells with non-overlapping (top) and overlapping (bottom) RFs for areas 17, 18, and 19 subserving central vision (0–5° eccentricity). For separation at different eccentricities see Table 4/1.

this procedure is independent of eccentricity. It is also noteworthy that, according to Ferster (1981), all cells having tuned excitatory binocular inter-actions have inhibitory sidebands.

On the plotting table we measure the RF *width as the width of the discharge region of a moving narrow slit of optimal length and orientation plotted with hand-held stimuli* (minimum discharge field). Of course as mentioned earlier RF width increases with RF eccentricity (Duysens et al., 1982 b; Orban and Kennedy, 1981; Wilson and Sherman, 1976) and the distinction between small and large fields is a function of eccentricity. Although we still have only small numbers of neurons, within each eccentricity class, the distributions of RF width of fields with overlapping and non-overlapping subregions are rather different, especially in areas 18 and 19 (Fig. 4/10). Most fields with non-overlapping subregions have small RFs (contributing to the first main mode of RF width distribution) while those with overlapping subregions have mainly large RF widths (contributing to the other modes of RF width distribution). The former are defined as S family cells and the latter

Table 4/1. Equations of lines separating B from C families and S from A families in the RF width (y) – eccentricity (x) plane

	B > < C	S > < A
Area 17	$y = 0.9 \ + 0.035\,x$	$y = 1.2 + 0.055\,x$
Area 18	$y = 0.75 + 0.158\,x$	$y = 1 \ \ + 0.192\,x$
Area 19	$y = 0.95 + 0.15\,x$	$y = 1 \ \ + 0.155\,x$

as C family cells. The small number of cells having large, non-overlapping fields are defined as A family cells and those having small, overlapping fields as B family cells. In all three areas the distinction between S and A families has been put at a larger RF width than between C and B families (Table 4/1).

4.2.4 End-Stopping or the Hypercomplex Property

Although Hubel and Wiesel (1965) initially described the hypercomplex property as an all or none phenomenon, it is now clear that there are *degrees of end-stopping* (Bodis-Wollner et al., 1976; Gilbert, 1977; Henry et al., 1978 a; Kato et al., 1978; Rose, 1977). The same authors have concluded that there is a continuum between end-stopped and end-free cells (Bodis-Wollner et al., 1976; Gilbert, 1977; Henry et al., 1978 a; Rose, 1977). These studies, however, either did not use sufficiently long stimuli (Bodis-Wollner et al., 1976; Henry et al., 1978 a) or relied on the ratio of responses to short stimuli and one long stimulus to calculate the proportion of end-stopping. Kato et al. (1978), on the contrary, used a multihistogram technique (interleaved stimuli) to test a large number of lengths including 10 values at the plateau level of the length-response (LR) curve. Before preparing the LR curve they measured quantitatively the orientation tuning of the cell and used the optimal orientation for the LR curve. They observed a *bimodal distribution* of the degree of end-stopping in area 17 subserving central vision, the dip separating the two populations occurring between 20 and 35% (Fig. 4/11). They also observed that there can be a substantial variability in the response at the plateau level of the LR curves (despite interleaved stimulus presentation not used in the other studies). This variability, together with the possible change in excitability between tests, probably explains the blurring of the bimodality in the other studies (Gilbert, 1977; Rose, 1977).

It should be noted that we (Orban, Kennedy and Duysens, unpublished) classified 36%, 21% and 63% of the cells as hypercomplex in areas 17, 18 and 19 respectively, the proportion being even higher in the visual regions subserving central vision. Therefore, *studies in which hypercomplex cells are excluded or only present in small amounts, may miss an important aspect of visual cortical processing.* Neglect of the hypercomplex property can also

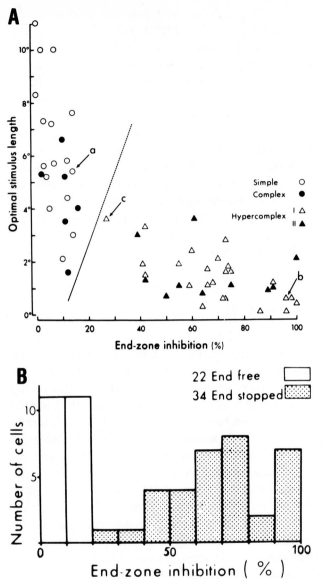

Fig. 4/11. End-stopped and end-free cells are distinct populations. A. Optimal stimulus length plotted as a function of end-zone inhibition. B. Distribution of various levels of end-zone inhibition. Adapted with permission from Kato et al. (1978).

cause problems. The suppressive zones which have been described outside the RFs (Fries et al., 1977; Maffei and Fiorentini, 1976) may well be neglected end-zones, the more so when the suppressive effects are orientation dependent, since it has been shown that the end-zones are orientation tuned (Hubel and Wiesel, 1965; Orban et al., 1979 b). Failure to distinguish end-stopped cells as a class may pose a problem, if one uses length summation as a criterion to subdivide complex cells (Berman et al., 1982; Ferster, 1981;

Gilbert, 1977). Failure to recognize end-stopping can also lead to wrong estimates of velocity sensitivity (Orban et al., 1981 a: Fig. 2).

According to Kato et al. (1978) the presence of an end-stopping of 40% or more can be detected on the plotting table. This is very close to the smallest degree of end-stopping in the second mode (mode of hypercomplex cells) of the end-stopping distribution (Fig. 4/11) of Kato et al. (1978). Therefore, every cell, for which after extensive qualitative testing (our hand-plotting procedure takes between half and one hour), we find end-stopping, is included among the end-stopped cells. From the distribution of end-zone inhibition of Kato et al. (1978) there is little reason to consider only cells as having at least 50% (Ferster, 1981; Toyama et al., 1981 b) or 80% inhibition (Henry, 1977) as end-stopped. The proportion of end-stopped cells (40%) we obtained with hand-plotting for area 17 subserving central vision ($0-10°$) is very similar to that (46%) of Kato et al. (1978) who used quantitative techniques, so that we feel confident in our hand-plotting methods.

4.3. The A, B, C, S Scheme (Fig. 4/12)

Most problems outlined in the first section are taken into account in the A, B, C, S classification scheme which has been in use in our laboratory for a few years. It has evolved from the scheme used by Kato et al. (1978) taking into account the suggestions of Henry (1977) and Henry et al. (1978 b) that intermediate types (A and B) may exist between complex-like (C) and simple-like (S) cells. The scheme as we use it, is similar to the one used by Henry et al. (1979). The differences between our scheme and that of Henry and his group concern the strength of end-zone inhibition necessary to define a cell as end-stopped or hypercomplex and the use of RF width to distinguish between B and C or between S and A families. It is important to note that our criteria do not involve functional properties such as degree of orientation selectivity or of velocity sensitivity, which may be different between areas. Indeed the scheme has been applied with success in areas 17, 18 and 19 of the cat (Duysens et al., 1982 b; Orban and Kennedy, 1981) and V1 and V2 of the monkey (Kennedy et al., 1981). The scheme has been primarily used on the plotting table but is now being quantified.

The A, B, C, S scheme uses *three criteria to classify cells* (Orban and Kennedy, 1981), the *spatial location of subregions* in the RF (i.e. overlap of ON–OFF subregions) (Figs. 4/13, 4/14, 4/15), the RF *width* (Figs. 4/8, 4/10) and the presence or absence of *end-zone inhibition* (i.e., the hypercomplex property). The first two criteria distinguish between the four families: A, B, C and S (Fig. 4/12). The third property distinguishes between members of these families: A, B, C and S cells (end-free, i.e. exhibiting no end-stopping

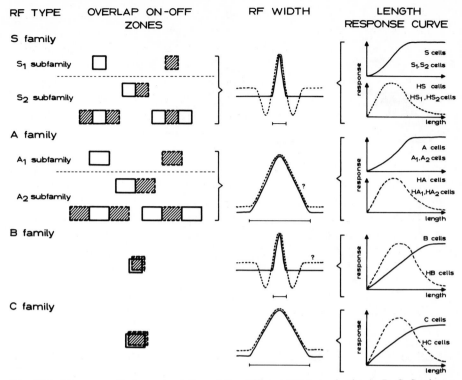

Fig. 4/12. Diagrammatical representation of the different RF types in the A, B, C, S scheme, using the 3 quantitative tests of Fig. 4/2. Open squares: ON subregions; hatched squares OFF subregions; the stippled profiles in the RF width columns indicate the PSTH with a conditioning stimulus to detect inhibitory sidebands. The presence or absence of inhibitory sidebands in the A and B families is uncertain.

or hypercomplex property) and HA, HB, HC and HS cells (end-stopped: i.e., having the hypercomplex property) (Fig. 4/12).

4.3.1 Properties and Distribution of Cell Types

Except for a small proportion of non-oriented cells and a few "rectangle" cells in area 19 (Duysens et al., 1982 b) *we could fit all cells in areas 17, 18 and 19 into one of the 4 families* (Table 4/2). In areas 17 and 18 the S family is the largest family (55%) followed by the C family (27%), while in area 19 the reverse is true (C family 36%, S family 21%). The other families represent only small proportions of the cells (5–15%). It must be stressed that in opposition to the initial observations of Hubel and Wiesel (1965) the RF types are very similar in areas 17 and 18 (Orban and Kennedy, 1981), an observation on which all recent studies, independently of the classification

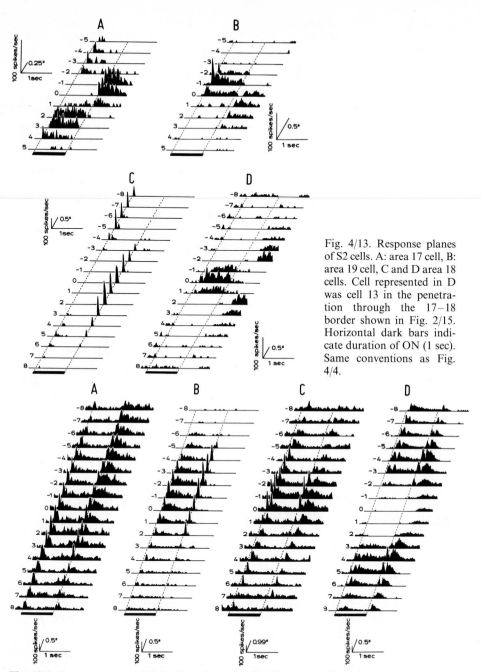

Fig. 4/13. Response planes of S2 cells. A: area 17 cell, B: area 19 cell, C and D area 18 cells. Cell represented in D was cell 13 in the penetration through the 17–18 border shown in Fig. 2/15. Horizontal dark bars indicate duration of ON (1 sec). Same conventions as Fig. 4/4.

Fig. 4/14. Response planes of C family cells in area 18 (A), area 19 (B) and area 17 (C and D). A, B and C show more typical examples: in A and C both ON and OFF responses are phasicotonic, in B the OFF response is phasic (see Fig. 4/4 for a C family cell with phasic ON and OFF responses). In D a less typical C family cell with a field in two parts: this cell was recorded just before the 17–18 border (cell 6 in the penetration shown in Fig. 2/15) and the edges of its RF extended more than 6° into the ipsilateral visual field. Same conventions as in Fig. 4/4.

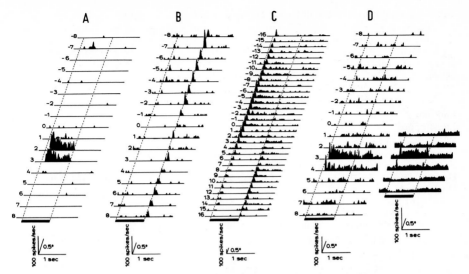

Fig. 4/15. Response planes of a S1 cell (area 17), A1 cell (area 17), A2 cell (area 18) and B cell (area 17) shown in A, B, C and D respectively. For the B cell, part of the response plane obtained while the cell was activated by a conditioning moving grating is also shown. Under these circumstances the ON/OFF responses become more phasic and inhibitory ON subregions are apparent at both sides of the excitatory subregions. Same conventions as Fig. 4/4.

scheme used, agree (Ferster, 1981; Hammond and Andrews, 1978; Harvey, 1980 a; Tretter et al., 1975). This cast doubt on studies (e.g. Movshon, 1975; Pollen and Ronner, 1975) which relied on the absence of simple cells as a distinguishing feature of area 18.

These different families of RF types show similar differences in properties in the 3 areas suggesting that they represent *fundamentally different populations* (Table 4/3). In each area S and B family cells have low spontaneous activity, in marked opposition to C family cells of which about 50% have spontaneous activity over 4 spikes/sec. In each area S and B cells have the narrowest orientation tuning. Their tuning is narrower than that of HS and HB cells and also than that of C and A family cells. In each area the S family is less binocular than the A or C family. In general end-stopped cells are more binocular than their end-free counterpart. With respect to velocity sensitivity S and B families of areas 17 and 19 respond mainly to slowly moving stimuli while A and C families have higher cut-off velocities. In area 18 this distinction does not hold, since almost all cells have upper cut-off velocities over 50°/sec. In each area S family cells have the largest proportion of direction-selective cells, markedly more, at least in areas 17 and 18, than C or A families.

These findings are in good agreement with those of Henry et al. (1979) and Harvey (1980 a) using a similar classification scheme. More broadly they are in agreement with former observations that area 17 simple cells were more

Table 4/2. Proportions of the different RF types in areas 17, 18 and 19

Area 17
Undrivable* = 11 (6%)
Unclassified = 12
Classified = 161

Non-oriented = 2
Oriented = 159

	S family	B family	C family	A family	Total
End-free	51	6	34	11	102 (64%)
End-stopped	38	2	12	5	57 (36%)
	89 (56%)	8 (5%)	46 (29%)	16 (10%)	159 (100%)

Area 18
Undrivable = 5 (3%)
Unclassified = 12
Classified = 151

Non-oriented = 2
Oriented = 149

	S family	B family	C family	A family	Total
End-free	64	10	28	16	118 (79%)
End-stopped	14	5	9	3	31 (21%)
	78 (52%)	15 (10%)	37 (25%)	19 (13%)	149 (100%)

Area 19
Undrivable = 24 (15%)
Unclassified = 27
Classified = 112

Non-oriented = 14
Oriented = 98

	S family	B family	C family	A family	Rect.	Total
End-free	7	4	18	7	–	36 (37%)
End-stopped	13	11	17	8	13	62 (63%)
	20 (21%)	15 (15%)	35 (36%)	15 (15%)	13 (13%)	98 (100%)

* No response to visual stimuli as tested with a battery of hand-held stimuli (1-hour search): long and short light and dark bars of different width, either flashed or moving, moving edges of different length, moving gratings of different spatial frequencies and moving noise fields.

narrowly tuned for orientation than complex cells (Albus, 1975 b; Hammond and Andrews, 1978; Heggelund and Albus, 1978; Henry et al., 1973; Kato et al., 1978; Leventhal and Hirsch, 1978; Rose and Blakemore, 1974; Sillito, 1977 b; Watkins and Berkley, 1974; Wilson and Sherman, 1976) and that area 17 simple cells are more often monocular than complex cells (Albus, 1975 c; Berman et al., 1982; Hammond and MacKay, 1977; Kato et al., 1978; Leventhal and Hirsch, 1978) and respond better to slowly moving stimuli in area 17 subserving central vision (Leventhal and Hirsch, 1978; Movshon, 1975; Pettigrew et al., 1968 a). They are in striking disagreement with those of Gilbert (1977) who observed no differences in orientation tuning or preferred velocity between his simple, standard complex and special complex cells and no difference in binocularity between his simple and standard complex cells.

The *laminar distribution* of the different families is also strikingly different (Fig. 4/16). The percentages indicated are percentages of a cell type in a given

Table 4/3. Functional characterists of the various cell families in areas 17, 18 and 19

Median orientation tuning width (degrees)

		S family	B family	C family	A family
Area 17	Free	44 (51)	61 (6)	80 (33)[oo]	65 (10)[++]
	Stopped	74 (38)	78 (2)	73 (12)	84 (54)
Area 18	Free	58 (61)	69 (10)	88 (28)[oo]	98 (16)[++]
	Stopped	76 (14)	63 (5)	91 (8)	126 (2)
Area 19	Free	65 (7)	55 (4)[§§]	107 (18)[oo]	85 (7)[+]
	Stopped	80 (13)	110 (11)	91 (17)	82 (8)

Binocularity (percentage of cells with ocular dominance classes 3-4-5)

	S family	B family	C family	A family
Area 17	36 (85)	25 (8)[§§]	57 (45)[o]	47 (15)
Area 18	25 (75)	57 (14)	59 (37)[oo]	50 (18)[+]
Area 19	37 (19)	47 (15)	60 (35)	80 (15)[++]

Spontaneous activity (percentage of cells > 4 spikes/sec)

	S family	B family	C family	A family
Area 17	4 (45)	0 (8)[§§]	47 (32)[oo]	17 (12)
Area 18	10 (52)	0 (6)[§§]	68 (22)[oo]	8 (13)
Area 19	7 (14)	18 (11)	38 (26)[o]	17 (12)

Velocity (percentage of cells with half height upper cut-off velocity* > 50°/sec)

	S family	B family	C family	A family
Area 17	29 (41)	14 (7)[§]	52 (38)[o]	73 (11)[++]
Area 18	82 (51)	100 (7)	74 (23)	100 (12)
Area 19	46 (13)	27 (11)[§]	68 (25)	82 (11)

Direction selectivity (percentage of DS* cells)

	S family	B family	C family	A family
Area 17	43 (44)	17 (6)	2 (38)[o]	9 (11)[+]
Area 18	56 (54)	29 (7)	36 (22)	8 (12)[++]
Area 19	25 (12)	9 (11)	13 (23)	20 (10)

Numbers between brackets are numbers of cells
* See Chapter 8 for definition
[+] A family significantly different from S family: [+] $p < 0.05$ [++] $p < 0.01$
[o] C family significantly different from S family: [o] $p < 0.05$ [oo] $p < 0.01$
[§] B family significantly different from C family: [§] $p < 0.05$ [§§] $p < 0.01$

lamina. This way of calculating the distribution offsets differences in sampling between layers, as e.g. layer IV cells are smaller and could therefore be less frequently sampled. In all three areas S family cells dominate in layer IV and VI. In addition in areas 17 and 18, S family cells also dominate in layers II and III. In all 3 areas, C family cells show a major peak in layer V and a smaller peak in the superficial layers (II–III). B family cells seem to occur somewhat more in the middle layers (IV and V). In all three areas hypercomplex cells occur in about the same proportions in all layers. Again these observations are in good agreement with the extensive studies of Henry et al. (1979) on area 17 and of Harvey (1980 a) on area 18. Both authors found S

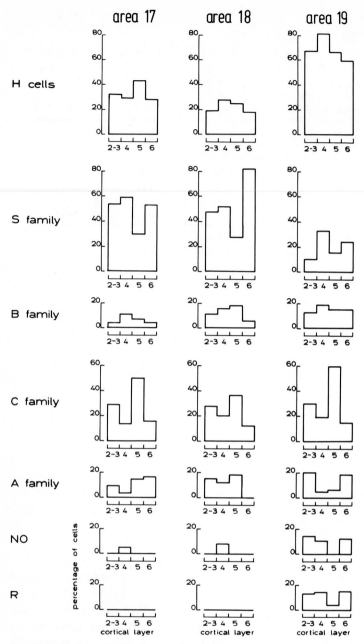

Fig. 4/16. Laminar distribution of different RF types in the 3 cortical areas. NO: non-oriented cells, R: rectangle cells (see Duysens et al., 1982 b).

family cells dominating in layers III, IV and VI, and C family cells dominating in layer V, and B family cells lying mainly on the III–IV borders and IV–V borders. It is worth pointing out that in their initial study on area 17 Hubel and Wiesel (1962) found simple cells in layers III, IV and VI and complex cells in layers II, III, V and VI. Of course, since they classified almost all cells in area 18 as complex, they could hardly observe any laminar difference in RF organization in area 18.

The *proportion of the different cell types changes with eccentricity* (Fig. 4/17). In areas 17 and 18, which have the largest proportion of S family cells, the proportion of S family seems to decrease with eccentricity from 65% to about 40%, the decrease being compensated by an increase in A family cells from 5–10% to 25%. Thus the total proportion of cells with non-overlapping subregions remains constant with eccentricity, in agreement with Berman et al. (1982) who consider all cells with non-overlapping subregions as simple. A similar decrease in proportion of S family cells was also observed by Wilson and Sherman (1976) in area 17. In addition the proportion of end-stopped cells decreases with eccentricity (Duysens et al., 1982 a; Orban and Kennedy, 1981). The change is the steepest in the area which has the largest proportion of end-stopped cells. In area 19 the proportion drops from 90% in the eccentricity class 0–5° to less than 30% for eccentricities over 20° (Fig. 4/17). In the two other areas the same trend is apparent, although the proportion of end-stopped cells in the eccentricity class 0–5° is smaller in those areas than in area 19.

4.3.2 The S and A Families

The S family is by far the largest group in both areas 17 and 18, and it includes RFs with different numbers of subregions. The most important distinction (Fig. 4/12) seems to be between cells with only one subregion (i.e., at most one subregion for dark or light edges and exclusively an ON or OFF subregion) which we label the *S1 subfamily* (members: S1, HS1 cells, Fig. 4/15) and cells with more than one subregion (i.e. at least two subregions disclosed by moving edges or flashed light slits) which we label the *S2 subfamily* (members S2, HS2 cells, Fig. 4/12). Berman et al. (1982) make a similar distinction between simple I and II cells of area 17. The S1 subfamily has been described first by Toyama and Takeda (1974) as type III and Singer et al. (1975) and Tretter et al. (1975) as class I. They also correspond to the eon and eoff cells of Toyama et al. (1981 b). Those cells were probably classified by Hubel and Wiesel as complex and almost certainly as standard complex by Gilbert (1977) and Ferster (1981). They have been included in the simple family (Kato et al., 1978) or in the S family (Duysens et al., 1982 b; Harvey, 1980 a; Henry et al., 1979; Orban and Kennedy, 1981; Palmer and Davis, 1981) since many S family cells have additional subliminal subregions

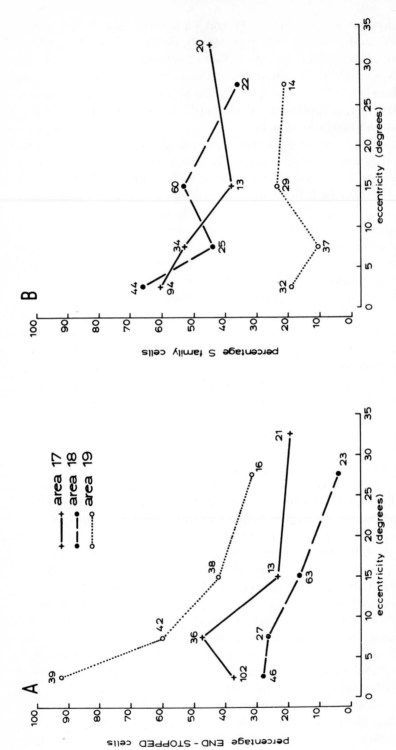

Fig. 4/17. Changes in RF type proportions with eccentricity. A) Proportion of end-stopped cells plotted as a function of eccentricity in the 3 areas. Note that the change with eccentricity is steepest in the area which has the largest proportion of end-stopped cells (area 19). B) Proportion of S family cells plotted as a function of eccentricity in the 3 areas. The numbers of cells at each eccentricity class (0–5°, 5–10°, 10–20° and over 20°) are indicated.

especially when tested with quantitative methods (Bishop et al., 1971 b, 1973); and since they were similar in all other respects to S cells having 2 or more subregions.

In both areas 17 and 18, S1 subfamily represents about one third of the S family. In area 17 the S1 subfamily outnumbers the S2 family in the superficial layers (II and III) while in the remaining layers (from bottom III to VI) the S2 subfamily occurs in larger numbers than its S1 counterpart, especially at the bottom of layer III and layer V. In area 18 the laminar distribution of S1 and S2 subfamilies is more even. While in area 17 the S1 subfamily cells are about equally dominated by ON and OFF, the OFF fields dominate among the area 18 S1 family in a ratio of 2/1 (see also Harvey, 1980 a; Tretter et al., 1975). We have reported before that in the portion of area 17 subserving central vision $(0-10°)$ only S cells (to the exclusion of HS cells) prefer horizontal and vertical orientation (Orban and Kennedy, 1981). The same observation holds for a larger sample of 42 S cells of which 25 preferred orientation within 15° from horizontal or vertical $(\chi^2 = 6.4,$ $p = 0.05)$. However separation of S1 and S2 cells shows that the trend is stronger among the S1 than the S2 cells, although both groups have a similar width of orientation tuning (medians 47 and 42° for S1 and S2 cells respectively) (see also Berman et al., 1981).

The S2 subfamily includes cells with 2 or 3 subregions (bi- and tripartite fields). Bipartite and tripartite S family cells probably correspond (Kulikowski and Bishop, 1981 a) to the odd and even symmetric simple cells of Robson (1975). It is worth noting that we observed more tripartite fields in area 18 than in area 17. In general area 18 responded better to stationary stimuli than area 17. Both observations may be simply a reflection of the greater responsivity of area 18 neurons (Fig. 8/4). The S2 subfamily includes cells which on the plotting table give no response to stationary stimuli or have only one ON or OFF area, but which have at least two separate subregions disclosed by moving edges. All these cells might have been classified as complex by Hubel and Wiesel (1962) and as standard complex by Gilbert (1977) and Ferster (1981). In both areas the latter cells occurred in layers II-III (except bottom III) or layer VI.

Among the A family cells one can also distinguish (Figure 4/12) between cells having only 1 subregion (A1 subfamily) and those having more subregions (A2 subfamily). In both areas 17 and 18 A1 subfamily cells are more frequent (about 60% of A family).

4.3.3 Responses to Other Stimuli

It seems interesting to report the responses of the different cell types to stimuli other than moving or stationary light and dark bars or edges. The effect of *flashing diffuse light* was tested both qualitatively and quantitatively

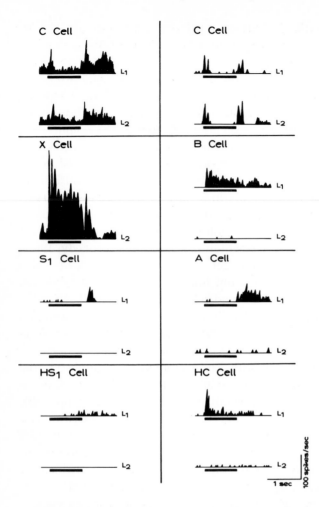

Fig. 4/18. Comparison of responses of different RF types to a flashing of an optimal slit (L1) and a whole field (L2). C cells and LGN cells (here X cell) do respond to whole field flashing, other cortical RF types not. Horizontal bars indicate duration of ON (1 sec).

on the different types. Of the 8 types only C cells were found to respond to whole field flashing (Duysens et al., 1982 b). In particular HC cells or B cells did not respond (Fig. 4/18). It is worth mentioning that at the LGN level both X and Y cells respond to diffuse whole field stimulation (Orban, Hoffmann and Duysens, unpublished, see Fig. 4/18). Thus the response of C cells to whole field stimulation, which they share with some non-oriented cells in area 19, is another functional difference between C and B cells, probably linked to the presence of inhibitory subregions in the latter.

Both in area 18 and in area 17 simple cells have been reported as being unresponsive to a *random pattern or a two-dimensional spatial visual noise pattern* (Hammond and MacKay, 1975, 1977; Orban, 1975; Orban et al., 1975; Burr et al., 1981), while a number of complex cells are very responsive. Bishop et al. (1980) also used noise as an effective stimulus for their complex and hypercomplex type II cells. Noise similar to that used by Hammond and

MacKay (1977), has been used to test A, B, C, and S families at least on the plotting table (Orban and Kennedy, unpublished). Both in areas 17 and 18 about 2/3 to 3/4 of the C family cells responded to visual noise while only 10 to 15% of the S family cells gave some response to moving noise. The A and B families in area 17 gave little response to noise but in area 18 a somewhat larger proportion (1/3) of cells of those families showed some response to moving noise.

The comparison of responses to *moving spots* and slits is a test for the degree of length summation of a cortical cell. The interest of this comparison stems from Palmer and Rosenquist's (1974) observation that corticotectal cells have complex RFs with as an additional property (in 31/34 cells) the absence of length summation i.e. an equal response to a moving spot and slits (Fig. 10/2). End-stopped cells, which incidently are only in the minority (4/43) among corticotectal cells according to Palmer and Rosenquist (1974), of course also respond very well to moving spots (Henry, 1977; Kato et al., 1978; Rose, 1977). Therefore, one should be careful when using the comparison of responses to moving spots and slits as a classifying characteristic of complex cells (Berman et al., 1982; Ferster, 1981; Gilbert, 1977). One should first remove the end-stopped cells from the complex or C family and then among the remaining cells distinguish cells responsive to spots and those responding only to long edges as done by Harvey (1980 b). It should be noted that, according to Harvey (1980 b) all corticotectal cells of areas 17 and 18 belonged to the C family, only 18% being end-stopped and about 45% responding well to moving spots.

We compared responses of area 17 and 18 cells to moving spots (Orban and Kennedy, unpublished). Significantly more area 18 than area 17 cells responded to a moving spot. In particular S family cells of area 18 were significantly more responsive to spots than their area 17 counterpart, despite the fact that area 17 has many more HS cells than area 18. It seems therefore that S cells of area 18 show much less length summation than their area 17 homologues. This may be the reason why Hubel and Wiesel (1965) who used summation as a defining characteristic of simple cells did not observe a single simple cell in area 18. In both areas almost all C family cells responded well to a moving spot which is in keeping with the dominance of the C family in lamina V, from which the corticotectal projection arises.

4.4 Correspondence of the A, B, C, S Scheme with Other Classification Schemes

Given the increasing discontent with the simple/complex/hypercomplex scheme, other schemes have been proposed, although most of these schemes have been applied only to that portion of area 17 subserving central vision.

Table 4/4. Comparison of A, B, C, S scheme with other classification schemes

A, B, C, S scheme 17 (0–45°)° 18 (0–35°) 19 (0–35°)	Kato et al., 1978 17 (0–10°) moving + edges ON/OFF inhibitory sidebands	Sherman et al., 1976 17 (0–70°) inhibitory sidebands	Palmer and Davis, 1981 17 (0–6°) excitatory and inhibitory subregions in response plane	Berman et al., 1982 17 (0–50°) moving edges ON/OFF	Singer et al., 1975 17 (5–10°) 18 (5–10°) ON/OFF	Gilbert, 1977 Ferster, 1981 17 (0–25°) 18 (0–25°) ON/OFF length summation	Sillito, 1977 17 (0–15°) ON/OFF iontophoresis of bicuculline	Leventhal and Hirsch, 1980 17 (0–15°) RF width velocity cut-off
S family								
S1	Simple		S1	Simple 1	Class I (and IV)	Standard complex	? Simple	
HS1	HC-I cell	Simple					Superficial layer hyper-complex cell?	SAS
S2	Simple		S2 and S3	Simple 2	Class II (and IV)	Simple and standard complex	Group 1 and 2 simple cell	
HS2	HC-I cell						Superficial layer hyper-complex cell	
B family								
B	Simple?			Complex (line ?)	Class III (and IV)	Standard complex	Complex type 1	
HB	HC-I?	Simple	C2?	Complex (spot?)			Superficial layer hypercomplex cell	SAS

C family							
C	Complex	C2	Complex (spot or line)	Class III (and IV)	Special and standard complex	Complex type 2	LAS and F
HC	HC-II					Complex type 3	
A family							
A1	?	C1	Simple 1	Class I (and IV)			
HA1	Complex				Special and standard complex	?	LAS and F
A2		S2?	Simple 2	Class II (and IV)			
HA2							

° Cortical areas and eccentricities where the scheme was applied
+ Main criteria used

In order to increase the understanding of the work done during the last decade on visual cortex it seems worthwhile to attempt a comparison between these proposals and the A, B, C, S scheme (Table 4/4) which has now been *applied to all three areas over a wide range of eccentricities* (Duysens et al., 1982 b; Orban and Kennedy, 1981).

The A, B, C, S scheme as we use it is essentially similar to that used by Henry and his group (Henry et al., 1979; Harvey, 1980 a, b; Bullier and Henry, 1979 a, b, c), with the two exceptions mentioned above. Our scheme is an evolvement of that of Kato et al. (1978) in which the intermediate groups had not yet been recognized. It is probable that B family cells would have been included in the simple family because of their inhibitory sidebands. Sherman et al. (1976) used as their only classifying criterion the presence or absence of inhibitory sidebands. Their simple cells, i.e. cells with sidebands, probably include both S and B family cells. Indeed among their simple cells there was a small proportion of cells with overlapping edges. The A family cells were probably included among their complex cells (i.e. those having no sidebands) as a number of their complex cells either had only one edge subregion (A1 subfamily) or separate edge subregions (A2 subfamily).

Palmer and Davis (1981 a) went back to the original methods of Hubel and Wiesel (1962) and used *stationary flashed slits but in a quantitative way producing response planes* (Fig. 4/19). They define simple cells (55%) as having spatially non-overlapping excitatory and inhibitory domains at light ON and light OFF. Their complex cells (43%) had one or two excitatory domains spanning the entire receptive field and usually had no inhibitory domains. They distinguish between C1 (9%) and C2 (34%) complex cells

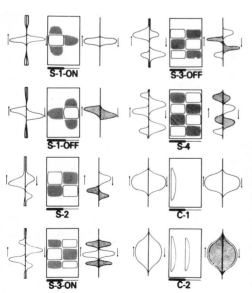

Fig. 4/19. Idealized summary of responses to moving and stationary stimuli for the major cell types seen in the study of Palmer and Davis (1981a). Each response plane summary diagram is accompanied by idealized responses to moving light slit (left) and moving light and dark edges (right). Stippled responses correspond to dark edge responses. Excitatory domains clear, inhibitory domains shaded. C-1-off cell not shown; it differed from the C-1-on cell only in that dark edges were effective rather than light edges. Adapted with permission from Palmer and Davis (1981 b).

having respectively one excitatory domain (at ON or OFF) or 2 excitatory domains (one at ON and one at OFF). These cells correspond to A1 family cells on the one hand and C and B families on the other hand. Among the simple cells they distinguished 4 types according to the number of excitatory domains: S1 (16%), S2 (22%) S3 (16%), and S4 (1%). They include S1 among simple cells because of their inhibitory domains, the smaller dimension of the excitatory domain than C1 cells and the sustained response throughout the 640 msec light cycle. Their S1 cell seems to correspond quite well to our S1 subfamily and their S2, S3 and S4 to our S2 subfamily. Unfortunately Palmer and Davis (1981 a) did not mention the hypercomplex problem. We do not know to what extent end-stopped cells were included in their analysis.

Berman et al. (1982) used criteria following those of Kato et al. (1978). Using *hand-held moving edges and stationary stimuli* they distinguish between cells with overlapping and non-overlapping subregions in the terminology used here and they labeled them as complex and simple cells. They further distinguish between simple 1 and simple 2 cells as having one or more subregions. Their simple cells correspond to both our S and A family which would explain why they failed to observe changes in the proportion of simple cells with eccentricity. They mention that they measured the degree of end-stopping but do not mention what proportion of cells were end-stopped and to what extent they are included in their cell types.

Singer et al. (1975) and Tretter et al. (1975) used mainly *hand-held stationary flashed* stimuli. They distinguished between class I cells giving only ON or OFF responses (corresponding to our S1 and A1 subfamilies), class II cells having separate ON and OFF regions (corresponding to our S2 and A2 subfamilies), and class III cells giving mixed ON and OFF responses (corresponding to our B and C families). Their class IV cells giving no response on the plotting table can belong to any of our categories.

Gilbert (1977) and Ferster (1981) also used *hand-held stationary flashed* stimuli and the strict Hubel and Wiesel (1962) criteria. They further subdivide the complex category into special and standard complex according to the agreement or disagreement between a differential (with a small stimulus tested at different positions) and in an integrated (with length-response curves) manner of measuring RF length.[3] The weakness of this classification, which gives results (proportion of cell types) different from all other studies of the visual cortex is due to the weakness of ON–OFF parcellation criterion when using just hand-held stimuli. Any of our cell types may have been considered by them as complex. Even S2 cells with separate responses to both light and dark edges but only one clear ON or OFF region would fall into the complex category. Furthermore their distinction between special and

---

[3] See also Chapter 7.

standard complex cells can at least partially be confused with the hypercomplex property. The length-activity profiles of cortical cells can be ill defined and the distinction between standard and special complex must be difficult to make with hand-plotting techniques and requires systematic quantitative measurement of integrated and differential length profiles.

Sillito (1977 b) uses the *effect of bicuculline on direction selectivity* of complex cells together with properties such as RF dimension, response to hand-held stationary flashed stimuli, spontaneous activity and degree of end-stopping, and degree of direction selectivity to subdivide complex cells into 3 categories (see Fig. 12/5). The clearest correlation seems to be between our B cells and his type 1 complex cells (see Orban et al., 1979 a). The correlation between his types 2 and 3 and our C and HC cells is more tentative.

Finally Leventhal and Hirsch (1980) distinguished between *small area slow* (SAS), *large area slow* (LAS) *and fast* (F) cells. They claim that SAS cells with small RFs (RF size < 2.25 deg^2 or RF width $< 0.8°$) and low upper cut-off velocity ($< 60°$/sec) correspond to X-recipient cells, LAS cells with large RFs (RF size > 2.25 deg^2 or RF width $> 0.8°$) and low upper cut-off velocity ($< 60°$/sec) to W-recipient cells, and F cells having high upper cut-off velocities ($> 100°$/sec) to Y-recipient cells. These associations seem to be questionable since both RF width and upper cut-off velocity undergo cortical transformations (see Chapter 11). Indeed Y geniculate afferents have slightly higher upper cut-off velocities than X geniculate afferents (Orban et al., 1981 c), but both types of afferents have much higher upper cut-offs than cortical cells. Therefore the upper cut-off velocity of cortical cells is determined to a large extent by intracortical processing and not by the type of afferents (Duysens et al., 1983). Indeed the data of Dreher et al. (1980) show that while 76% of the cells with upper cut-off velocities over 100°/sec received Y input (as shown by their OX−OR latency difference), only 70% of the cells receiving Y input had an upper cut-off velocity over 100°/sec. With respect to RF width, large cortical RF widths may be due to the type of afferents (Y or W afferents instead of X afferents) or to convergence onto the same cell of several rows of LGN cells (see above for arguments). Indeed electrical stimulation experiments show that in area 17 both X and Y afferents can provide input to cells with small and large RFs (Bullier and Henry, 1979 b; Henry et al., 1979). According to Dreher et al. (1980), area 17 cells with X input (OX−OR latency difference between 1.6 and 2.2 msec) have significantly narrower RF width than cells with Y or W input (OX−OR latency < 1.5 ms or > 2.2 msec). However, as can be judged from their Fig. 8 E the best separation is at 1.2° RF width and not at 0.8° used by Leventhal and Hirsch (1980), and the probability of error either way is about 10 to 15%.

There is however a good correspondence between the Leventhal and Hirsch (1980) scheme and our scheme in the sense that Orban et al. (1981a) observed that in area 17 subserving central vision (0−5°) nearly all S and B family cells had low velocity cut-offs and thus correspond to SAS cells while A and C families split about equally in cells having low and high upper cut-off velocity corresponding to LAS and F cells respectively.

4.5 Conclusion

The A, B, C, S scheme is in the opinion of the author a major improvement in the *taxonomic differentiation* of cortical cells. It is clearly defined, has no hierarchical connotations and implements solutions to the major difficulties encountered for 20 years with the previous scheme. In this sense it continues the efforts of Hubel and Wiesel (1962, 1965), Henry (1977) and Palmer and Davis (1981). It has been successfully used in the 3 major cortical areas of the cat (17, 18 and 19) as well as in V1 and V2 of the monkey (Kennedy et al., 1981). In all those areas there is a good correlation with laminations indicating correlations with afferent and efferent projections. The classification also isolates cell types with clearly different functional properties, in the orientation, velocity and binocular interaction domain. These differences indicate that A cells are not just large S cells nor B cells or small C cells. It seems, therefore, worthwhile to pursue the effort and to translate the present criteria which are mainly criteria for hand-held stimuli into quantitative criteria, in order to improve the scheme. This process has been started (Duysens et al., 1982 b) and is now in progress in our laboratory.

RF organization is much *more similar in the 3 cortical* areas than Hubel and Wiesel (1965) initially suggested. Areas 17 and 18 seem to have almost the same RF types although some functional properties of these cells are markedly different. Area 19 differs more in that it has less S family cells and more end-stopped cells. However, all three areas seem to share the same basic RF types. Therefore, there is little experimental support left for Hubel and Wiesel's proposal of a serial processing between the 3 cortical areas. This together with anatomical and physiological evidence of direct thalamic input to the 3 areas clearly suggests that the 3 areas operate to a large extent in parallel, as argued in Chapter 2.

The different RF types, rather than being serially linked, seem to *represent parallel chains or streams* in which the information reaching the cortex is funneled. Indeed just as there seem now to be six different streams (X, Y and W cells each combined with ON or OFF centers) reaching the cortex, new parallel streams (most of the different RF types) seem to emerge at the cortical level. These streams are likely to analyze different aspects of visual information. In particular S and C families seem to operate in parallel as witnessed by the absence of response to diffuse flash and moving noise in S family cells and their presence in C family cells. Also the different velocity characteristics of some of the C family cells point in the same direction. These arguments however do not preclude the possibility that some of C family cells would be second-order cells receiving afferents from the S family. It is important to notice that moving noise fields will only stimulate a limited number of RF types (mainly the C family). One can therefore expect differences in psychophysical experiments between line and noise stimuli, since one is addressing different sets of cells.

Chapter 5. Parameter Specificity of Visual Cortical Cells and Coding of Visual Parameters

As will be shown in the subsequent chapters, the study of response properties of visual cortical cells has clearly shown that, compared to subcortical cells, cortical cells have a large number of parameter specificities. As a result of cortical transformations of the afferent geniculate input, cortical cells will respond only over limited ranges of a number of parameters. Hence these cells can, by their activity signal the values of these parameters. The relationship between neuronal activity and stimulus parameter values is called neuronal coding. Before reviewing the different parameters for which cortical cells are specific and hence the parameters they can encode, it is worthwhile to describe in general terms the different types of specificities and thus the different ways of encoding parameters. The significance of parameter specificity of cortical cells for the ultimate goal of visual perception, the identification of visual objects, will be taken on in the final chapter.

5.1 The Tuned Cells as Bandpass Filters: The Multichannel Representation of a Parameter

The most obvious form of parameter specificity of a neuron is the *tuning* to an optimal value (Fig. 5/1). A tuning curve implies that the neuronal response is maximal at a given value of a parameter and falls off to zero (or the spontaneous activity level) at both sides of the optimum.[1] Such a parameter response curve may be considered as that of a *bandpass filter*[2] and can be described by its optimum and its bandwidth (provided the curve is symmetrical). The latter is often measured by the half-width at half-height (X in Fig. 5/1A), since stronger responses can be measured with more accuracy. However it may well be that the total range of parameter values (passband

---

[1] Here a tuning curve is defined by considering the response as a function of a parameter. It can also be defined by measuring the threshold intensity necessary to activate the neuron as a function of a parameter: if this function has a minimum the neuron is tuned to the parameter value producing that minimum. Both definitions are equivalent as the optimal parameter values defined by the minimum threshold and by the maximal response are usually the same.

[2] Both terms, filter, and bandpass, are used here in a broad, descriptive sense: a filter meaning a device operating only over a limited range of a parameter and a bandpass filter meaning that the range of the parameter values does not include one of the extremes.

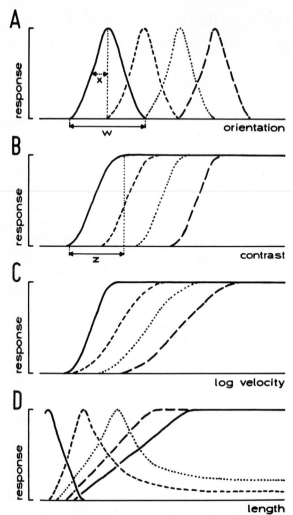

Fig. 5/1. Different types of filtering in cortical cells: A, bandpass filtering, B and C, high-pass filtering and D, mixed filtering: low-pass, bandpass, and high-pass filtering. Filtering properties are derived here from parameter response curves; parameter threshold curves would give a similar result. x: half-width at half-height, w: passband, z: dynamic range.

W in Fig. 5/1A) over which the cell responds is more important (see below). In order for a set of cells to be able to signal the value of a parameter, the cells not only have to be specific for that parameter, they also have to cover the range of parameter values to which the visual system is sensitive. This means for a set of tuned cells that they need to have different optima covering the whole parameter range to which the system is sensitive. For example cat cortical cells are tuned for orientation (see Chapter 7). In order for a set of such orientation-tuned cells to code for orientation, the cells of this set have to be tuned to different orientations ranging from 0 to 180° since cats, like humans, can perceive all orientations.

In a way however, cortical tunings are deceptive: the *bandwidth is quite broad*. It seems therefore that the information conveyed by a single cell is very limited. For example the narrowest orientation tuning of cat visual cortical cells has a half-width at half-height of 5 or 6°. This means that the cell responds well over a range of at least 15°. Given the response variability of single cells (Heggelund and Albus, 1978), such a cell, which is almost certainly a S cell, could correctly resolve an orientation difference of 5.75° in 75% of the trials. The average area 17 cell (HW at HH 25.6°) could only achieve this performance for an orientation difference of 23°. Yet the comparable[3] behavioral thresholds for orientation discrimination in the cat are 2.9° for principal (horizontal and vertical) orientations and 4.7° for oblique orientations (Vandenbussche and Orban, 1983). Hence in the cat the performance of the whole system is better than the performance of a single cell.[4] It is, therefore clear that the value of a parameter is not signalled by the activity of one cell[5] but by the activity of a group of cells. More precisely, the value of the parameter is specified by comparing the outputs of the different cells (Westheimer, 1979; Regan, 1982): this is the *multichannel system*. In such a system the resolution of the set depends not only on the tuning width, but also on the *number of tuned cells*. This is shown in Fig. 5/2, for an idealized set of bandpass filters. They are supposed to be triangular in shape, to have equal tuning width and to be equally spaced. We only consider the simplest possible code which just depends on whether the cell is active or not,[6] and not the levels of its activity. In the simplest case where the whole parameter range is covered by non-overlapping filters (Fig. 5/2A), the resolution is equal to the tuning width. As soon as the filters overlap, which supposes an increase in their number to cover the same range, the resolution improves. Each resolvable interval of the parameter is signalled by a simple combination (by "and" and "and not" operations) of a small number of filters (in fact only 3 filters). In this idealized situation the resolution equals $W/(N+3-2R/W)$, where W is the parameter range values over which one filter operates (i.e., the passband of the cell), R the parameter range to be covered, and N is the number of filters. Hence the visual system can improve its resolution either by making more narrow tunings or by increasing

---

[3] The performance level of 75% correct in a 2 alternative forced choice situation corresponds to a level halfway between the best performance (100% correct) and the worst performance (random choice: 50% correct). With the behavioral method (go-on go) used by Vandenbussche and Orban (1983) the performance halfway between best (0% go responses) and worst (100% go responses) performances is 50% go responses. This level was used to calculate the differential orientation thresholds.

[4] In the monkey the discrepancy is likely to be greater, in as much as jnds in orientation of monkeys are similar to those of humans. Human jnds are a factor 1.8 to 3 smaller than those of the cat. On the other hand, De Valois et al. (1982 a) have shown that orientation tuning width of area 17 cells is similar in cats and monkeys.

[5] Another reason is that the activity of a single cell depends on several stimulus parameters.

[6] If the subsequent neuron has a threshold for firing, this condition can be relaxed to active above a given level or not.

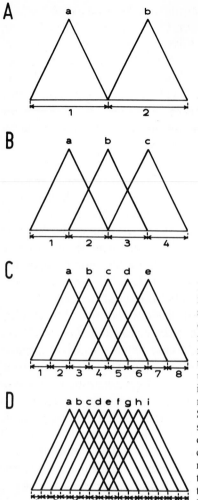

Fig. 5/2. The resolution of a set of idealized bandpass filters. A) Set of 2 non-overlapping filters (a and b) spanning the whole range of parameter values. B) Set of 3 overlapping filters (a, b, and c) spanning the same range. C) and D) Sets of 5 respectively 9 filters spanning the same range. The horizontal segments between arrows indicate the interval of parameter values that can be distinguished by the set of cells e.g. interval 1 in B, C and D could be signalled by "a and not b", meaning that cell a is active and cell b is not. Similarly intervals 2 and 3 in C and D would be signalled by "a and b and not c" and "a and c and not d" respectively. Any interval can be signalled by the combination of at most 3 filters. In A the intervals resolved by the set of cells equal the passband (w) of the cell, in B, C and D the intervals are fractions of the passband. These fractions are w/2, w/4 and w/8 in B, C and D respectively.

the number of filters involved.[7] Increasing the number of filters is more efficient than decreasing the tuning width but increases the distance between the filters which have to be combined. The upper bound of this distance equals W in the idealized situation of Fig. 5/2. Due to the limited extent of horizontal intracortical connections, there can be constraints on this upper

---

[7] A similar reasoning allows us to understand that despite the large dimension of cortical RFs (about 10 x cone separation in the monkey, see Chapter 14) the minimum angle resolvable by the monkey is equal to the cone separation. Indeed if the different RFs overlap, the minimum overlap can be the width of a cone so that two objects differing in location by one cone diameter can be distinguished. Taking into account the spatial sensitivity profile of the cones, it is conceivable that the minimum overlap between cortical RFs is less than a cone diameter. Such an interpolation process could explain the hyperacuities (Westheimer, 1981).

bound if the parameter is systematically mapped on the cortical surface e.g. in a columnar fashion as is the case for orientation (Hubel and Wiesel, 1963). With respect to this columnar organization, considerations of coding make a continuous representation of orientation (Albus, 1975 b) much more attractive than a discrete one (Hubel and Wiesel, 1974 a). In the latter case, the number of different optima would be reduced ($\pm$ 12) and the resolution under the assumptions made here would be limited to W/11. This would thus require a very narrow tuning width to achieve the behaviorally measured differential orientation thresholds.

The coding illustrated in Fig. 5/2 is a very simple one in which the neurons are considered as digital devices (active or not). While such a coding scheme would perform quite well when the stimuli to be discriminated are presented either sequentially in the same position or simultaneously in different positions, the scheme could fail when the two discriminanda are so close in time and space that they activate the same sets of cells. Under these circumstances more complex codes, in which the activity levels of the cells are compared (i.e. considering the neurons as analogue rather than digital devices) (Westheimer, 1979; Regan, 1982), would perform better. It is also possible that with the latter codes a greater resolution could be achieved for a given number of filters and width of tuning. A potential problem however, is that cortical cell activity depends on several parameters. Therefore a code depending on a comparison of activity *levels* in different filters would require that all cells used in the comparison are equally affected in their response *level* by changes in another parameter. The more simple code using presence or absence of activity, only requires that the tuning width remains unaffected by changes in another parameter. The limited data available suggest that the latter condition could be verified: orientation tuning width is invariant with contrast (Sclar and Freeman, 1982) and spatial frequency tuning is invariant with contrast (Tolhurst and Movshon, 1975; Albrecht and Hamilton, 1982).

The performance of a set of overlapping filters as shown in Fig. 5/2 depends not only on the tuning width W and the number of filters but also on the *variability* of the neuronal elements. The larger the variability, the larger the number of neurons needed to produce one of the deterministic curves shown in Fig. 5/2. Hence the behavioral performance (resolution) of a system will depend on three factors: response variability, tuning width and number of cells. These considerations on variability suggest that the activities of single cells can be combined in two ways: pooling and differentiation. In the pooling operation, the outputs of different filters with similar preferences are summated to produce a mean tuning curve with reduced variability (reduced by the square root of the number of filters pooled). This pooling could also ensure that the other parameters have about an equal effect on the different mean tuning curves. A pool of filters (neuronal elements) would appear as a single entity in psychophysical experiments and could correspond to the "channel" as measured by this type of experiments. The differentiation could then in a second step operate on the mean tuning curves resulting from pooling. In this differencing operation elements with different preferences are compared in a subtractive or divisive manner.

The idealized set of overlapping filters shown in Fig. 5/2 allows us to understand the kind of information different types of psychophysical experiments provide. Adaptation experiments allow the estimation of tuning width. Indeed provided adaptation is proportional to the degree of activation, adaptation to a parameter value will maximally affect the filters with an optimum at the adaptation value and not all the filters which do not respond to the adaptating parameter value. Hence the range of values over which the subject adapts correspond to the tuning range. The discrimination-detection experiments estimating the minimum number of channels will estimate the number of non-overlapping filters spanning the parameter range.[8] Finally, experiments measuring differential thresholds or just noticeable differences estimate the resolution of the system which depends as discussed above on the tuning width, the number of cells, and the neuronal variability.

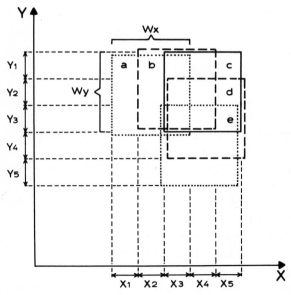

Fig. 5/3. A cortical cell can participate in the encoding of 2 parameters. The squares a, b, c, d and e represent the range of values of parameter X and Y to which the cells respond. Their passband for each parameter (W_x and W_y) are supposed to be equal. Logical combination of outputs of cells a, b and c allow the distinction between 5 intervals (X_1 to X_5) of parameter X. Similarly combinations of outputs of cells c, d, and e distinguish between 5 intervals (Y_1 to Y_5) of parameter Y. It should be noted that the coding of parameter Y by cells c, d, and e is invariant for X over a range of values of X corresponding to W_x. This may be a reason why cortical tuning should not be too narrow.

---

[8] It should be mentioned that discrimination-detection experiments suppose that a parameter range is covered by only one set of more or less overlapping tuned filters. This assumption is not necessarily verified. Indeed the study of velocity-response curves in the cat visual cortex (Orban et al., 1981 a) shows that the same range of velocity is covered as well by velocity-tuned cells as by other types of cells (velocity high-pass and velocity broad-band cells). Hence it is possible that for discriminations only the velocity tuned cells are used, while for detection any velocity type would be used. This would ruin the assumptions of the discrimination-detection experiments which suppose that the same set of filters is used for discrimination and detection.

As mentioned above, *visual cortical cells are influenced by many parameters* and cells can be tuned for different parameters. This has little effect on the coding of a parameter, if the tuning width for one parameter is not affected by changes of the other parameter. In fact if a system has to encode a large number of parameters, this dependence of cortical cells on many stimulus parameters may be an advantage. Indeed a single cell can participate in the encoding of several parameters, thereby reducing the total number of cells required. This is illustrated in Fig. 5/3 for the two-dimensional case and the digital code discussed above. The squares represent the range of the two parameters over which the cells respond. In the example shown the filter c participates both in the encoding of parameter X (by combination with filters a and b) and of parameter Y (by combination with filters d and e).

5.2 Are All Tuned Cells Simple (Passive) Bandpass Filters or Are Some of them Active Filters?

Up to now we have considered the tuned cells as simple passive bandpass filters, i.e. devices which extract the energy in their passband. Such a device responds when the parameter value is within its passband and *is not affected* by values outside its passband. Such a passive filter can be modelled in first approximation by a two-state logical unit which is 0 outside its passband and 1 inside (Fig. 5/4). This logical model was used in the simple coding of a stimulus parameter formalized in previous paragraphs.

There is however evidence that for some parameters such as e.g. orientation, the tuned cells are activated by values within their passband and *inhibited* outside this band (cross orientation inhibition of Morrone et al., 1982). For such a parameter the cell does not act as a simple passive filter but responds to the difference or ratio of energy within and outside its passband. However in its coding capacities such a cell can still be described as a two-state logical unit since the inhibition usually does not show in the output due to the low spontaneous activity level. The main consequence is that the parameter-response curve gives only an incomplete description of behavior of the cell, namely the behavior for a single stimulus. To describe the behavior of the cell completely, a parameter-excitability curve is needed which plots activation and inhibition as a function of the parameter (Fig. 5/4). Such a curve will predict the response to multiple stimuli.

The mere possibility that tuned cells are inhibited by stimuli outside their passband calls for caution in the interpretation of psychophysical experiments on the interactions of two stimuli. Psychophysical interactions may be due to interactions within the filters (or channels, as a collection of filters with similar optima) rather than between filters (or channels). In as much as the inhibition from outside the passband is divisive (Morrone et al., 1982), the psychophysical correlates of this inhibition must be suprathreshold effects.

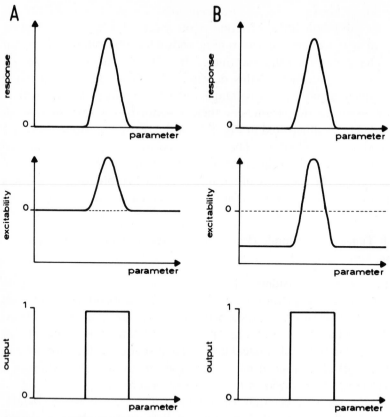

Fig. 5/4. Comparison of passive (A) and active (B) bandpass filters. Both types of filters cannot be distinguished by their parameter-response curves as the spontaneous activity of cortical cells is usually extremely reduced. Parameter-excitability curves however do distinguish both types. Two stimuli experiments are necessary to derive such curves: one (conditioning or activation) stimulus is used to raise the activity of the cells and the other (test) stimulus is used to probe the effect of different parameter values. For coding purposes both passive and active filters are equivalent, since only the output of the filters, indicated by the parameter-response curves, influences subsequent cells.

5.3 Cells with Thresholds as High-Pass Filters: Single or Multichannel Representation of a Parameter

Not all parameters are represented by bandpass filters at the cortical level. Indeed for some parameters the parameter response curves do not show a tuning but rather *a threshold and a saturation*. Such a curve can be described by its threshold and dynamic range (i.e. the parameter range over which the cells response increases Z, in Fig. 5/1B). This is e.g. the case for contrast-response curves. Visual cortical cells can be considered as high-pass filters for

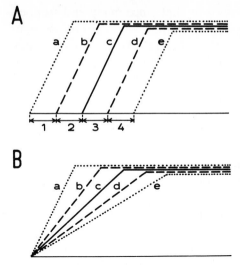

Fig. 5/5. Coding for a parameter with a set of high-pass filters. A multichannel system requires that the dynamic range of the cells are differently positioned along the parameter range. In the set shown in A, logical combinations of the type "a and not b", meaning that cell a is active and cell b is not active, can be used to encode a parameter. The resolution will depend on the distance between thresholds: the numbered horizontal segments indicate the parameter intervals that can be distinguished by the set of cells. A single channel model only requires that the different cells reach saturation at different parameter values. Hence it could operate as well with cells with different thresholds (A) as with cells with the same thresholds (B). a, b, c, d, e represent different filters.

contrast. These cells, however, show a wide range of threshold and saturation values. A set of high-pass filters could encode a parameter in two completely different ways. With the first way (single channel model) the activities of the different cells are pooled together and the parameter is represented by the gradation of activity in the whole set of filters. The changes in pooled activity of the whole set will occur over a wider range than changes in activity of a single cell. Such a coding has been suggested for coding of velocity by the velocity high-pass the cells (Orban et al., 1981 a) (see Fig. 5/1 C). The other way of encoding with same set of filters (multichannel model) is the combination of filters with differently positioned dynamic range (Fig. 5/5). One possible combination could be that a minimum change in any of the filters would be considered as a signal. Such a coding has been proposed by Albrecht and Hamilton (1982) to underly jnds in contrast. Another way of combining the different high-pass filters is very similar to that discussed for bandpass filters: comparison of activity in the different channels, e.g. an "and not" combination of filters with almost completely overlapping dynamic ranges could provide quite good resolution of the parameter. The latter coding requires a rather large spread of thresholds (Fig. 5/5). In opposition, the single channel model requires only spread of saturation values (see Fig. 5/5). It is worth mentioning that human subjects can both estimate the magnitude of and discriminate between values of the parameters for which threshold curves have been observed. It could well be that one performance (magnitude estimation) relies on a single channel code while the other one (jnds) uses some multichannel code.

Finally for some parameters e.g. stimulus length, a combination of curves can be found (Fig. 5/1D). It could be that such a parameter is encoded in a mixed way. It should be mentioned however that since many end-stopped cells have only partial inhibition (see Chapter 4), they would not be useful in a 'digital' length coding scheme (considering only activity or not) since they keep responding to all stimulus lengths.

5.4 Conclusion

Given the width of tuning of cortical cells and their variability, the *discriminative abilities of single cells are far inferior to those of the whole system.* This fact, together with the observation that many stimulus parameters affect cortical cell responses, implies that a set of cells, rather than a single cell, codes for a stimulus attribute. It is likely that differencing operations – in digital or analog terms – between tuned cells allow the fine discriminations of the system. Sets of cells with threshold and saturation for a stimulus parameter could also encode a parameter either by differencing or by pooling operations.

Chapter 6. Influence of Luminance and Contrast on Cat Visual Cortical Neurons

Two types of stimuli have been used to investigate the influence of stimulus contrast on cortical cells. Studies using sinusoidal gratings have been restricted to area 17. On the contrary, area 17 and 18 neurons have been investigated with stationary or moving slits. Both types of studies have reached 3 conclusions: (1) the relevant parameter for almost all cortical cells is contrast and not luminance (2) the contrast-response (CR) curve exhibits both a threshold and saturation contrast and (3) the contrast threshold decreases with increasing background luminance.

Our own data show that at the 18-19 border neurons are especially sensitive to small luminance increments, in keeping with their large RFs. We also have preliminary evidence that at some of the levels of the 17-18 border the contrast sensitivity may change quite abruptly.

Finally a few studies have investigated the influence of contrast and luminance on other response properties of cortical cells.

6.1 Contrast-Response Curves Obtained with Sinusoidal Gratings

Several studies have used drifting sinusoidal gratings to study the contrast-response (CR) curves of area 17 cells. The advantage of such a display is that mean luminance remains constant while changing contrast. Contrast is defined for gratings as

$$c = \frac{L_{max} - L_{min}}{L_{max} + L_{min}} \times 100,$$

where L_{max} and L_{min} are the maximum and minimum luminance in the pattern (see Fig. 7/1). Defined in this way c varies between 0 and 100%. All studies (Maffei and Fiorentini, 1973; Tolhurst and Movshon, 1975; Tolhurst et al., 1981; Dean, 1981; Albrecht and Hamilton, 1982) agree that response is a monotonic function of contrast with a contrast threshold and a saturation at high contrast. There has been considerable disagreement on the shape of the curve. As pointed out by Albrecht and Hamilton (1982) these disagreements result from the exploration of a too narrow range of contrasts (usually between 0 and 30%). Albrecht and Hamilton (1982) have studied a large

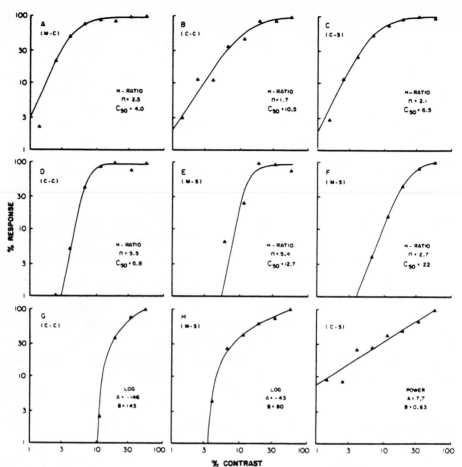

Fig. 6/1. Contrast-response functions for nine representative striate neurons: percent response (relative to the maximum response) is plotted on log-log coordinates as a function of the luminance contrast of spatio-temporal sine-wave grating patterns. The smooth curve drawn through responses of each cell is the best-fitting function of four candidates (H ratio, log, linear, power). As can be seen, there is a great deal of variation from cell to cell with respect to the exact shape and relative position of each cell's contrast response. Some cells are best fitted by a log function, others by a power function; however, most are best fitted by the hyperbolic ratio. Note the variation in the position (along the contrast axis) where the dynamic response range is distributed. Animal type (monkey or cat) and cell type (simple or complex) are specified in the upper left corner of each graph (animal type-cell type). Adapted with permission from Albrecht and Hamilton (1982).

number of area 17 cells both in the cat and monkey over a large range of contrasts (1 to 56%) and concluded that the CR curve is best fitted by a *hyperbolic function* (H ratio): $R = R_{max} \cdot (C^n/(C_{50} + C^n))$ where R_{max} is the maximum response, C_{50} the semi-saturation contrast (i.e., contrast producing 50% of the maximum response) and n the exponent characterizing the rate of change (Fig. 6/1). In fact such a function provided the best fit for 70%

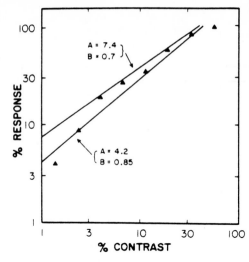

Fig. 6/2. Data points show the average response of the entire population of 247 cortical cells (striate cortex of cat and monkey); the normalized contrast-response functions from each and every cell were averaged together across contrast to provide some indication of how a large population of visual cortical cells might respond during the course of a typical behavioral contrast-discrimination task. To derive the two power functions shown, 2 SE of each population mean were added and subtracted; these upper and lower bounds were then analyzed for a least squares fit (the saturated response at 56%, primarily from the cat cells, was excluded from this analysis; if 56% is included, values of the high and low parameters become: A = 9.7, 6.2, B = 0.6, 0.7). These estimates of the slope of the population contrast-response function (the average being 0.77) are all well within the range of estimates found for behavioral contrast discrimination. Adapted with permission from Albrecht and Hamilton (1982).

of the cells (same percentage for simple and complex cells and for cat and monkey cells), the logarithmic function giving the best fit in 20% of the cells, and the remaining percentage being split between linear and power functions as best fit. Although the hyperbolic function provided the best fit for CR curves of individual neurons, pooling all neurons together (single channel model of coding, see previous chapter) produces an average CR curve for the striate population which is a power function with exponent between 0.7 and 0.85 (Fig. 6/2). This relationship may explain why just noticeable differences (jnds) in contrast increase with contrast of the background grating (Campbell and Kulikowski, 1966). In fact the exponent of the behavioral discrimination function is 0.77, a close fit to the estimate for the whole striate population. According to Tolhurst et al. (1981) the variance of the response increases with contrast and this may contribute to the increase in jnds (see previous chapter).

It is important to realize that the CR curve depends on the *mean luminance* (i.e. the retinal adaptation level). This has been shown by Hess and Lillywhite (1980) (see Fig. 6/3). This explains why the thresholds measured by the Cambridge group (Tolhurst et al., 1981; Dean, 1981) who use a high mean luminance (300 cd/m²) are lower (around 1% or 2%) than those reported by others: about 1 log unit lower than those reported by Maffei and Fiorentini (1973) who use a mean luminance of 2 cd/m² and about half a log unit lower than those reported by Albrecht and Hamilton (1982) who use 27 cd/m² as mean luminance.

There is another reason why contrast thresholds are relative measures: Ohzawa et al. (1982) have recently reported that for a substantial number of

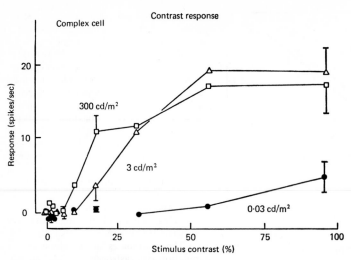

Fig. 6/3. Contrast-response curves at three luminances from an area 17 complex cell. Error bars represent standard deviations from 100–150 presentations of a 1c/deg grating moving at 2 Hz. Mean spontaneous activity (0–4 Hz) has been subtracted from responses. Error bars represent standard deviations. Adapted with permission from Hess and Lilliwhite (1980).

area 17 cells the CR curve changes with *adaptation of the cell to a given contrast level* (Fig. 6/4). This would be a cortical analogue of retinal adaptation to the ambient luminance level, the difference being that presumably all retinal cells adapt to ambient luminance while not all cortical cells adapt to ambient contrast. This adaptation is a cortical phenomenon and Ohzawa et al. (1982) suggest that this adaptation to contrast may explain the cortical contrast threshold. While this adaptation will certainly affect the estimate of the contrast threshold value, other evidence suggests that cortical cells have a genuine contrast threshold. Indeed CR curves obtained with slits, which stimulate the RF of the cell for too brief a time for the contrast adaptation to occur, also exhibit a contrast threshold (see below). Dean (1981) insists on the importance of the existence of a cortical contrast threshold which in his opinion results from a cortical transformation (probably due to a threshold for firing). Indeed Dean (1981) argues that thresholds have not been demonstrated for retinal ganglion cells and, at least as regards X cells, are not characteristic of geniculate neurons (Barlow and Levick, 1969; Robson, 1975). It should, however, be mentioned that Galletti et al. (1979) using slits, have reported contrast thresholds for geniculate cells, unfortunately without specifying their X, Y classification. At any rate it would be useful to compare CR curves obtained under the same experimental conditons at all 3 levels of the retino-geniculo-striate system to identify the site at which the threshold originates.

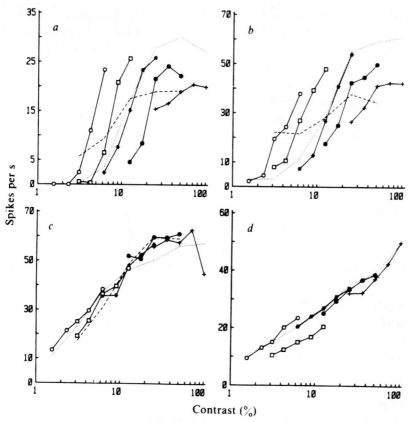

Fig. 6/4. Adaptation to contrast. Amplitudes of the responses of cortical neurons to drifting grating stimuli plotted as functions of contrast. Solid lines represent contrast-response functions when the neurons were adapted to different levels of contrast. The curves were measured in the order: open circle, asterisk, plus sign, filled circle, open square. The dashed curve shows the steady state response which is derived from the last 40 sec of impulse data to 80 sec of continuous stimulation at fixed contrasts. We assume here that the first 40 sec of data contain transient components of the response when adaption is still in progress. The cut-off of 40 sec was determined empirically and was based on our observation that most transients decayed well within this period. The dotted curve shows the contrast response when all the contrasts ranging from 1.56 to 100% were randomly interleaved. In all the following cases temporal frequency was 2 Hz. a) Gives contrast-responses (first harmonic) for a simple cell which showed substantial contrast adaptation; spatial frequency was $0.8 \, c \cdot deg^{-1}$. b) Gives results (d.c. component) of a similar experiment for a complex cell; spatial frequency was $0.3 \, c \cdot deg^{-1}$. c) Represents results from another complex cell which did not show adaptation (d.c. component); spatial frequency was $1.2 \, c \cdot deg^{-1}$. d) Illustrates results (d.c. component) for LGN fibre (ON-centre, Y-cell) recorded in the striate cortex; spatial frequency was $0.5 \, c \cdot deg^{-1}$. With permission from Ohzawa et al. (1982).

Two studies have investigated the CR curves at spatial frequencies different from the optimal spatial frequency. Dean (1981) reports a decrease in gain of the initial part of the CR curve, while Albrecht and Hamilton (1982) mainly found a vertical shift of the function (i.e. R_{max} was changed, while C_{50} and n were little affected). Both studies clearly show that with non-optimal spatial frequencies the response saturates at much lower levels (contrast set gain rather than response set gain in the Albrecht and Hamilton, 1982 terminology). Both studies also show that the threshold increases for non-optimal spatial frequencies.

6.2 Contrast-Response Curves Obtained with Slits

Slits are small localized stimuli and the mean luminance of the stimulation (and hence the retinal adaptation level) is here in first approximation equal to the background illumination. Changes in contrast can be obtained by modifying the slit luminance, but this implies that one has to use at least two background luminances to make sure that the response changes observed are due to changes in contrast rather than to changes in stimulus luminance. While some authors use the formula

$$c = \frac{L_{max} - L_{min}}{L_{max} + L_{min}} \times 100$$

to characterize the contrast of a slit (Orban et al., 1981 a; Henry et al., 1978 a) it seems more appropriate to use $\log \frac{\Delta I}{I}$ where ΔI is the difference between slit and background luminance and I the background luminance. Indeed, as mentioned above, the mean luminance is approximatively equal to I when the slit is small. Both the work of Galletti et al. (1979) using stationary slits and of Kennedy and Orban (unpublished) using moving slits has shown that the cortical response *is a function of stimulus contrast and not of stimulus luminance* (Figs. 6/5 and 6/6A). The CR curves obtained with slits also exhibit threshold and saturation contrasts. There seems to be a decrease in response at the very high contrast levels (Fig. 6/5A, B). It is possible that the same is true when gratings are used (see Fig. 6/4). Galletti et al. (1979) have shown that the contrast threshold obtained with slits also increases with decreasing background illumination (Fig. 6/5C). We (Orban and Kennedy, 1981) define the contrast threshold as the intersection of the significance level (i.e. mean spontaneous activity +2 SD) and the CR curve obtained by fitting a spline function [1] through the data points. This procedure yields thresholds $\left(\log \frac{\Delta I}{I} \right)$

---

[1] Spline function is a piecewise polynomial function.

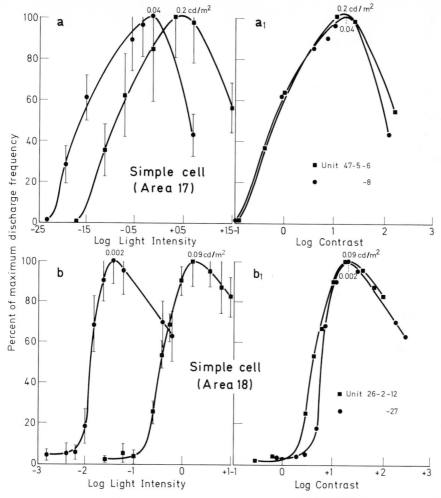

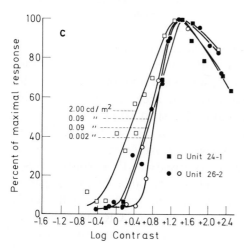

Fig. 6/5. A, B. Stimulus-response curves of an area 17 and of an area 18 simple cell obtained at different levels of light background. Each unit was activated at two different levels of light background (indicated around the top of each curve). A and B: neural response (expressed in percent of the maximum discharge rate) versus log light intensity of the stimulus. A_1 and B_1: the same stimulus-response curves shown in A and B, plotted versus log contrast of the stimulus. C. Stimulus-response curves of two simple cells obtained at different levels of light background. Each unit was activated at two different levels of light background (indicated along the curves). The standard deviations of data points have been omitted for the sake of clarity. Adapted with permission from Galletti et al. (1979).

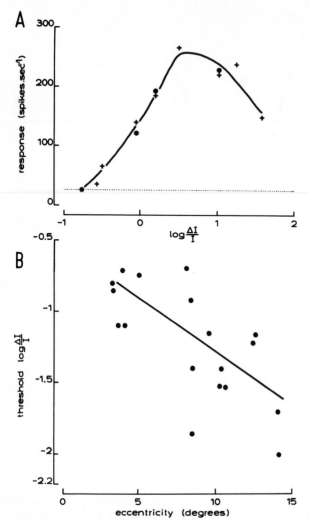

Fig. 6/6. Contrast-response curves of area 18 neurons. A. Contrast-response curve of an area 18 HS cell (eccentricity 4°). Crosses: response with 0.045 cd/m² background illumination, *dots:* responses with 0.9 cd/m² background. Horizontal stippled line: significance level. B. Contrast threshold plotted as a function of eccentricity for 18 area 18 cells. The linear regression indicated a correlation of −0.7 (Orban and Kennedy, unpublished).

around −0.65 for area 17 cells, which is in close agreement with the thresholds measured by Galletti et al. (1979). Although we explored only a small range of eccentricities (0–10°) in area 17, we found little or no evidence for a change in contrast threshold with eccentricity in area 17. This is in keeping (if admittedly contrast sensitivity depends on RF size) with the shallow slope of the RF width-eccentricity relationship in area 17 (see Chapter 4). We found however a striking *correlation between contrast threshold and eccentricity in area* 18 (Fig. 6/6B). An increase in eccentricity of 15° corresponds to a tenfold (1 log unit) decrease in threshold. This is probably the counterpart of the steep increase in RF width with eccentricity in area 18 (see Chapter 4). Together with a decrease in threshold, the slope of CR curve becomes shallower and the saturation becomes less marked and disappears. As a con-

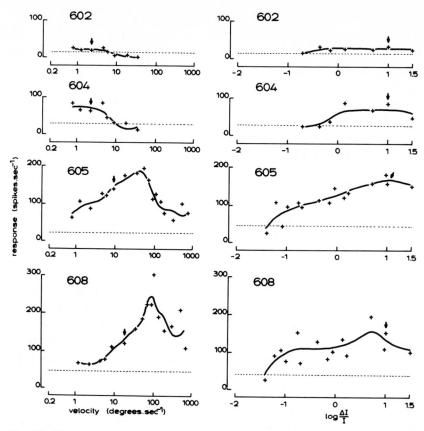

Fig. 6/7. Changes in contrast sensitivity at the 17–18 border. Lefthand side: velocity-response (VR) curves and righthand side: contrast-response (CR) curves. The arrows indicate at which velocity the CR curve and at which contrast the VR curve were taken. Stippled lines: significance levels. Cells 604 and 605 at each side of the 17–18 border were only separated by 200 μ in a penetration illustrated in Fig. 1 of Orban et al. (1978) (Orban and Kennedy, unpublished).

sequence of these different contrast threshold-eccentricity relationships in areas 17 and 18, one can expect a change in contrast threshold at the 17–18 border, at least in penetrations sufficiently far away from the fixation point. This is exactly what we observed. In a fortunate penetration, 9–10 degrees below the area centralis, we observed a sudden decrease in contrast threshold (from −0.7 to −1.3) as the electrode penetrated from area 17 into area 18 as witnessed by the change in velocity sensitivity (Orban et al., 1980). In this penetration the change in velocity sensitivity and contrast sensitivity occurred between the two same cells, less than 200 μ apart (Fig. 6/7). These changes are all the more remarkable in that the electrode remained in the same layer (III) and that both cells belonged to the same RF family (S family). This, together with the evidence presented in Chapter 2, strongly suggests that the 17–18 border is functionally a sharp border, much sharper than the histologically defined border. We have shown (Orban et al., 1980), that the differences in velocity sensitivity between areas 17 and 18 are the most marked at small eccentricities and that velocity sensitivity is useful as a criterion to locate the 17–18 border for penetrations within 10° of the fixation point. It seems that in this respect contrast sensitivity could be the complement of velocity sensitivity in that for penetrations more than 10° from the fixation point, monitoring of contrast thresholds may allow a precise location of the border.

6.3 The Extreme Contrast Sensitivity at the 18–19 Border

We (Orban and Duysens, unpublished) have recently made additional observations on the extreme contrast sensitivity of neurons near the 18–19 border. Since area 19 has a RF width-eccentricity relationship almost identical to that of area 18 one can therefore expect area 19 neurons with eccentric RFs to be as sensitive as area 18 neurons in the same region of the visual field. Figure 6/8 illustrates the *extreme sensitivity of an area 18 neuron* with a RF 24° from the area centralis. The neurons responded to a flashed slit at contrast up to −2. Note also the increase in latency at lower contrast levels. This neuron responded at all stimulus durations tested (12.5 to 3298 msec) at higher contrast levels. At the lowest contrast levels however the neuron failed to respond to stimuli shorter than 50 msec. Non-oriented cells in area 19 as well as C cells in all three areas respond to diffuse light stimuli (Chapter 4). Cells near the 18–19 border also exhibited *great sensitivity to small changes in luminance of a whole field stimulus* ($25 \times 25°$). Figure 6/9A shows a non-oriented area 19 neuron responding to extremely small changes in illumination. While the neuron in Fig. 6/9A showed a transient response to changes in diffuse illumination, a number of area 19 neurons near the 18–19 border also responded with tonic changes in firing rate (Fig. 6/9B). Although we routinely tested these neurons with changes in illumination lasting only 5 sec, it is possible that they represent luxotonic cells[2] which were reported to be virtually absent in the cat visual cortex (DeYoe and Bartlett, 1980). It is also possible that a large number of cells responding to diffuse illumination occur in the cortical region lateral to area 19 (Orban, Duysens and van der Glas, unpublished observation). Our results therefore clearly show that area 18 and 19 neurons with eccentric RFs have an extreme sensitivity to low contrasts

---

[2] Luxotonic cell: cell of which the maintained discharge depends of the overall illumination level (see Chapter 14).

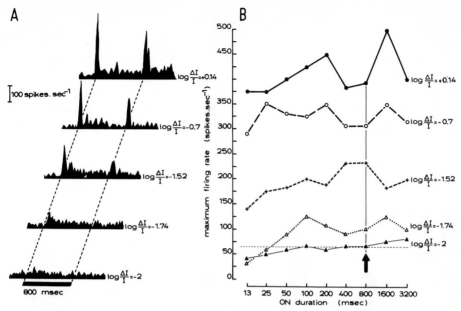

Fig. 6/8. Responses of an area 18 C cell (eccentricity 24°) to different ON durations of a slit flashed at different contrast levels. The different durations were tested with the multihistogram method (Henry et al., 1973). The multihistograms at different contrast level were taken separately. A. PSTHs corresponding to a single ON duration (800 msec) indicated by *horizontal bar*. The OFF duration was kept constant at 1 sec. B. Response-duration curves for ON response at different contrast levels. Horizontal stippled line: significance level. Note that at log $\frac{\Delta I}{I} = -1.74$ the cell stops responding at short ON durations. Arrow indicates duration for which the actual PSTHs are shown in A. (Orban and Duysens, unpublished).

and to small changes in whole field luminance. This is probably due to their large field dimensions. Parts of areas 18 and 19 subserving peripheral vision, are crowded together in the islands of the 18–19 border and receive their main bulk of afferents from MIN (see Chapters 2 and 3). MIN cells are almost all Y cells, with a larger RF diameter than Y cells in the laminated part of the LGN (Kratz et al., 1978). We therefore suggest that the main function of the MIN – areas 18–19 islands system is *the analysis of low contrast objects and small changes in luminance*, a function which is of great significance for a nocturnal predator. This may explain why the MIN is a particular feature of the carnivore LGN, without counterpart in monkeys (Rodieck, 1979). It would be of great interest to know whether other nocturnal animals have homologous system. Some of the responses of cells at the 18–19 border, especially the tonic changes to diffuse illumination, may be due to W afferents. Meyer and Albus (1981 b) have provided anatomical evidence that the proportion of W afferents in area 18 increases with eccentricity.

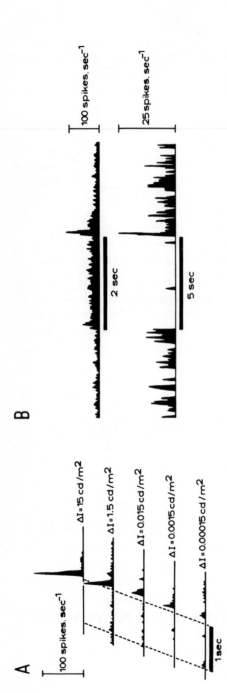

Fig. 6/9. Responses of area 19 cells to diffuse illumination. A. PSTH giving average responses of area 19 C cell (eccentricity 19°) to a diffuse flash (1 sec ON – 1 sec OFF) for different intensity increments (ΔI). B. PSTHs giving average responses to a long lasting change in diffuse illumination: upper PSTH, non-oriented cell near 18–19 border (eccentricity 10°); lower PSTH, non-oriented cell deeper into area 19 (eccentricity 6°). Horizontal bars indication diffuse light ON (Orban and Duysens, unpublished).

6.4 Influence of Contrast and Luminance on Other Response Properties

A number of studies have been concerned with the influence of contrast and luminance on other functional properties of cortical neurons. Tolhurst and Movshon (1975) and Albrecht and Hamilton (1982) have shown that spatial frequency selectivity of area 17 cells is little affected by changes in contrast. However Henry et al. (1978 a) have shown that the linearity of width summation in area 17 cells disappears for contrast levels over 40%. Sclar and Freeman (1982) have shown that the width of orientation tuning is invariant with stimulus contrast. Kulikowski et al. (1979), Grusser and Grüsser-Cornehls (1973), and ourselves (Orban and Kennedy, unpublished) have shown that direction selectivity of areas 17, 18 and 19 neurons is unaffected by changes in contrast (Fig. 6/10). Large changes in contrast have an influence on velocity-response curves. Most marked is the influence of contrast on velocity high-pass cells (see Chapter 8 for definitions). Strong reduction in stimulus contrast will decrease the response at fast velocities (Duysens et al., 1982 c). The reduction of responses to fast velocities may actually be a benefit for area 18 velocity tuned cells with eccentric RFs: at low contrast levels the velocity tuning will become sharper. This, together with the invariance of direction selectivity, may indicate that the cells of the areas 18–19 islands do not merely detect the stimuli, but also analyze them.

Finally, it should be mentioned that Bisti et al. (1977) have reported the invariance of orientation tuning with large changes in background luminance. Bisti et al. (1977) also observed that the spatial frequency tuning of

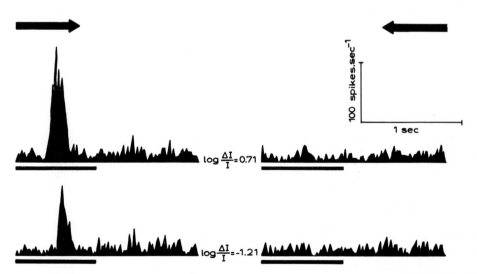

Fig. 6/10. Average responses of a direction-selective (DS) area 18 cell to movement in opposite directions at 2 contrast levels (indicated). Horizontal dark bars indicate movement duration (Orban and Kennedy, unpublished).

simple cells did not change with luminance while that of complex cells shifted slightly towards lower spatial frequencies as did that of LGN fibers. However the low frequency attenuation in complex cells was unaffected in opposition to the situation for retinal ganglion cells. Hess and Lillywhite (1980) briefly reported that spatial and temporal tuning were unaffected by large changes in background luminance. We (Duysens, Orban and Cremieux, unpublished) have recently obtained evidence that decrease in background luminance can alter the RF organization.

6.5 Conclusion

Stimulus contrast and not luminance is the stimulus attribute determining cortical cell responses. Visual cortical cells display a contrast threshold, function of the background luminance and of cortical area. Some cells display a contrast adaptation. The area 18–19 border region seems to be especially sensitive to low contrast and to small luminance changes. This may be related to the dense MIN projections to this region, typical of carnivores.

Chapter 7. Coding of Spatial Parameters by Cat Visual Cortical Neurons: Influence of Stimulus Orientation, Length, Width, and Spatial Frequency

Hubel and Wiesel (1959, 1962) introduced the use of *elongated* edges and light and dark bars as stimuli for visual cortical cells. Edges and bars are characterized by an orientation and a length (dimension parallel to orientation). Bars in addition have a width (dimension orthogonal to the orientation) (Fig. 7/1). Campbell et al. (1968) introduced *gratings* in visual cortical physiology. Gratings all have a given length and orientation. Gratings can have different luminance profiles. Sinusoidal gratings are mathematically the simplest. A sinusoidal grating is characterized by its spatial frequency (cycles/degree) which is the inverse of the spatial period (sp), and its amplitude or modulation depth (contrast, see Chapter 6). Other gratings used are square wave gratings or rectangular gratings of different duty cycles (ratio of light and dark parts). Two-dimensional *noise fields* were introduced by Hammond and MacKay (1975) and Orban (1975). Although one can produce noise fields with different spatial frequency content, the influence of the spatial parameters (e.g. pixel size) describing this pattern have not yet been studied. One-dimensional noise has recently been used by Burr et al. (1981). The spatial parameters characterize a stimulus whether stationary or moving. When elongated stimuli move, it is customary that their axis of movement is orthogonal to their orientation. The influence of stimulus orientation, a parameter ranging over 180°, will be described first.

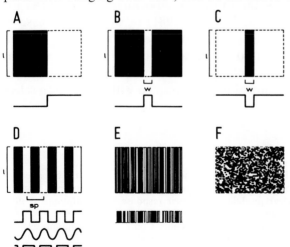

Fig. 7/1. Stimuli used in cortical visual physiology: edges (A), light (B), and dark (C) bars, gratings (D) and uni (E) and two (F)-dimensional noise fields. In A to E the patterns have a vertical orientation. Other spatial parameters are indicated length (l), width (w), and spatial period (sp) of a grating. The spatial frequency (cycles/degree) of a grating is the inverse of the spatial period (degrees). The luminance profiles are drawn below patterns A to E. For the gratings 3 luminance profiles are indicated: square, sinusoidal and rectangular.

7.1 Orientation Tuning of Cortical Cells

7.1.1 Definitions and Criteria

In their initial study of area 17 Hubel and Wiesel (1959, 1962) discovered the orientation tuning of cortical neurons (Fig. 4/1). They used stationary flashed stimuli and qualitative[1] single sweep recordings to demonstrate *orientation selectivity*.[2] In fact orientation is a spatial parameter which can be the attribute of both a stationary and moving stimulus. Since it has long been believed that moving stimuli are more powerful than stationary flashed stimuli (see Chapter 4 for evidence to the contrary), most subsequent studies have used moving stimuli and in fact investigated *axial selectivity*.[3] However, in as much as the optimal axis is always orthogonal to the optimal orientation of the stimulus, the axial selectivity of most cells is entirely the reflection of their orientation selectivity. This is attested by the almost perfect identity between axial selectivity tested with a moving slit and orientation selectivity tested with a stationary slit (Fig. 7/2). It is also confirmed by the observation that longer moving slits produce much narrower axial tuning than do short moving slits or spots (see below). In the normal adult animal the most notable exception seems to be a small number of C cells (Orban and Kennedy, unpublished) which display no orientation tuning for a stationary flashed bar and an equally wide axial tuning for a moving spot and long moving bar. It should be noted that in young animals or in animals raised in abnormal environments the situation may be different and that *in order to conclude that orientation selectivity is present* in such animals one should either use stationary flashed stimuli (in those animals, as in normals, one can expect flashed stimuli to be as powerful as moving stimuli provided that one uses quantitative tests and this has been demonstrated at least for strobe-reared animals, Duysens and Orban, 1981) or show an increase in sharpness of axial tuning with length. The mere observation that the cell responds better to a long slit than to a spot cannot be taken as evidence that the cell is orientation specific; it only shows that it has length summation, which happens in the normal animal to be associated with orientation selectivity.

---

[1] Qualitative technique: using hand-held stimuli and listening to cell discharges.

[2] Orientation selectivity requires that there is at least one orientation to which the cell does not respond. Otherwise, cells have to be considered not orientation selective and can then be either orientation biased, if there is a clear modulation of their response by orientation, or non-oriented, if all orientations yield about the same response level.

[3] Axial selectivity: selectivity for axis of motion of a stimulus. Contrary to orientation selectivity, which requires an elongated stimulus for characterization, axial selectivity can be tested both with elongated moving stimuli and with moving spots.

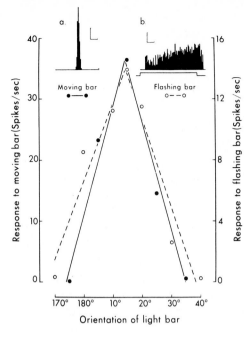

Fig. 7/2. Orientation and axial selectivity compared. The same simple cell (G25–1–8) has been used to obtain orientation specificity curves for a moving bar of light and for a stationary flashing bar. Each datum point averaged 30 responses for the moving bar and 150 responses for the flashing bar. Straight regression lines have been fitted in each case. Inserts: (a) response to optimally oriented moving bar; abscissa: 500 ms (0.8°); ordinate: 10 spikes/sec. (b) ON response to optimally oriented stationary flashing bar; abscissa: 100 msec; ordinate: 10 spikes/sec. Adapted with permission from Henry et al. (1974 a).

7.1.2 Quantitative Determinations: Orientation-Response Curves

Orientation-response curves have been quantified in two ways (Fig. 7/3): by fitting two straight lines to both legs of the tuning curve (Albus, 1975 b; Campbell et al., 1968; Hammond and Andrews, 1978; Leventhal and Hirsch, 1978; Rose and Blakemore, 1974) or by computing a smoothed Gaussian weighting function through the data points (Henry et al., 1973; Nelson et al., 1977). The former procedure is simpler but may be less precise. It creates the false impression of a sharp selectivity, while in fact the responses to orientations within a few degrees of the optimum are very similar so that the function is bell shaped rather than triangular (Henry et al., 1973, 1974 a, b). It may also be that the linear regression lines tend to overestimate the asymmetry between the parts of the curve at both sides of the optimum (Hammond and Andrews, 1978; Rose and Blakemore, 1974). Orientation-response curves yield an *optimal or preferred orientation* and a measure of selectivity which is the *half-width of tuning at half-height* (Fig. 7/4). Most quantitative studies have been devoted to area 17 subserving central vision (see Table 7/1). The narrowest tuning reported (usually for a simple cell) has a half-width (HW) at half-height (HH) between 5° and 7°, while the widest tuning (usually a complex cell) has a HW at HH between 40° and 67°. Simple cells have a significantly narrower orientation tuning than complex cells (Table 7/1). The only quantitative study for area 18 cells is that of Hammond and Andrews

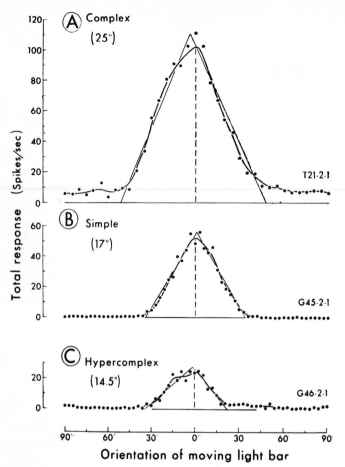

Fig. 7/3. How to fit orientation tuning curves. Orientation specificity curves (multihistogram method) for three cells, each characteristic of its class, using the broadside movement of a long narrow bar of light angled to successive settings at intervals of 5° (complex) or 3° (simple, hypercomplex). Data points have been fitted both with straight regression lines and with a smoothed curve using a Gaussian weighting function. The half-width of curves at half-height are indicated in parentheses for each cell. The optimal orientation (smoothed curve) in this and subsequent figures has been arbitrarily set at 0° in each case. Adapted with permission from Henry et al. (1974 b).

(1978): they report a mean half-width at half-height of 22° for simple-like cells and 27° for complex cells.

It has been claimed that the orientation preference of cortical neurons changes (Donaldson and Nash, 1975 a). However, with the multihistogram technique (i.e., interleaved stimulus presentation) which offset slow changes in responsiveness (Henry et al., 1973), it has been shown that the *orientation tuning curve is extremely stable* (Hammond et al., 1975; Henry et al., 1973). The difference in reproductibility of orientation-response curves with and

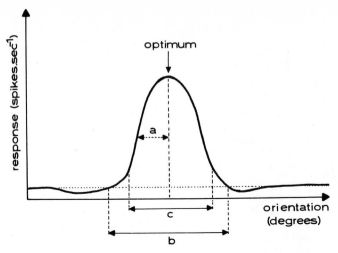

Fig. 7/4. Measures of orientation selectivity shown on a theoretical tuning curve: a: half-width at half-height; b: range of orientation to which the cell responds or passband (quantitative measure on the curve); c: width of orientation tuning determined by hand-plotting. Horizontal stippled line spontaneous activity level. Note: some authors use bandwidth at half-height which equals 2a.

Table 7/1. Orientation tuning (half-width at half-height in degrees) in area 17 of the cat (0–10° eccentricity)

Investigators	Overall population			Simple cells		Complex cells		Difference between simple and complex
	smallest	largest	N	mean	N	mean	N	
Henry et al. (1973)	5	40[+]	(56)	17	(40)	27.5	(11)	S (p < 0.01)
Rose and Blakemore (1974)	5*	55	(88)	14	(39)	19	(40)	(p < 0.1)
Watkins and Berkley (1974	5*	56[+]	(28)	13.9	(14)	26.9	(14)	S (p < 0.01)
Nelson et al. (1977)	7.2*	62[+]	(75)	16.7	(37)	29.2	(31)	S (p < 0.01)
Hammond and Andrews (1978)	7*	51[+]	(32)	15.3	(–)	26.6	(–)	–
Heggelund and Albus (1978)	7	67	(84)	19.5	(41)	31.6	(31)	S (p < 0.01)
Kato et al. (1978)	5.4*	54	(54)	17.1	(17)	23.2	(9)	(p < 0.1)
Leventhal and Hirsch (1978)	–	–		22	(59)	30	(79)	S (p < 0.02)

* This cell had a simple RF
[+] This cell had a complex RF

A. Sequential method

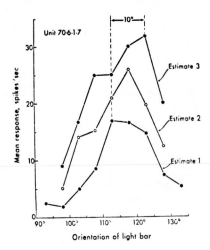

B. Multihistogram method

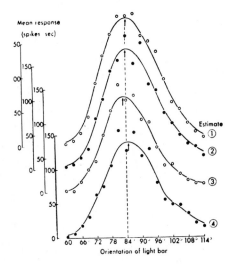

Fig. 7/5. Multihistogram technique offsets orientation tuning variability. A) Sequential method. Three separate estimates of the optimal stimulus orientation for the one simple cell. Each data point was derived from an average response histogram in response to a light bar moved over the receptive field. The histogram for each data point summed 30 responses. The recording of each histogram was completed before moving on to a new orientation setting. Mean response: firing rate averaged over the duration of the five analyser bins centered on the bin containing the maximum count. B) Multihistogram method. Four separate estimates of the optimal stimulus orientation of cell G28−1−8 with curves fitted by the Gaussian smoothing function method. The ordinate scales have been displaced upward to correspond with their respective curves. The total recording time for all the data points (multiple histogram method) was 100 min. The vertical arrows indicate the optimal orientation in each case and the vertical broken line corresponds to the mean estimate (84.0°). Adapted with permission from Henry et al. (1973).

without stimulus interleaving is illustrated in Fig. 7/5. *The far greater stability obtained with the multihistogram technique makes the use of this technique mandatory for parametric studies of visual cortical cells.*

It has been shown that orientation tuning curves depend on *slit length* in the sense that while the optimum nearly always remains the same, the curve becomes more sharply tuned with larger lengths. A very small number of cells

of the complex family have a different optimum for short and long slits
(Bishop et al., 1980). According to Henry et al. (1973), Orban et al. (1979 a)
and Rose (1977), sharpness in orientation tuning increases with slit length in
the simple family (both simple and hypercomplex I cells). Many cells in the
complex family have the same behavior (Henry et al., 1974 b; Rose, 1977) but
a few (especially hypercomplex II cells) show the same sharpness of tunings
for moving spots and slits (Henry et al., 1974 b; Orban et al., 1979 a). The
latter group of cells probably correspond to the C family cells seen by Orban
and Kennedy (unpublished) as being only axis and not orientation selective.
Unfortunately, not enough data are available to know up to what length the
orientation tuning sharpness increases. As a rule one should use the optimal
stimumus length of the cell (up to 8 or 10° for some S cells but only 1 or 2°
for an end-stopped cell) for determining the orientation tuning width.

7.1.3 Qualitative Determination: Hand-Plotting

Most data on orientation selectivity outside area 17 subserving central
vision, have been obtained with hand-held stimuli. The selectivity of the cell
is then measured by the *width of orientation tuning* (Fig. 7/4), which is the
range of orientations to which the cell responds, and the preferred orientation
then corresponds to the orientation in the middle of that range. There is a
good agreement between preferred orientations measured quantitatively and
qualitatively (Blasdel et al., 1977). The range of orientations is *underestimated*
by about 20% (Wilson and Sherman, 1976) or 30% (comparison of our
median hand-plotted width of tuning for S cells in area 17 (44) with the mean
half-width of simple cells in Kato et al.'s (1978) study). As mentioned earlier
(Chapter 4) all cortical cells, with the exception of less than 2% of the cells
in areas 17 and 18 and less than 12% of the cells in area 19, are axially
selective, which means that, with the exception of a few C cells, they are
actually selective for orientation.

Cells in area 17 are more narrowly tuned than cells in area 18 and those
in turn are more narrowly tuned than area 19 cells (median hand-plotted
orientation tuning widths: 65° in area 17, 70° in area 18 and 91° in area 19)
(Fig. 7/6). This is in keeping with Albus' (1979) recent observation that the
orientation "bands" labelled with deoxyglucose are wider in V3 (area 19)
than in V1 (area 17). Considering different cell types (Table 4/2), *S cells of
area 17 are the most narrowly tuned of all cell types in the 3 areas*. In particular
area 17 S cells are more narrowly tuned than area 18 S cells (Hammond and
Andrews, 1978; Orban and Kennedy, 1981). It should also be stressed that
in the 3 areas, but most clearly in area 17, HS cells had wider tuning than S
cells (median hand-plotted orientation tuning width 44° and 74° for S and
HS cells of area 17). This underscores the differences between end-free and

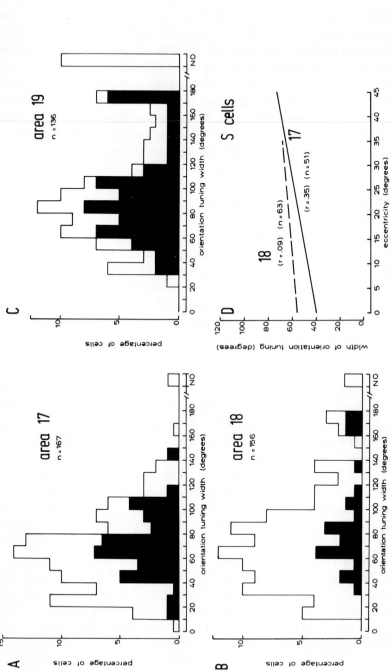

Fig. 7/6. Orientation tuning width of cortical cells (hand-plotting). A through C: distributions for area 17, 18 and 19: filled columns end-stopped cells, top curve all cells. Medians of the three distributions were 65, 70 and 91° for area 17, 18 and 19 respectively. D: linear regression line indicating increase of orientation tuning width of S cells with eccentricity: in area 17 the correlation was significant, in area 18 not. (In area 19 the number of S cells was too small to estimate the relationship.)

end-stopped cells of the same family. To some extent, this is also true for B and HB cells.

We found a small but significant correlation between width of orientation tuning and eccentricity for S cells in area 17 but not in area 18 (Fig. 7/6D). With a change in eccentricity of 30° the width of tuning increases 50% for area 17 S cells. Wilson and Sherman (1976) failed to observe such a relationship for simple cells. There seems to be a correlation in their data (Fig. 7A of Wilson and Sherman, 1976), except for the datapoint corresponding to the eccentricity class 0–5°. It could be that, given the difficulty of localizing the 17–18 border, (see Chapter 2), some of the 0–5° cells were actually area 18 cells, which would explain the wider tuning for the eccentricity class 0–5°. For area 17 Leventhal and Hirsch (1978) mention that there is a change in degree of selectivity of complex cells with lamination: complex cells in the deeper layer are less selective. This fits with our observation that C family cells which have the broadest orientation tuning largely dominate in layer V. It also fits with Hubel and Wiesel's (1965) observation that orientation columns in area 17 were less clear in the deeper layers.[4]

7.1.4 Distribution of Preferred Orientations

As initially pointed out by Hubel and Wiesel (1962) the preferred orientations of cortical cells span the whole 180° range. This is the neuronal mechanism by which cats, and probably humans, see all orientations. It now seems established that in the cat there is no overrepresentation of any orientation in any of the three areas. In particular in area 17 there is *no significant overrepresentation of horizontal and vertical orientations, at least if one considers the overall population* (Henry et al., 1979; Hubel and Wiesel, 1962; Orban and Kennedy, 1981; Rose and Blakemore, 1974). This seems to be at variance with the monkey where there is a small overrepresentation of horizontal and vertical orientations in the overall population at least for eccentricities below 2° (see Chapter 14). However it now seems established that in the cat *a subset of area 17 cells* with RFs within 10° from fixation point is preferentially tuned to horizontal and vertical: simple cells according to Pettigrew et al. (1968 a), small area slow (SAS) cells according to Leventhal and Hirsch (1980), S cells according to Orban and Kennedy (1981), and simple I according to Berman et al. (1981). Wilson and Sherman (1976), Henry et al. (1974 b) and Rose and Blakemore (1974) reported no orientation preference among simple cells. Rose and Blakemore (1974) however reported

---

[4] It has been claimed (Bauer, 1982) that in vertical (i.e., orthogonal to the cortical surface) penetrations, there is a change in preferred orientation of the neurons at the transition between layers IV and V.

a narrower tuning for simple cells preferring horizontal and vertical orientations. Nelson et al. (1977) also reported that simple cells, but not the complex cells, were more narrowly tuned when preferring vertical or horizontal orientation. We have now found a similar correlation for our S cells (Fig. 7/7) in a sample somewhat larger than previously published (Orban and Kennedy, 1981). Figure 7/7 confirms our previous report (Orban and Kennedy, 1981) that S cells of area 17 (0–10° eccentricity) are not homogenously distributed over the whole orientation range but rather prefer horizontal and vertical orientations. Consideration of S1 and S2 cells separately shows that the preference for horizontal and vertical is significant only for S1 cells, in keeping with Berman et al.'s (1981) observation. As shown in Fig. 7/7, S cells of area 18 or HS cells of area 17, do not show preferences for horizontal and vertical and are not more narrowly tuned when preferring horizontal and vertical orientations. These observations show that the contradiction in reports on orientation anisotropies in the cat visual cortex can at least partially be explained by the difficulties of classifying RF types and of distinguishing area 17 from area 18.

7.1.5 Orientation Columns

The preferred orientations are not randomly scattered over the surface of the cortex. As noted by Hubel and Wiesel (1962, 1963) cells (and background activity) in the same vertical (i.e. orthogonal to the surface of the cortex) penetration (especially in the superficial layers) have *the same preferred orientation* and neurons in oblique penetrations *change their preferred orientation in a systematic way*. Hubel and Wiesel (1963) used the term "columns" introduced by Mountcastle (1957) in his study of the somatosensory cortex, to describe this organization, despite the fact that, due to their irregular shape (as projected on the cortical surface, see Fig.4 Hubel and Wiesel, 1963), they looked more like "*slabs*" than "*columns*". Hubel and Wiesel (1963) estimated that the orientation "columns" could be as thin as 100 μ. The term column suggests that there are clear separations between the preferred orientations of the different columns. Subsequent studies with quantitative techniques have shown that orientation is systematically represented on the cortical surface but the scatter of the preferred orientations is too large (Albus, 1975 b; Lee et al., 1977 a) to admit columns in the strict sense. There seems to *be a gradual change in orientation over the cortical surface* (Albus, 1975 b) and not a change in discrete steps as suggested by Hubel and Wiesel (1963). Recently Albus (1979) and Schoppmann and Stryker (1981) have confirmed the systematic changes of preferred orientation over the cortical surface of area 17 with deoxyglucose labelling experiments. While these experiments show that the changes affect all layers of the cortex, they do not show whether orienta-

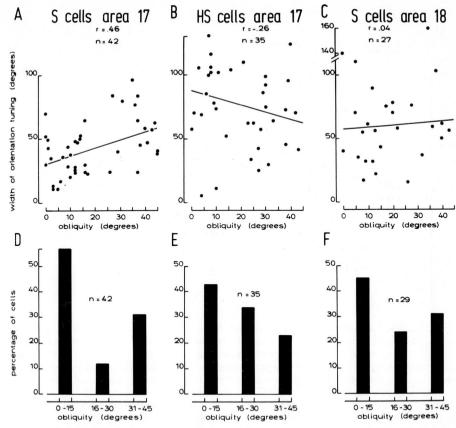

Fig. 7/7. Meridional variations in orientation preference and selectivity of different RF types. A through C width of orientation tuning plotted as a function of preferred orientation relative to principal meridians (obliquity) for S cells in area 17 (A), HS cells in area 17 (B), S cells in area 18 (C). D to F proportion of cells having given preferred orientation relative to principal meridians (obliquity). D: area 17 S cells, E: area 17 HS cells, F: area 18 S cells. All cells had RFs within 10° from fixation point. Only area 17 S cells showed significant meridional variations in tuning width (correlation with obliquity significant at .01 level) and in number of cells ($\chi^2 =$ 10.7, p < 0.005).

tion columns are discrete entities or whether orientation varies continuously across the cortical surface. Schoppmann and Stryker (1981) could correlate the deoxyglucose labelled "bands" with the preferred orientations of cells recorded in penetrations through those bands. The half width at half height of the radioactive band [5] is approximatively 30° which corresponds approximatively to the average orientation tuning of cells in area 17 (see Table 7/1). Single-cell recordings have shown that a total orientation shift of 180° took place over a cortical distance of 800–1200 μ in area 17 (Albus, 1975 b; Hubel

---

[5] Measured on the plot of the radioactivity (indicating density of labelling) – preferred orientation relationship (Fig. 3 b in Schoppmann and Stryker, 1981).

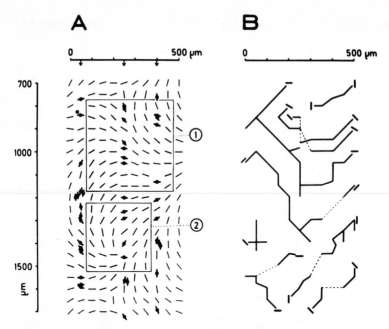

Fig. 7/8. Spatial organization of the orientation domain. A) Plan view of an extended surface of the postlateral gyrus in the cat. Striate cells were recorded along three tangential electrode tracks indicated by the arrows coming from the scale at the *top*. The cell positions (filled circles) are projected onto the surface and their preferred stimulus orientation indicated by a line in each case. The area (orientation matrix) selected is 1 mm long in an anteroposterior direction and 0.5 mm wide in a mediolateral direction. The gaps between the experimentally recorded cells have been filled in with hypothetical neurons located at regular spacings of 50 μm and with their preferred orientations set to be 10° different from that of the preceding cell. Two arbitrarily selected regions (1, 2) each contain almost the full range of preferred orientations. B) Positions of cells having the same preferred orientation and not more than 50 μm apart as shown in A are connected by continuous lines. The broken lines interconnect cells which were between 50 and 100 μm apart. The orientation represented by each iso-orientation line is indicated at one or both ends of the line. Adapted with permission from Albus (1975 b).

and Wiesel, 1963) and in area 18 (Orban et al., 1980). This is in keeping with the distance between "bands" labelled with deoxyglucose (700 μ – 1200 μ) (Albus, 1979; Schoppmann and Stryker, 1981). Thus a region of cortex approximatively 1000 μ wide will represent all orientations. However as shown by Fig. 7/8 the representation of orientations over the cortical surface cannot spread equally in all directions and there are several breaks and twists in the "slabs" representing orientations. These twists express themselves in jumps in otherwise regular sequences of preferred orientations. We have noticed a tendency for these jumps to involve horizontal and vertical orientations (Orban and Kennedy, unpublished), a tendency also present in the data of Albus (1975 b). This may explain a slightly larger occurrence of cells preferring horizontal and vertical orientations. On the other hand the existence of orientation "columns" or "slabs" make the demonstration of orientation preferences difficult at least when the overall population of a cortical area is involved. Indeed any overrepresentation of orientation may be due to sampling bias. This objection however cannot hold when the preference for horizontal and vertical is only observed among a single cell type representing a mere 30% of the overall population, as we reported for S cells in area 17 (Orban and Kennedy, 1981).

7.1.6 Conclusion

In conclusion almost all cortical cells (of areas 17, 18 and 19) can be considered as bandpass filters[6] for orientations. The average bandwidth of the filters at half-height is about 30 to 50°. The optima of the filters cover the entire range of orientations, allowing the system to "represent" all orientations. The filters in a piece of cortex about 1000 μ wide cover the whole range of orientations at a given retinal locus. Among those orientation filters, one set (S cells of area 17 subserving central vision) is remarkable by being the most sharply tuned and by its preference for horizontal and vertical orientations.

7.2 Influence of Stimulus Length on Cortical Cells

Although often neglected in studies involved in spatial frequency coding (e.g. in De Valois et al., 1979; Burr et al., 1981) stimulus length (measured in degrees of visual angle) is an important *attribute of nearly all visual stimuli used* (slits, dark bars, edges and gratings), except noise fields and spots. It is thus useful to know how stimulus length affects the cortical responses. Hubel and Wiesel (1965) in their initial accounts on area 18 and 19, suggested that a group of cells (hypercomplex cells) may be specific for length. Preparation of length-response curves can tell us how specific cortical cells are for length and whether a subset of them can code for stimulus length.

All quantitative studies on the influence of stimulus length are restricted to area 17 subserving central vision (0–10°) except for a short report on area 18 (Camarda, 1979). Our qualitative observations (Orban and Kennedy, unpublished) suggest that in area 18 there is less length summation than in area 17, even in S cells. This is indicated by the relative efficiency of moving spots compared to moving slits (see Chapter 4) in area 18. All studies agree that area 17 cells show a substantial length summation (Bodis-Wollner et al., 1976; Gilbert, 1977; Henry et al., 1978 a; Kato et al., 1978; Orban et al., 1979 a; Rose, 1977). In one study (Henry et al., 1978 a) length summation

---

[6] See Chapter 5 for definition.

was shown to be much stronger than width summation. It is trivial to say that length summation is non-linear in hypercomplex or end-stopped cells. The question is less trivial for end-free cells. The shapes of the length-response curves are quite variable (Fig. 7/9). The ascending part can be linear (Bodis-Wollner et al., 1976; Rose, 1977), S shaped (Kato et al., 1978), linear with two different slopes (Rose, 1977), or even logarithmic (Gilbert, 1977). Thus for many cells the ascending part can be considered as close to linear especially if one accepts some slowing down of the slope close to the saturation point. However, most cortical cells are non-linear when one compares the length-response curves to the length activity profile[7] (Fig. 7/10). Indeed in many cases length summation extends over a larger range of lengths (7° for the simple cells in Fig. 7/10C) than the activity profile (4° for some cells, Fig. 7/10A) and the response reaches higher levels in the length-response curve. As shown by Henry et al. (1978 a) this non-linearity[8] can be removed by accepting a *neuronal threshold for firing* (around 5–10 impulses/sec).

Except for a few cells for which a spot or small square is the best stimulus, the length-response curve of end-stopped cells increases steeply with length reaching a maximum between 0.5 and 4° (Kato et al., 1978; Rose, 1977). In area 17 subserving central vision the mean optimal length was about 1.4° with little difference between different types of hypercomplex cells (Kato et al., 1978; Rose, 1977). There is a good *correlation between strength of end-stopping and optimal length* (Fig. 4/11): more strongly stopped cells prefer shorter stimuli (Kato et al., 1978; Rose, 1977). Qualitatively the same has been found to be true for area 19 end-stopped cells (Duysens et al., 1982 a). The optimal lengths of end-free cells are much longer than those of end-stopped cells (Kato et al., 1978; Rose, 1977). These optimal lengths are seriously underestimated in the hand-held stimuli (Kato et al., 1978). Kato et al. (1978) found longer optimal lengths for simple (6.4°) than for complex cells (mean 4.4°) but Rose (1977) (mean 3.8° and 3.8°) and Gilbert (1977) did not. It is noteworthy that a number of cortical cells have optimal lengths over 8°. According to Kato et al. (1978) they all belong to the simple family, according to Gilbert (1977) they can be either simple or standard complex (which is not necessarily a contradiction, see Chapter 4) but occur mainly in layer VI.

---

[7] Length-response curves are obtained by measuring responses for different stimulus lengths, the shortest stimulus being centered on the RF center. In unilateral length-response curves the length increases only at one end of the stimulus, while in bilateral length-response curves length increases are produced by extension at both sides. Length-activity profiles are measured with a short stimulus (just long enough to produce a reliable response). The response is measured as a function of the position of the stimulus across the length of the RF. RF length can be estimated from the LR curves: (integrated manner) and from the length-activity profiles (differential manner). Both estimates are not necessarily equal (Fig. 7/10) (see Chapter 4 for the relevance of this for RF classification).

[8] Non-linearity here means that the length-response curve cannot be simply obtained by integration of the length-activity profile.

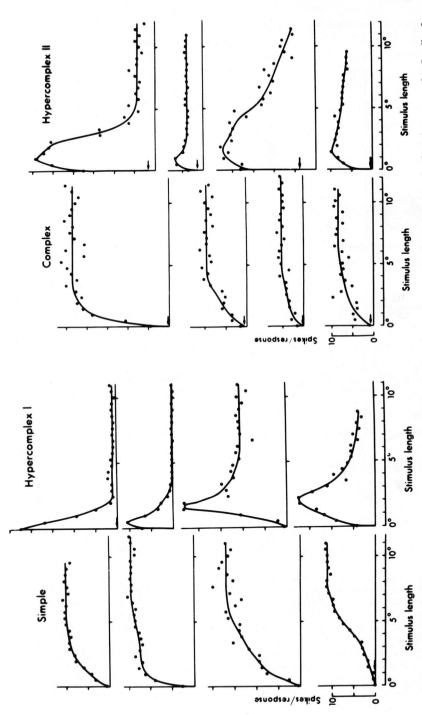

Fig. 7/9. Sample length-response curves. From left to right: bilateral length-response curves from four simple, four hypercomplex I cells, from four complex and four hypercomplex II cells. The horizontal arrows, indicating the level of the spontaneous activity, mark the zero on the ordinate scales used for estimating the percentage of end-zone inhibition. Adapted with permission from Kato et al. (1978).

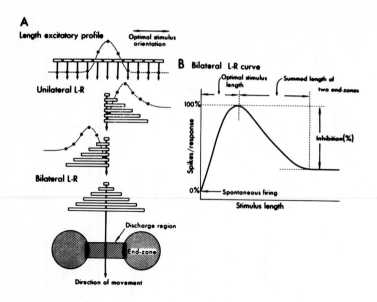

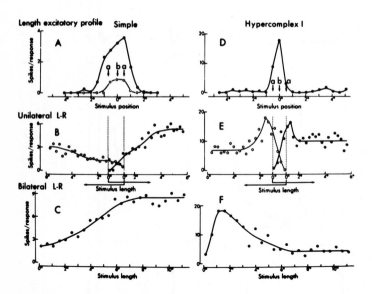

Fig. 7/10. Length-activity profiles and length-response curves compared. Top half: A. Diagram of experimental procedures used to prepare a length-excitatory profile and unilateral and bilateral length-response curves. The filled circles are data points for the respective curves (dashed lines). B. Diagram of bilateral length-response curve showing how the various parameters are measured. The curves illustrated were prepared with moving bar stimuli. Bottom half: Response curves as indicated obtained from a simple cell (A, B, C) and a hypercomplex I cell (D, E, F). A. Two length-excitatory profiles were prepared with bar lengths of 1.0° (open circles) and 2.9° (filled circles), respectively. A, D: a, initial locations of bar stimuli used for unilateral length-response curves in B and E; b, initial locations of bar stimuli used for bilateral length-response curves in C and F. Adapted with permission from Orban et al. (1979 a).

The mean percent of end-zone inhibition was about 70% in the study of Kato et al. (1978). In the data of Gilbert (1977) and Rose (1977) the mean was somewhat lower, about 50 and 55%, due to differences in techniques and calculation mentioned earlier (Chapter 4). It seems therefore that hypercomplex or end-stopped cells should not be considered as coding stimulus length, because their range of optima is too narrow and their attenuation at longer lengths is too weak. However the whole cortical population of area 17 could signal length, shorter lengths being signalled by end-stopped cells and longer lengths (up to 16°) being signalled by end-free cells. In any respect the results reported above clearly show that one will stimulate different populations when using short or long stimuli. This should be kept in mind when comparing responses to checkerboards and gratings (e.g. in psychophysics or visual evoked pontential studies).

7.3 Selectivity of Cortical Neurons for Spatial Frequency and Stimulus Width

7.3.1 Selectivity for Spatial Frequency

Following up the psychophysical experiments of Campbell and Robson (1968) and of Robson and Campbell (1964) suggesting the existence in the visual system of a number of channels each selectively sensitive to a limited range of spatial frequencies, Campbell et al. (1969) have shown that area 17 (eccentricity 0–15°) cortical cells, when *tested with sinusoidal grating patterns are selective for spatial frequency*. The selectivity is similar whether one measures the response strength at a given contrast, producing response – spatial frequency curves or the contrast sensitivity (i.e., the inverse of the threshold contrast for a given spatial frequency) yielding the contrast sensitivity curve which plots the contrast sensitivity as a function of spatial frequency. The same authors showed that the LGN fibers had less low frequency attenuation than the cortical cells. This fits with the observation reported in Chap. 4 (Fig. 4/18) that all LGN neuron respond to flashing a whole field while hardly any cortical cell responds to this stimulus.

This spatial frequency tuning (Fig. 7/11) has now been repeatedly confirmed for area 17 cells (Albrecht and De Valois, 1981; Andrews and Pollen, 1979; Bisti et al., 1977; Ikeda and Wright, 1975 b; Kulikowski and Bishop, 1981 a, b; Maffei and Fiorentini, 1973; Movshon et al., 1978 c; Tolhurst and Movshon, 1975) and for area 18 cells (Movshon et al., 1978 c). Maffei and Fiorentini (1973) confirmed that the low frequency attenuation is stronger in cortical cells than in LGN and retinal cells. Movshon et al. (1978 c) and Kulikowski and Bishop (1981 b) have confirmed the similarity between

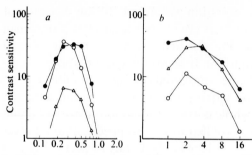

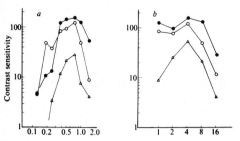

Spatial frequency (cycles per degree) Temporal frequency (Hz)

Fig. 7/11. Contrast sensitivity functions of cortical cells. Upper half: Spatial and temporal contrast sensitivity functions of a simple cell. Contrast sensitivity is the reciprocal of the contrast at threshold. a) Spatial frequency tuning. The cell's contrast sensitivity as a function of the spatial frequency is shown for gratings drifting at three temporal frequencies: ●, 1 Hz; ○, 4 Hz; △, 16 Hz, b) Temporal frequency tuning. The contrast sensitivity as a function of temporal frequency is shown for gratings of three spatial frequencies: ○, 0.13 cycles per degree; ●, 0.25 cycles per degree; △, 0.5 cycles per degree. Lower half: Spatial and temporal contrast sensitivity function of a complex cell. a) Spatial frequency tuning. ○, 1 Hz; ●, 4 Hz; △, 16 Hz. b) Temporal frequency tuning. ○, 0.38 cycles per degree; ●, 0.75 cycles per degree; △, 1.5 cycles per degree. Conventions as in upper half. Adapted with permission from Tolhurst and Movshon (1975).

curves using contrast sensitivity and those using response amplitude. Some authors have used constant velocity[9] (Andrews and Pollen, 1979; Kulikowski and Bishop, 1981 a, b; Maffei and Fiorentini, 1973; Maffei et al., 1979) while Movshon et al. (1978 a, b, c) and Albrecht et al. (1980) used constant temporal frequency.[10] It has however been shown that at least for area 17 simple cells (eccentricity 0–10°) both methods yield similar curves (Andrews and Pollen, 1979).

In order to be able to code the parameter spatial frequency, cortical cells must not only be selective, but be *selective to different spatial frequency ranges*. Campbell et al. (1969) reported that the upper frequency cut-off (i.e., spatial frequency above optimum at which the response was half maximum) of area 17 cells ranged from 0.2 to 3.8 cycles per degree for fields within 0–15° of the fixation point. In subsequent studies the optimal spatial frequency has been used as an indication of the position of a cell in the spatial frequency range. According to Movshon et al. (1978 c) the optima range from 0.3 to 2.2 cycles/degree in area 17 subserving central vision (0–5°). Ikeda and Wright (1975 b) report an even wider range (0.5–4 cycles/degree) for the same area. Thompson and Tolhurst (1979) reported a range of 0.25 to 2.5 c/deg for area

---

[9] Since temporal frequency equals spatial frequency times velocity this implicates that changes in spatial frequency also induced changes in temporal frequency.
[10] For the same reason, changes in spatial frequency now imply changes in velocity.

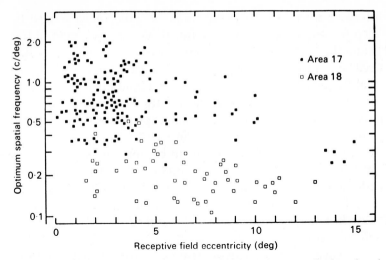

Fig. 7/12. The optimal spatial frequency (c/deg) for 238 neurons is plotted against the eccentricity (deg of visual angle). Note that, in this figure, eccentricity is the radial distance from the area centralis. Neurons recorded in area 17 are represented by filled symbols; neurons recorded in area 18 are represented by *open* symbols. Excluded from this figure are four neurons recorded in area 18 which had no low spatial frequency decline in sensitivity. Adapted with permission from Movshon et al. (1978 c).

17 cells within 3° of area centralis. With *increasing eccentricity the optima* decrease, which can be expected given the excellent inverse correlation between RF width and optimal spatial frequency (Maffei and Fiorentini, 1977) and the increase of RF width with eccentricity (see Chapter 4). In area 18 subserving central vision (0–5°) the range of optimal spatial frequencies observed by Movshon et al. (1978 c) was 0.1 to 0.5 c/deg. It should be noted that Movshon et al. (1978 c) only recorded cells well in area 18. This may explain the large difference in optimal spatial frequencies between areas 17 and 18, since the area 18 cells close to the border have RF width not very different from those of area 17 cells (Orban et al., 1980, see Fig. 2/16). According to Movshon et al. (1978 c) the selectivity of area 18 cells is similar to that of area 17 cells (1.5 octave bandwidth at half-height). Considering areas 17 and 18 together, optimal spatial frequencies in the parts subserving central vision, span a spatial frequency range of more than 4 octaves and as eccentricity increases this range narrows and shifts to low spatial frequencies (Fig. 7/12).

Since simple and complex cells have been attributed different roles in spatial analysis, it is important to compare their spatial selectivity. Initially Maffei and Fiorentini (1973) reported that complex cells were more widely tuned than simple cells. This was denied by Movshon et al. (1978 c) and Albrecht et al. (1980), who both used constant temporal frequency as opposed to Maffei and Fiorentini (1973) who used constant velocity. This may explain the difference since at low spatial frequency, the velocity must be increased to keep temporal frequency constant. If one uses a temporal frequency of 2 Hz and the optimal spatial frequency is as low as can be expected for a complex cell with a large field, one may have to use a velocity of 20°/sec to reach a spatial frequency of 0.1 c/deg. The attenuation attributed to that spatial frequency may then actually be a velocity attenuation if the cell is a velocity low-pass cell (Orban et al., 1981 a). Other explanations are of course the differences in criteria for RF classification (see Chapter 4). Movshon et al. (1978 c) found simple and complex cells to be tuned to similar ranges (0.3 to 2.2 cycles/deg). Andrews and Pollen (1979) report a range of 0.3 to 1.8 c/deg for simple cells and Kulikowski and Bishop (1981 b) a range of 0.5 to 2.3 c/deg for the simple cell family (hypercomplex I cells included). Recently Kulikowski and Bishop (1982) have described silent periodic cells similar to B cells, which have a similar range of optimal spatial frequencies as simple cells but have especially narrow bandwidth (mean bandwidth at half-height of 0.75 octave), narrower than that of any simple cell (narrowest bandwidth at half-height 0.96 octave) in their comparison study.

Since spatial frequency selectivity may be a fundamental parameter handled by the visual system, various authors have looked for *systematic change in optimal frequencies in the cortex at a local level* (i.e. other than changes with eccentricity). Maffei and Fiorentini (1977) have reported systematic changes with depth in the cortex (area 17) launching the idea of constant spatial frequency "horizontal" rows orthogonal to the "vertical" orientation columns [11]. Berardi et al. (1979) reported the same observation for area 18. This view is disputed by Thompson and Tolhurst (1980 a) who favor a vertical (i.e. column like) organization of optimal frequency. Thompson and Tolhurst (1980 b) and Tootell et al. (1981) also presented evidence from deoxyglucose labelling experiments for spatial frequency "columns". According to Tootell et al. (1981), for each of the spatial frequencies tested (ranging from 0.3 to 2 c/deg), density labelled columnar patterns were seen, extending throughout all layers of area 17. The distance between the spatial frequency "bands" was approximately 1000 μ. According to Silverman et al. (1981) the spatial frequency bands are correlated with the optimal spatial frequencies of cells recorded in penetrations in the same hemisphere. Furthermore Silverman et al. (1981) showed that the three "columnar" systems (ocular dominance, orientation and spatial frequency) run over the cortical surface (area 17) independently of each other [12].

---

[11] Horizontal and vertical here mean parallel and orthogonal to the cortical surface.

[12] This supposes that the functional architecture of area 17 is more complicated than initially suggested by Hubel and Wiesel (1977). In their diagram of the functional architecture of area 17 they drew their 2 columnar systems (ocular dominance and orientation) at right angles to each other to mean independence of both systems (see Fig. 15/1).

7.3.2 Spatial Frequency and Coding of Stimulus Dimensions

From the above reported data it is clear that, tested with sinusoidal gratings, cortical cells show a selectivity for a limited range of spatial frequencies. This could be the counterpart of the psychophysically measured spatial frequency channels (Ginsburg, 1981).[13] While these data allow us to understand a vast psychophysical literature they do not necessarily prove that the *visual system uses this selectivity* and decomposes the visual objects into to their spatial frequency spectrum. Before embarking on the review of the evidence for or against this hypothesis it must be mentioned that feature extraction by bar and edge detectors is not the only alternative as some spatial frequency champions have suggested (Albrecht et al., 1980). Indeed there are many other ways in which spatial dimensions could be encoded, for example coding of orientation and width or coding of orientation and length.

A first type of experiments uses stimuli which can be either described in terms of edges or bars or in terms of spatial frequencies and tries to demonstrate that the cortical response is *function of the spatial frequency and not of the edges.* DeValois et al. (1979) measured responses of cortical cells to checkerboards which have their spatial frequency components oriented differently from their edges. There was however a confounding variable in these experiments: the length of the stimuli. While edges were always short, the spatial frequency components were always long. Thus these experiments show that the cortical cells are linear (MacKay, 1981), which is surprising since some of the cells were complex which are reputedly non-linear (Movshon et al., 1978 b), and that cortical cells show considerable length summation. They do not show that cortical responses are dictated by spatial frequency rather than by edges. If De Valois et al. (1979) had tested checkerboards on hypercomplex cells the result of their test might have been the reverse.

Another experiment in the same vein is the comparison of responses to gratings with luminance profiles other than sinusoidal gratings, e.g. rectangular gratings with different duty cycles, missing fundamental gratings (Maffei et al., 1979; Pollen and Ronner, 1982). These elegant experiments show that *when the fundamental of the non-sinusoidal pattern is within the spatial tuning domain of the cell,* the response is dictated by the spatial frequency component and not by the edges (Fig. 7/13). Under those circumstances both simple and complex cells respond equally well to rectangular and sinusoidal gratings

---

[13] This correspondence has to be qualified. There is a continuum in the range of optimal spatial frequencies of cortical cells (De Valois, 1982 b). In fact this means that there are an infinite or very large number of spatial frequency "filters". Psychophysical experiments, in particular discrimination-detection experiments report a small finite number of spatial frequency channels (3 or 4). This is in fact the minimum number of non-overlapping filters covering the range of spatial frequencies to which humans are sensitive (see Chapter 5).

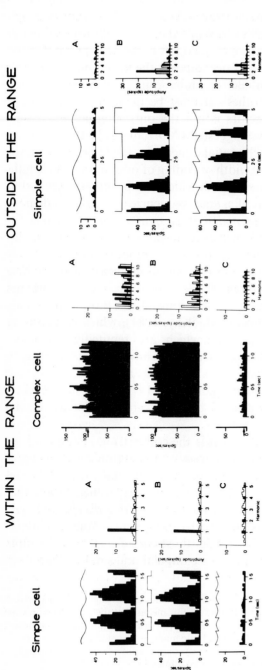

Fig. 7/13. Cortical cells are only sensitive to spatial frequency components in their working range. Left: Average responses (thirty sums) of a simple cell to drifting gratings of different profiles: sinusoidal (A), square (B) and missing fundamental (C). The profiles are reported on top of each response. Spatial frequency of the grating 0.5 c/deg, velocity 2.3 deg/sec, contrast 20% for the sinusoidal grating and 15.7% for the squarewave grating and average luminance 5 cd/m². The width of the bin in the histograms is 50 msec. On the right of the histograms the fast Fourier (amplitude spectrum) transforms of the corresponding responses are reported; these transforms were computed in a temporal series with four periods of average responses. The black vertical bars are the amplitudes of the harmonics. Harmonic no. 1 corresponds to the fundamental periodicity of the response. Middle: Average responses (forty sums) of a complex cell to drifting gratings of different profiles: sinusoidal (A), square (B) and missing fundamental (C). Spatial frequency of the grating 0.5 c/deg, velocity 3.2 deg/sec, contrast 20%, luminance 5 cd/m². The width of the bin in the histogram is 19 msec. On the right of the histograms the fast Fourier transforms of the corresponding responses are reported. The arrows on the ordinates indicate the average discharge. In C the average discharge is equal to the spontaneous discharge. Right: Average responses (forty sums) of a simple cell to drifting gratings of very low spatial frequency outside the range of response of the cell to sinusoidal gratings. The three gratings had the same spatial frequency 0.12 c/deg, velocity 3.2 deg/sec, contrast 15% and average luminance 5 cd/m² in B. B: response to a square-wave grating. C: response to a missing fundamental grating. Fast Fourier transforms of the corresponding responses are reported on the right of the histograms. The location of the receptive field was within 5 deg of the area centralis. The width of the receptive field was 2 deg. Adapted with permission from Maffei et al. (1979).

but not to a grating with a missing fundamental which has edges with about the same spacing as the rectangular grating. There is however a fundamental difference between simple and complex cells: the output of the simple cells contains the same harmonics as the stimulus, that of complex cells does not (Fig. 7/13). Maffei et al. (1979) elegantly showed that the output of simple cells very closely matches the harmonics at the input (i.e. in the stimulus) when one remains in their operating range. Pollen and Ronner (1982) in a similar experiment have shown that with rectangular gratings there is a secondary peak in the sensitivity curve of simple and complex cells at 1/3 the spatial frequency of the optimal one. However outside the spatial tuning domain of the cells, defined by Maffei et al. (1979) as spatial periods smaller than twice the RF width, the response of the cells can solely be accounted for by the edges (Fig. 7/13). This is also evident, although they do not mention this, from the data of Pollen and Ronner (1982) (their Figs. 2 G, 3 G and 5). Thus the *cortical cells have a working range of spatial frequency*. The lower boundary of this range is the spatial frequency corresponding to the spatial period equal to twice the RF width and the upper boundary the acuity of the cell i.e. the upper spatial frequency at which the cell fails to respond. Within this working range the cells are selective to spatial frequency components and not to edges. Outside this range the cells respond to the edges of the patterns and we know that almost all cortical cells respond to single edges (Kennedy and Orban, unpublished). At first glance then the output of cortical cells seems to be ambiguous – a price for having small RFs and thus to be able to localize the stimuli – but several considerations reduce the impact of this observation. Firstly most visual objects are finite and not infinite as are gratings for a cell with small RF field. Secondly the message of a single cell may be ambiguous but that of a set of cells will be less ambiguous especially if it includes cells with large and small optimal spatial frequencies. This notion of limited operating range due to finite spatial dimensions will be taken up in the discussion of Gabor functions[14] as model for cortical RFs.

Another "crucial" experiment aimed at demonstrating the use of spatial frequency selectivity by the visual system compares the *selectivity of cortical cells to sinusoidal gratings and bars* (Albrecht et al., 1980). Such experiments show that while all cortical cells are bandpass filters for spatial frequency very few cortical cells have a bandpass function for slit width. Pollen and Ronner (1975), Watkins and Berkley (1974) and Sherman et al. (1976) mention a few. Most cortical cells are high-pass filters for slit width (Fig. 7/14). This is not to say that the visual system may not use width instead of spatial frequency as spatial parameter, using e.g. the pooled output of the cells as suggested in Chapter 5. In this respect the "crucial" experiment would be to show that at a given eccentricity all the neurons have the same threshold and saturation

---

[14] A Gabor function is the product of a sinusoidal function with a Gaussian function.

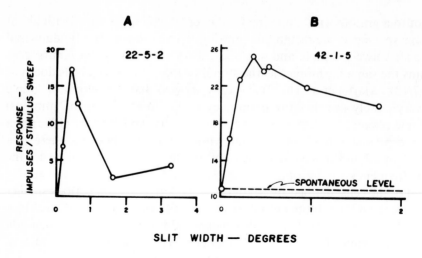

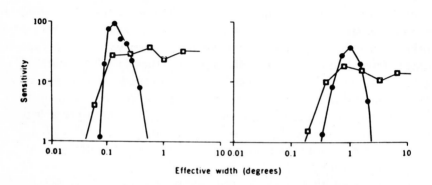

Fig. 7/14. Influence of slit width on cortical cells. Upper half: Effect of slit width on the response of two single units of cat striate cortex. The data of A (left) are from a simple cell. The stimulus was a slit of light oriented at 30° the preferred orientation – and moved across the receptive field at 8.4°/sec. The data of B (right) are from a complex receptive field. The stimulus was a slit of light oriented at 181° – the preferred orientation – and moved across the receptive field at 1.5°/sec. Adapted with permission from Watkins and Berkley (1974). Lower half: Selectivity functions for bars (squares) and gratings (circles) of two striate neurons. (A) Macaque monkey simple cell. (B) Cat complex cell. Contrast sensitivity (the reciprocal of the contrast required to reach a constant response criterion near threshold) is plotted as a function of effective width (for gratings, the effective width is equal to the width of one half of one period). There is little selectivity for bars and essentially no drop in the sensitivity as bar width increases. In contrast, the cells are sensitive to only a limited range of spatial frequencies and are therefore selective for gratings. Note that the bar has edges and the grating does not. Hence these results are eventually similar to those of Maffei et al. (1979) (Fig. 7/13) showing that the cells are sensitive to spatial frequency components inside their working range and to edges outside this range. Adapted with permission from Albrecht et al. (1980).

width and thus cannot code for width.[15] Both hypotheses are not mutually exclusive. A bandpass coding supposes a multichannel system and usually requires more cells than a single channel system. It could therefore be that the spatial frequency bandpass system is used in visual areas representing central vision (high magnification) and the width high-pass system in areas representing peripheral vision (low magnification).

7.3.3 Linearity of Cortical Cells

Once it has been established that at least in a certain working range cortical neurons are spatial frequency selective we can consider a more ambitious hypothesis that the cortex works as a Fourier analyzer of the light distribution (Maffei and Fiorentini, 1973; Pollen et al., 1971). A necessary condition for the latter hypothesis is that the neurons *behave linearly*.[16] This linear behavior can and has been assessed in two different ways.[17] All these experiments reach the same conclusion: most simple (or better S family) cells behave linearly, complex cells (or C family cells) do not. A first way of testing linear behavior is to look at the response to a drifting sinusoidal grating. A linear cell should have an output which is a *copy of the input:* firing rate

---

[15] The absence in area 17 of bandpass filtering for width and length is often used by the defendants of spatial frequency analysis as a key argument in favor of their hypothesis. In addition to the possibility that width is encoded in another way than by bandpass filters, it could also be that width and length are encoded further up in the visual cortical system. In this respect it is worth mentioning that both in V4 of the macaque and in area DL of the owl monkey such tunings have been reported (Desimone, 1982; Petersen et al., 1980).

[16] More precisely that the response of a neuron to a visual stimulus is predictable according to linear system theories (Pollen and Ronner, 1982).

[17] These tests have to be distinguished from tests of linearity of spatial summation. Linearity of summation has been tested by examining the responses to stationary gratings presented in different phases. The grating can either be flashed (this is the celebrated null test of Enroth-Cugell and Robson, 1966) or be modulated with a temporal square wave (counter phase) or sine wave (Movshon et al., 1978 a). According to Movshon et al. (1978 a, b) the majority of simple cells (17/25) showed a linear spatial summation, either since they had a null position (13/17) i.e. phase where the grating elicited no response (Fig. 7/16C), or since the neuron although responding to all phases, still showed a behavior (Fig. 7/16B) that need not indicate non-linear spatial summation (4/17). According to the same criteria about 1/3 of the simple cells (8/25) are non-linear (Fig. 7/16A). Movshon et al. (1978 a) showed that these cells which were non-linear for this phase test (which measures harmonic distortion) behaved linearly when RF profiles were compared with the inverse Fourier transforms of their spatial frequency selectivity functions. Complex cells are invariably non-linear for this test (Fig. 7/16D). These observations were confirmed by Kulikowski and Bishop (1981 b) who found that 9/12 cells of the "ordinary" simple family (simple and hypercomplex I) were linear by the null test, while all 6 fast simple cells (a type for which Kulikowski and Bishop give no precise definition) failed to show a null point. Expressing the response at the phase where there is frequency doubling (i.e. where the cell responds at each half of the temporal period) as a percentage of the maximum response one can evaluate the degree of non-linearity for spatial summation. According to Kulikowski (personal communication) simple cells (and hypercomplex I) are 0% non-linear, fast simple and A cells are 20% non-linear, B cells 60% and complex cells 90%.

should be a sinusoidal function of time (luminance sinusoidal function of time). Simple cells fulfil these requirements (Andrews and Pollen, 1979; Movshon et al., 1978 a) with the exception of a truncation non-linearity: the firing rate cannot decrease below zero (Fig. 7/15). This minor non-linearity reflects a threshold for firing similar to the one mentioned before for the length-response curves. Complex cells do not fulfil the requirements as they show an unmodulated increase in firing rate except sometimes for lower spatial frequencies (Movshon et al., 1978 b). Fig. 7/15 however, shows that the separation between linear simple cells and non-linear complex cells is not as sharp as one would like to think.

The most stringent test of linear behavior is the *comparison of the RF profiles* with the *inverse Fourier transform of the spatial frequency selectivity curve* (or the reverse: Fourier transform of the RF profile with the actual selectivity curve). All studies (Andrews and Pollen, 1979; Kulikowski and Bishop, 1981 b; Maffei et al., 1979; Movshon et al., 1978 a) agree that there is a reasonable fit (indicating linearity) for the simple cells or simple cell family (simple and hypercomplex I) (Fig. 7/17). According to Kulikowski and Bishop (1981 b) the agreement is better when one uses the RF profile obtained with moving stimuli rather than that obtained with stationary stimuli as used in the first studies (Andrews and Pollen, 1979; Movshon et al., 1978 a). Among the RF profiles of simple cells two kinds can be distinguished: odd and even symmetric (Robson, 1975) corresponding to the bi- and tripartite simple cells described by Hubel and Wiesel (1962) (Fig. 4/12). According to Kulikowski and Bishop (1981 b) both types occur in equal proportion. Movshon et al. (1978 a) reported a slightly higher proportion of odd symmetric simple cells (62%) than of even symmetric simple cells (38%). For complex cells the inverse Fourier transform of the selectivity curve does not fit the RF profile but the subunit within this profile (Movshon et al., 1978 b). One can thus safely conclude that a majority of simple and hypercomplex I cells behave linearly the other simple cells being only weakly non-linear, while complex cells do not behave linearly. Daugman (1980) has recently criticized the experiments comparing RF profile and spatial frequency selectivity for considering only one dimension of the RF (across the width). RFs should be considered as two-dimensional and should allow spatial frequency tuning to be independent of orientation. Daugman (1980) has proposed such two-dimensional RF profiles.

The relationship between RF profile and spatial frequency tuning, has implications for the *relationship between bandwidth and optimal spatial frequency*. The optimal frequency is related to the width of a subregion (say ON or OFF regions) and the width of the spatial frequency selectivity to the number of subregions (Fig. 7/18). If the width of the field is constant (i.e. same position uncertainty for all cells whatever their spatial frequency characteristics) then the bandwidth should increase exactly as the optimal spatial

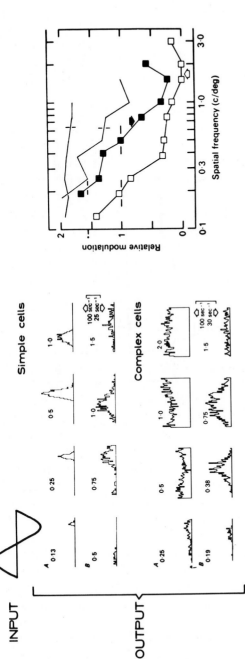

Fig. 7/15. First test of linear behavior of cortical cells: the output of the cells should be a copy of the input (inset). Top left: The responses of two simple cells to sinusoidal gratings of different spatial frequencies, moving over their receptive fields at 2 Hz. Each histogram represents the average response of the neuron to the passage of one cycle of the grating across its receptive field; the number above each histogram indicates the grating's spatial frequency in cycles per degree. The contrast of all the gratings was 0.5. Neither neuron had any maintained discharge in the absence of stimulation. Bottom left: The responses of two complex cells to sinusoidal gratings of different spatial frequencies, moving over their receptive fields at 2 Hz. Each histogram represents the average response of the neuron to the passage of one cycle of the grating across its receptive field; the number above each histogram indicates the grating's spatial frequency in cycles per degree. The contrast of all the gratings was 0.5. Neither neuron had any maintained discharge in the absence of stimulation. Right: Relative amplitudes of modulated and unmodulated components in the responses of three cortical neurons to moving gratings of different spatial frequencies. Relative modulation was determined by calculating the frequency components of the neurons' average responses by Fourier analysis, and then by dividing the amplitude of the component corresponding to the frequency of movement (f1) by the amplitude of the component at zero frequency (f0). The asterisk on the ordinate indicates a value of 1.57, which corresponds to the value obtained for a precisely halfwave rectified sine wave. The two complex cells whose responses are illustrated in bottom left are shown; open symbols for neuron A, filled symbols for neuron B. The arrows indicate each neuron's optimum spatial frequency. The solid lines without symbols reproduce the data from two simple cells from top left: upper curve cell A, lower curve cell B. Adapted with permission from Movshon et al. (1978 a, b).

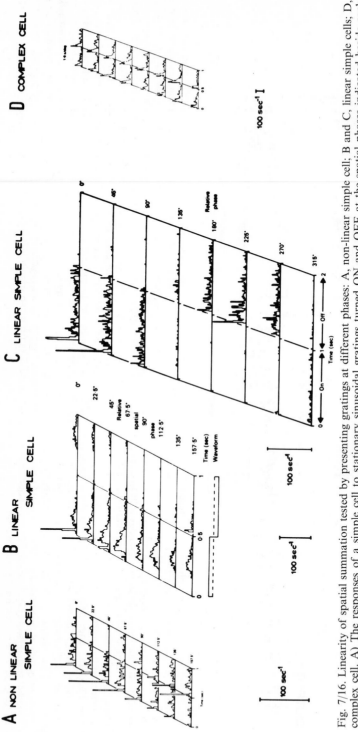

Fig. 7/16. Linearity of spatial summation tested by presenting gratings at different phases: A, non-linear simple cell; B and C, linear simple cells; D, complex cell. A) The responses of a simple cell to stationary sinusoidal gratings turned ON and OFF at the spatial phases indicated beside each histogram. The spatial frequency of the grating was 0.75 c/deg, they all had a contrast of 0.5, and were turned ON for 1 sec every 2 sec. B) The responses of a simple cell to stationary sinusoidal gratings modulated in time with either a square wave at 1 Hz, at the spatial phases indicated. The spatial frequency of the gratings was 0.5 c/deg, and they all had a contrast of 0.5. The neuron had no maintained discharge in the absence of stimulation. C) The responses of a simple cell to stationary sinusoidal gratings modulated in time with a 1 Hz square wave at the spatial phases indicated. The spatial frequency of the gratings was 0.75 c/deg, and they all had a contrast of 0.72. D) The responses of a complex cell to stationary sinusoidal gratings modulated in time with a 1 Hz square wave at the spatial phases indicated. All the gratings had a spatial frequency of 1 c/deg and a contrast of 0.5. Adapted with permission from Movshon et al. (1978 a, b).

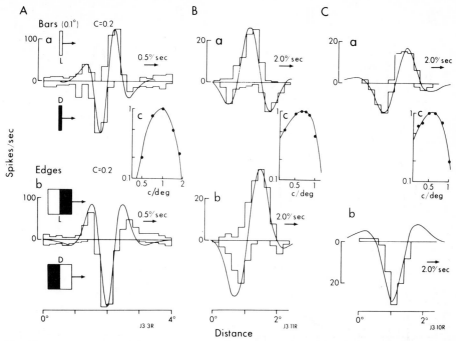

Fig. 7/17. Second test of linear behavior of cortical cells: comparison of RF profile and inverse Fourier transform of contrast sensitivity function. Average response histograms from 3 simple striate cells (A, B and C) to moving bars (a) and edges (b) showing the predictability of these responses from the inverse Fourier transformation (continuous lines) of the respective contrast sensitivity tuning curves (c). The shapes of these tuning curves are chosen to produce the best fit to the data points, thereby testing the predictability of responses to bars and edges (essential for the proper classification of simple cells). However, the fitted tuning curves are not much different from the ideal Gaussian functions for tuning curves with medium and narrow band widths ($B_{df} < 1$). Cell A is fitted best by an antisymmetrical profile (sinusoidal Fourier transform), whereas cells B and C are pair fitted with symmetrical and antisymmetrical profiles respectively. Adapted with permission from Kulikowski and Bishop (1981 a).

frequency decreases (slope -1). If on the contrary units should have the same band width (same uncertainty for spatial frequency) whatever their optimal spatial frequency, then the width of the field should increase as the spatial frequency decreases (and position uncertainty should increase). Thompson and Tolhurst (1979) measured optimal spatial frequency and bandwidth for 232 area 17 cells within $3°$ from the area centralis. They observed a negative correlation between log bandwidth and log optimal spatial frequency with a slope of -0.46. Kulikowski and Bishop (1981 b) report a similar negative correlation for simple cells with a slope of -0.3. Thus it seems that cells with lower optimal spatial frequency, increase their band width, but only to some extent, so as to keep their bandwidth within useful limits. This requires in counterpart that the width of their RF also increases to some extent with decreasing optimal spatial frequency.

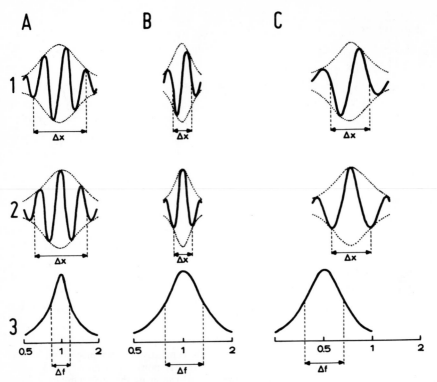

Fig. 7/18. Analogues in the spatial domain of Gabor's sampling functions of (1) 'sine' and (2) 'cosine' type with their corresponding (3) spatial frequency spectra (adapted from Gabor, 1946). Comparison of (A) with (B) shows the reciprocal relationship between 'spreads' in space (Δx) and in spatial frequency (Δf): the Δf decreases with the number of subregions. Comparison of (B) and (C) shows the relation between optimal frequency and width of subregions.

7.3.4 The Visual Cortex as a Fourier Analyzer

The hypothesis that the cortex acts as a Fourier analyzer was proposed by Pollen et al. (1971) and by Maffei and Fiorentini (1973). While Pollen et al. (1971) considered complex cells as the substrate, Maffei and Fiorentini (1973) attributed this role to simple cells. From the above reported experiments on linearity behavior, it is plain that while complex cells can contribute to a spatial frequency analysis, only simple family cells can be the substrate of a Fourier analysis. The "Fourier" hypothesis *supposes that the visual image is broken down into its spectral components at different orientations, each represented by the activity of a cell, and that by recombining the activities of these cells the system can reconstruct the image.* It is noteworthy that this hypothesis has at least the advantage of specifying how the messages of the cortical cells have to be recombined. The hypothesis as such is not tenable since the cortical cells have only a limited RF. Therefore, the hypothesis has been reformulated by Robson (1975) who followed a suggestion of Pollen et al. (1971) and proposed *a patch by patch Fourier analysis* where a piece of the visual image is analyzed by a set of cells with RFs of same location and extent, of which the activity constitutes the representation of the spatial frequency spectrum of the patch filling the RFs. In this hypothesis each patch would only be analyzed into its first three harmonics, each harmonic being represented by a series of pairs of simple cells (one odd and one even symmetric representing the sine or consine coefficients of the Fourier sum) having different orientations (minimum 2). The requirement that all the fields have the same extent may be too stringent (and leads to a representation by only 3 harmonics) and unnecessary. In a more modern version of this localized Fourier analysis (Pollen and Ronner, 1982) the simple cells are considered as *Gabor elements*[18]: a pair of simple cells (one odd and one even symmetric) would represent a harmonic at a given locus and a given orientation. In this respect the recent observation by Pollen and Ronner (1981) that a pair of simple cells recorded together are 90° out of phase would suggest that the elements of a pair representing the harmonic are grouped together in the cortex (Fig. 7/19). In fact, given the truncation in the output of simple cells (see above), a harmonic should be represented by 2 pairs: one pair for light ON (each cell 90° out of phase) and another pair (each cell also 90° out of phase) for light OFF. Thus the four cells each represent a phase (0, 90, 180, 270°) of the harmonic at an orientation. Contrary to the general Fourier hypothesis, this view of simple cells as Gabor elements, is compatible with the observation that cortical cells represent spatial frequency only in their working range. One should also not forget that most of the stimuli that the visual system must analyze are localized objects so that a localized system with Gabor elements should perform almost as well as a general Fourier analyzer. However, the theory needs a second modification in order to accommodate the bandwidth of the spatial frequency selectivity of cortical cells which is often quoted as an objection (MacKay, 1981). Indeed it is likely that a harmonic at a given orientation and one phase (0, 90, 180 or 270°) is not represented by the activity of a single cell, but rather *by the activities of a set of cells* all with the same phase and orientation. This is exactly similar to saying (see Chapter 5) that one orientation is not represented by the activity of a single cell but can be derived from the comparison of the activities in a given set of cells. This comparison of simple cell outputs incorporates into the theory the reciprocal inhibitory influences on cortical cells of a fundamental frequency (F) and its high harmonics (4F or 5F) (Albrecht and De Valois, 1981). This modification also takes into account the recent observations of Petrov et al. (1980) and Morrone et al. (1982) who showed interaction between gratings of different orientations. The grating of non-optimal orienta-

---

[18] According to Gabor (1946) the amplitude and phase at any given frequency can be derived from the amplitudes of the sine and consine terms at any given instant in time.

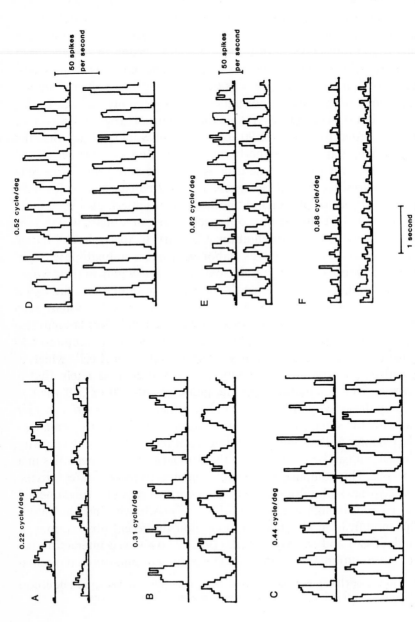

Fig. 7/19. Pairs of simple cells are 90° out of phase. Responses of two adjacent simple cells to six different spatial frequencies. The cells were recorded simultaneously from the same micro-electrode placement. The upper tracings in each section represent the responses of one cell, and the lower set represents the responses of the other. The calibration in (D) applies to (A) to (C) and (F) as well. Adapted with permission from Pollen and Ronner (1981).

tion inhibits the response of cortical cells to an optimally oriented grating. If the output of a single cell were to represent the harmonic at a phase and orientation, the reconstructed image produced by combining the output of these single cells will be distorted. If however a comparison of outputs of different cells, represents the harmonic at a phase and orientation, then the results of this comparison may remain unchanged even if all the cells are affected [19] and so the recombined signal using this comparison of outputs may remain undistorted.

It is probable that even more modifications, in addition to those accommodating the localized RF and the bandwidth will have to be made. For example, it will probably be necessary to extend the concept of a working or operating range of the cell so as to include the possibility that the simple cells do not respond to some patterns (as two-dimensional visual noise). Burr et al. (1981) have recently shown that area 17 simple cells do not respond to two-dimensional noise but do respond to one-dimensional noise. This can be interpreted as evidence that simple cells perform a two-dimensional Fourier decomposition by analyzing orientation and spatial frequency along the axis orthogonal to the orientation (i.e. across the width of the RF). Given their strong length summation (Kato et al., 1978) simple cells integrate over the other axis (parallel to the orientation). This length summation property probably explains why simple cell respond to one-dimensional noise and not to two-dimensional noise [20] and also explains why simple cells can extract long contours so well from such a complex pattern as a checkerboard (De Valois et al., 1979) or a slit embedded in visual noise (Hoffmann et al., 1980). Furthermore the theory will probably have to be relaxed so that non-linear elements (at least the non-linear simple cells, but maybe also other types) can contribute to the representation of spectral components of the image. It is indeed likely that under certain circumstances (fast moving objects) area 18 cells will take over the analysis of the visual objects from area 17 cells. These cells are probably all non-linear (this has to be verified experimentally), yet they most likely contribute to some form or spatial vision (van der Glas et al., 1981).

7.3.5 Spatial Frequency: Conclusion

Cortical cells are selective for spatial frequency when tested with sinusoidal gratings and within a working range they can encode spatial frequency.

---

[19] The comparison rules given in Chapter 5 would have this virtue.

[20] Morrone et al. (1982) explain the absence of response of simple cells to two-dimensional noise by cross orientation inhibition (i.e. inhibition by orientation outside the range of preferred orientation). Their argument rests upon the assumption that a bright spot evokes the same response from a simple cell as a dim long line (with same lengthwise integral of contrast). Recent results reported by Schumez and Movshon at the '83 ARVO meeting support this assumption but also underscore the length summation of simple cells.

That the visual system uses spatial frequency rather than width or length to measure the spatial dimension of visual objects is by no means proven. While the hypothesis that the cortex acts as a simple Fourier analyzer is certainly not verified, a modified version, taking into account the localized RFs, the rather large band width, and possibly other properties of simple cells cannot be rejected at the present stage.

It should be noted that the spatial frequency selectivity of cortical cells can be given *a function other than encoding of spatial frequency*. In this theory on vision D. Marr has developed a theory in which visual object segregation and identification is performed in three stages. The first stage results in the raw primal sketch: a rich but primitive description of the light intensity distribution on the retina (Marr, 1982) and could be carried out by striate cortex neurons. According to Marr simple cells act as zero crossing detecting devices acting on channels of different sizes. The important point is that the theory supposes that in order to assume the presence of an edge, zero crossings of the same orientation have to be present in independent channels of adjacent sizes. Hence this theory requires channels of different optimal spatial frequency, although according to this theory, spatial frequency is not handled as a parameter by the system. It should further be noted that the physiological realization of zero crossing detector proposed by Marr would be orientation dependent and spatial frequency tuned.

The primitives of the raw primal sketch are edges, bars, blobs and discontinuity or termination primitives, while the attributes of these primitives are orientation, contrast, length, width, and position. Hence from such a viewpoint it is easier to find a functional role for end-stopped cells which amount to about 40% of the cells in cat visual cortex. These cells respond poorly to elongated stimuli and it is not clear what function they may have in a Fourier-like processing hypothesis. Also in view of D. Marr's theory, the observation of Bishop et al. (1971 a) that cortical cells respond to single edges of the slit rather than the body of the slit is important.

The idea that cortical cells process primarily *information about edges* (in a Marr type of hypothesis) and the Fourier hypothesis that cortical cells process *spatial frequency components are not necessarily mutually exclusive*. Indeed we have seen that inside their operating range cortical cells are responsive to the spatial frequency components and outside that range they respond to single edges. It could thus be that cortical cells participate in two analyses: one of contour based on its responses to the edges and one of texture based on its responses to spatial frequency components. In the center of the visual field most cells have small RFs and rather high optimal spatial frequencies. Many visual objects in the center of the visual field will have their outline outside the operating range of most cells who will analyze the contour of the objects by their edge function. The texture of the objects will be analyzed by the spatial frequency component function of the cells. In the periphery of the visual field most objects would fall within the operating range of cortical cells which have much coarser RFs and hence lower optimal spatial frequencies. Thus in the periphery of the visual field very few objects will be analyzed by their contours but almost all of them will be analyzed (and seen) as texture.

7.4 Spatial Parameters: Conclusion

With respect to the coding of spatial parameters, area 17 subserving central vision seems to enjoy a large superiority compared to the rest of area 17 and to areas 18 and 19. Only this cortical region contains neurons tuned to a wide range of spatial frequencies (including high spatial frequencies) and neurons sharply tuned for orientation. Indeed area 18 and 19 neurons have large RFs and are tuned for lower spatial frequencies and are less sharply tuned for orientation. Within area 17 subserving central vision the *simple or S family plays a major role in the spatial analysis of visual objects*. Indeed "central" area 17 S cells are the most sharply tuned for orientation and the S family with its sharp RF profile carries precise position information. While HS cells seem to have only a small contribution to orientation coding they can contribute to spatial frequency analysis or edge detection.[21] Among the S cells it may be useful to distinguish between S1 cells (Fig. 4/12) which may be more involved in orientation coding (because of their preference for vertical and horizontal) and S2 cells which correspond to the odd and even symmetric fields and may be more involved in spatial frequency coding. This may explain why behaviorally spatial frequency and orientation tasks seem to be underlied by separate mechanisms (Vandenbussche and Orban, 1983). Both S1 and S2 cells could also participate in edge detection. While C family cells may be involved in orientation and spatial frequency analysis, it could well be that they play a completely different role and are involved in the subject-related analysis of *the visual background*. This would fit with the sensitivity of C family cells to noise texture, with the orientation distribution of complex cells (Berman et al., 1981) which make them maximally sensitive to radial flow patterns, and with their uniform distribution over the different cortical parts representing the visual field.

---

[21] Edge detection is used here to designate a zero crossing processing a la Marr leading to a raw primal sketch.

Chapter 8. Coding of Spatio-Temporal Parameters by Cat Visual Cortical Neurons: Influence of Stimulus Velocity, Direction and Amplitude of Movement

The *retinal image is constantly shifting*. This movement can be caused by movement in the visual world, movement of the subject, or movement of the eye. The latter movements give rise to swift displacement resulting from saccadic or pursuit eye movements or to slow drifts as during fixation. The dynamic nature of the retinal image underlines the importance of studies devoted to the influence of spatio-temporal parameters. The movement parameters most commonly investigated are angular velocity and direction of movement. Both parameters describe completely the movement of a stimulus. An alternative description is given by direction and amplitude of movement.

All visual cortical cells *respond to moving stimuli*. This is not too surprising since even during fixation the eyes are moving slowly and hence the images drift over the retina (see Grüsser and Grüsser-Cornehls, 1973). In the paralyzed and anesthetized cat the cortical cells respond equally well to moving and stationary flashed stimuli (see Chapter 4). Hence the preference of moving stimuli over stationary ones cannot be used as an indication that a cell recorded in such a preparation is *involved in movement perception*. It is from the way that the cells are influenced by movement parameters that one can reach such a conclusion (Orban et al., 1981 a). It must be stressed that the visual cortical cells are not analyzing movement but moving objects. Moving objects have two types of attributes: those related to their spatial pattern or shape (spatial attributes, which they share with stationary objects) and those related to their motion (spatio-temporal attributes). The present chapter deals with the influence of the latter attributes on cortical cells.

8.1 Influence of Stimulus Velocity

Study of the influence of velocity can answer two questions (1) to *what range of velocities* are the neurons sensitive and (2) are there neurons responding only over a limited range of velocities so as to be *specific for velocity*? Answering the first question will indicate the range of velocities over which cortical cells, many of which are not concerned with the analysis of velocity, can operate. The answer to the second question will tell us whether some cells are able to encode stimulus velocity and are concerned with the analysis of velocity. In contrast to spatial parameters, the study of spatio-temporal parameters is difficult with hand-held stimuli and often leads to incorrect observations (Orban et al., 1981 b; Wilson and Sherman, 1976). Therefore little reliance can be put on the older work carried out on spatio-temporal parameters using exclusively or mainly hand-held stimuli (Gilbert, 1977; Hubel and Wiesel, 1962, 1965; Pettigrew et al., 1968 a; Tretter et al., 1975). Semiquantitative studies determining only upper cut-off velocity (Dreher et al., 1980; Leventhal and Hirsch, 1980) give only limited information. A misleading, but often used measure, is the optimal velocity (Gilbert, 1977; Leventhal and Hirsch, 1978; Movshon, 1975; Pettigrew et al., 1968 a; Wilson and Sherman, 1976). As will be shown most cortical neurons, especially in areas 17 and 19, are not sharply tuned for velocity and it thus makes little sense to talk about their optimal velocity, the only meaningful measure being their optimal range of velocities.

We have determined with a multihistogram technique the *velocity-response* (VR) *curves* of areas 17, 18 and 19 neurons over a wide range of eccentricities (Duysens et al., 1982 a; Orban et al., 1981 a, b). The *response measure* is maximum firing rate measured on post-stimulus time histograms (PSTHs) compiled with a 8 msec bin width. The reasons for adopting this measure have been given in Orban et al. (1981 a). Briefly, the number of spikes cannot be adopted since this measure depends on stimulus duration, which changes with velocity. Mean firing rate supposes that the shape of the response remains unchanged for the different velocities, a hypothesis not always verified as witnessed by the difference in VR curves obtained with maximum and mean firing rate (Fig. 2 B in Orban et al., 1981 a). Finally when using maximum firing rate as a measure (which is evaluated from the number of spikes in one bin of the PSTH) the VR curve depends on the bin width, which has to be short in order not to distort short responses to fast velocities. Since the shortest cortical cell responses measured about 20 msec, a 8 msec bin width is optimal (further reduction tends to increase the scatter of the VR curve). Between to and fro movements the stimulus stands still for 5 or 6 sec. This is important as it disentangles velocity and rate of presentations. Some area 18 cells fail to respond to fast movements (over 300°/sec) if there is no pause between to and fro movement (Dinse and von Seelen, 1981 a). Finally the stimulus (a narrow light slit) has to be *optimal* (best eye, optimal orientation and length). Stimulus width is important but not critical. As long as stimulus width exceeds some threshold value velocity curves will be little affected (this fits with the high-pass functions for slit width reported in Chapter 7). The importance of stimulus width depends on the RF structure of the neurons: dominant ON center cells respond to light edges and the width of a light bar is more critical than that of a dark bar; the reverse is true for OFF center cells which react to dark edges (see Fig. 7 in Duysens et al.,

1982 c). In the eccentricity studies stimulus width was increased for testing more peripheral cells: from 0.2 or 0.3° for neurons with central RFs to 1° or 2° for area 17 neurons with eccentric RFs and to 3° to 5° for area 18 and 19 neurons with eccentric RFs. A more critical parameter is stimulus length, at ·least for end-stopped cells, (see Fig. 2A, Orban et al., 1981 a). Finally, we used high contrast ($\log \Delta I/I = 1$) stimuli, but the VR curves are largely unaffected by contrast changes unless the contrast is sharply reduced (below $\log \Delta I/I = -0.4$ see Duysens et al., 1982 c). The first second of rest after the to or fro movement is included in the post-stimulus time histogram (PSTH) in order to evaluate the spontaneous activity. A set of interleaved PSTHs each corresponding to a to or fro movement at a given velocity (typically 20 velocities ranging between 0.18 or 0.35 and 700 or 900°/sec), constitute a velocity test (Fig. 8/1). The *significance of responses* was tested by comparison with the mean plus twice the standard deviation of the spontaneous maximum firing rate. VR curves were compiled by spline interpolation through the smoothed data points (Orban et al., 1981 a). Two sets of measurements were made on the VR curves for the preferred direction of motion. Comparison of the VR curve with the level of significant response (average maximum spontaneous firing rate plus twice its standard deviation) yields (Fig. 6/2): lower cut-off velocity (v_1), the lower velocity value at which the VR curve intersects the significance level; upper cut-off velocity (v_2) the higher velocity value at which the VR curve intersects the significance level. Comparison of the VR curve with the average maximum spontaneous firing rate defines (Fig. 8/2): *optimal velocity* (v_4), the velocity corresponding to the maximum of the VR curve; *response strength* (a), half the maximum response (i.e., the difference between the maximum of the VR curve and the average maximum spontaneous firing rate); *half-height upper cut-off velocity* (v_5), the higher velocity value at which the response is half the maximum response; *full width of velocity tuning* (v_5/v_3), the ratio of the two velocities corresponding to the intersection of the VR curve with the half-maximum response level; *response to slow movement* (100b/2a), the response (b) to the slowest movement tested (0.35°/sec or 0.18°/sec) expressed as a percentage of the maximum response. The full width of velocity tuning can be undetermined if the VR curve does not drop below the half-maxium response level at low or fast velocities.

In order to evaluate the velocity sensitivity of a group of cells, their *velocity-sensitivity profile* was compiled. For each cell, the part of the VR curve above the significance level was divided into three equal intervals (Fig. 8/2). For a given velocity a cell was given a score of 0, 1, 2 or 3 depending on whether for that velocity the VR curve was below the significance level or was contained in the lowest, middle, or highest interval above that level. The scores of the different cells of the group for a given velocity were summated. These sums for the different velocities were then ex-

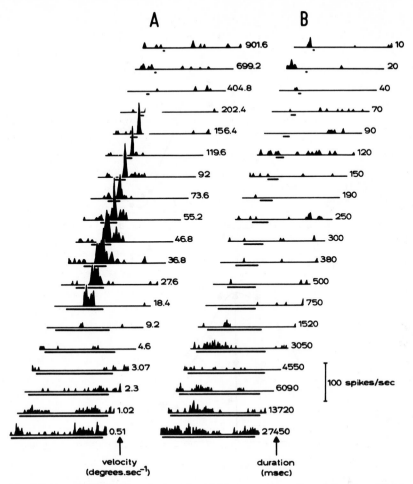

Fig. 8/1. Set of PSTHs of a velocity test. A) Movement in preferred direction. B) Movement in non-preferred direction. The cell was an area 18 cell (eccentricity 12.5°) classified as velocity tuned (optimum 60°/sec, tuning width 6.5) and direction selective (MDI = 81). The cell was recorded in the penetration shown in Fig. 2/15A (cell 19). Velocities and movement duration (the same in A and B) are indicated next to each pair of PSTHs. Horizontal dark bar indicates movement duration.

pressed as a percentage of the highest sum, yielding the velocity-sensitivity profile (Fig. 8/3).

The *range of velocities at which the different areas* operate is given by their velocity-sensitivity profiles (Fig. 8/3). For cortical parts subserving central vision both areas 17 and 19 respond best to slowly moving stimuli while area 18 responds best to medium fast velocities (5–30°/sec). With increasing eccentricity the responses to fast stimuli improve in all three the areas, but more so in area 18. Also the response to slow movement decreases at least in areas 17 and 18. The range of velocities to which a single cell is responding

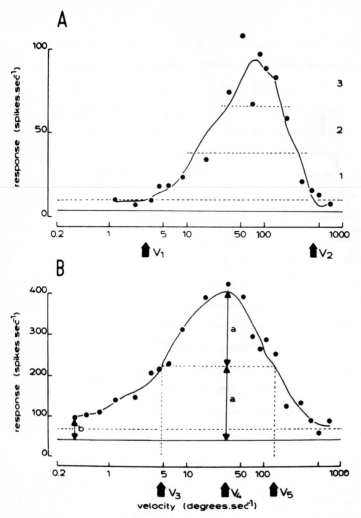

Fig. 8/2. VR curves of two cortical cells: an area 17 cell (A) (eccentricity of RF 5.1°) and an area 18 cell (B) (eccentricity of RF 2°). All characteristics are calculated on the interpolated curve. Horizontal lines indicate average maximum, spontaneous firing rate (full line) and significance level (long dashed line). A) definition of lower cut-off velocity (v_1, 3.1°/s) and upper cut-off velocity (v_2, 320°/sec). The short dashed lines divide the significant part of the VR curves into three equal intervals: parts of the VR curve in these intervals are given different scores (1, 2, 3) for the construction of velocity-sensitive profiles (see text). B) Definition of optimal velocity (v_4, 32°/sec), response strength (a, 182 spikes/sec), half-height upper cut-off velocity (v_5, 128°/sec), full width of velocity tuning (v_5/v_3, 27), and response to slow movement (100b/2a, 27%). Adapted with permission from Orban et al. (1981 a).

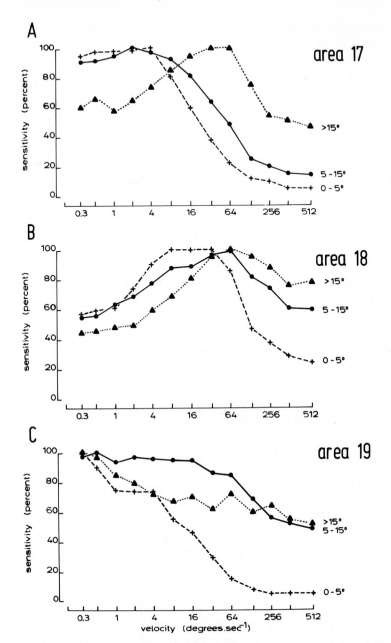

Fig. 8/3. Velocity profiles for 3 eccentricity classes in the 3 cortical areas. Eccentricity classes: 0–5°; 5–15° and > 15° (15 to 45° in area 17 and 15 to 35° in areas 18 and 19). Number of cells in each eccentricity class: 0–5°: n = 56 (17), n = 30 (18), n = 25 (19), 5–15°: n = 33 (17), n = 41 (18), n = 42 (19), > 15°: n = 17 (17), n = 26 (18), n = 20 (19).

is given by its upper and lower cut-off velocities. However very few cells had a lower cut-off velocity (1 out of 106 in area 17, 10 out of 97 in area 18 and 4 out of 87 in area 19). Most area 18 cells subserving central vision had upper cut-off velocities over 100°/sec while most cells of areas 17 and 19 subserving central vision had upper cut-off velocities below 100°/sec. However, a large proportion of area 18 cells (60 out of 97), about 20% of area 17 cells (23 out of 106) and about 30% of area 19 cells (31 out of 87) had no upper cut-off velocity in the range of velocities tested. Therefore, the range of velocities to which a cortical cell responds is best described by the half-height upper cut-off velocity and response to slow movement. Area 17 and 19 neurons give larger responses to slow movement (Fig. 8/4) and area 18 have higher half-height upper cut-off veloicities and stronger responses (large response strength). These differences are most striking in the regions representing central vision (0–5°). This explains why these characteristics can be used as criteria to distinguish area 17 from area 18 cells in penetrations through the 17-18 border (Orban et al., 1980). *In all three areas half-height upper cut-off velocity and response strength increase with eccentricity while response to slow movement decreases.*

Almost all cells (278 out of 290) could be fitted into one of four *velocity types*. Representative examples of each of these types are shown in Fig. 8/5. *Velocity tuned* cells have an optimal velocity and their response decreases on either side of the optimum. Velocity tuned cells have a full width of velocity tuning of 50 or less and half-height upper cut-off velocities below 200°/sec. *Velocity broad-band* cells have no optimum velocity, but respond over a wide range of velocities (width of velocity tuning > 80). *Velocity low-pass* cells repond very well to low velocities and have a half-height upper cut-off velocity below 20°/sec. *Velocity high-pass* cells have a velocity threshold around 2–14°/sec. Their response increases with velocity up to a saturation velocity. This increase can be fitted by a power function, as described previously (Orban and Callens, 1977 b; Grüsser and Grüsser-Cornehls, 1973). Their response remains at a very high level at velocities exceeding the saturation velocity, and at 700°/sec their median response level is 80% of the maximum response (range 40–100%).

By definition, velocity tuned and velocity high-pass cells give little or no response to low velocities (Table 8/1). Both velocity broad-band and velocity low-pass cells gave strong responses to slow movement (Table 8/1). Velocity low-pass cells were the least responsive and velocity high-pass cells the most responsive (Table 8/1). Velocity tuned cells occurred mainly in layer V (65%) in area 18 and throughout all layers in area 17. Velocity high-pass cells were found almost exclusively in the superficial layers (II and III) in area 17 and in layers II-IV in area 18. Velocity broad-band cells were found predominantly in layer VI in area 18 and in layers III and V in area 17. Velocity low-pass cells were found throughout the cortex in area 17 but reached 70%

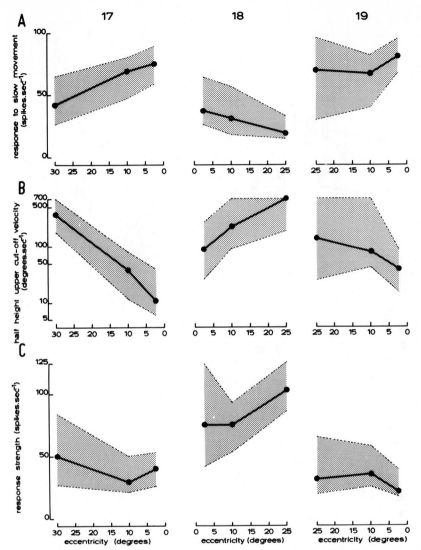

Fig. 8/4. Characteristics of VR curves in the 3 cortical areas. Responses to slow movement (A), half-height upper cut-off velocity (B), and response strength (C) plotted as a function of eccentricity in all 3 areas (17, 18 and 19). Median (solid line) and first and third quartiles (dotted lines) are plotted. Number of cells, see Fig. 8/3.

in layer IV. In area 19 velocity broad-band cells made up more than half the cells in each layer.

The *relative proportions of the 4 velocity types* in the 3 cortical areas are given in Fig. 8/6. Velocity tuned cells dominate in area 18 subserving central vision and decrease in proportion with eccentricity. In areas 17 and 19 small proportions (about 10%) of velocity tuned cells are found at all eccentricities.

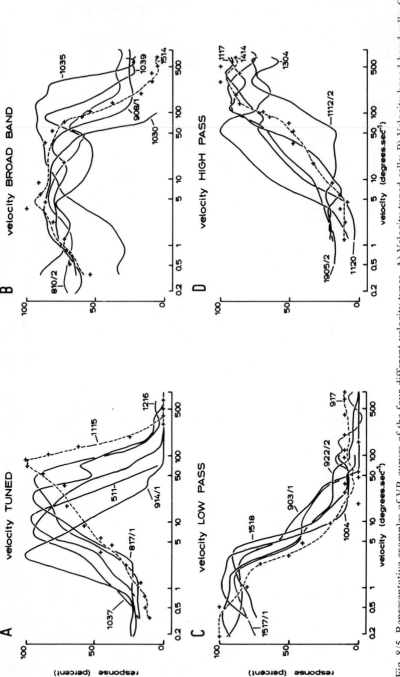

Fig. 8/5. Representative examples of VR curves of the four different velocity types. A) Velocity tuned cells; B) Velocity broad-band cells; C) Velocity low-pass cells; D) Velocity high-pass cells. Response is plotted in percent of maximum response. Data points of only one VR curve (dotted lines) are shown. The significance levels ranged from 2 to 10% for velocity tuned cells, 5 to 20% for velocity broad-band cells, 10 to 35% for velocity low-pass cells, and 2 to 15% for velocity high-pass cells. Adapted with permission from Orban et al. (1981 a).

Table 8/1. Properties of velocity types (medians)

	n	Response to slow (percent)	Response strength (spikes/s)	n[+]	RF width (degrees)
Velocity low-pass[0]	62	90	29	54	0.9
Velocity broad-band[0]	120	68	37	108	2
Velocity tuned[0]	46	25	65	44	1.5
Velocity high-pass[0]	50	20	103	40	5.1
Velocity broad-band[0]					
area 17	35	67	30	30	2.1
area 18	31	55	71	27	1.55
area 19	54	75	28	51	2.5
Velocity low-pass*					
area 17	46	84	31	38	0.8
area 19	14	99	18	14	2.6

* Two VLP cells were recorded in area 18
[+] Bimodal cells were excluded
[0] All 3 cortical areas pooled

Velocity high-pass cells are virtually absent in area 18 subserving central vision and increase in proportion with eccentricity. A few velocity high-pass cells are found in areas 17 and 19, mainly in cortex subserving peripheral vision, where they reach 20%. Velocity low-pass cells dominate (63%) in area 17 subserving central vision and occur in a fair number (30%) in area 19 subserving central vision. In both areas their proportion decreases with eccentricity. Velocity low-pass cells are virtually absent in area 18. Velocity broad-band cells occur in small proportions in area 17 subserving central vision and increase in proportion with eccentricity reaching over 60% in area 17 subserving peripheral vision. In areas 18 and 19 their proportion changes little with eccentricity and they represent about 35% and 60% of the cells in areas 18 and 19 respectively. While areas 17, 18 and 19 tend to be more similar in parts subserving peripheral vision (except for higher proportion of high-pass cells in area 18), their regions subserving central vision are strongly different regarding the proportion of velocity tuned, velocity low-pass, and velocity broad-band cells (see Table 8/2).

Velocity low-pass cells only respond to low velocities. This is probably the price [1] for having a response which is almost *completely invariant with velocity* (Fig. 8/7). Response strength, latency, and shape hardly change with velocity in a velocity low-pass cell and the duration of the response decreases exactly as does stimulus duration. For these cells spatial and temporal parameters can be used interchangeably and the firing of the cell securely represents the convolution of the stimulus with the spatial sensitivity profile of the

---

[1] Velocity low-pass cells acquire the benefit of response invariance at the "expense" of the range of velocities over which they operate.

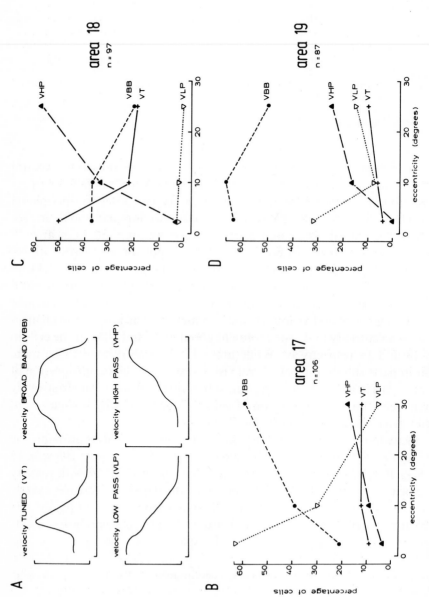

Fig. 8/6. Proportion of the four different velocity types plotted as a function of eccentricity in areas 17 (B), 18 (C) and 19 (D). The velocity-response curves are schematically indicated in (A). Number of cells, see Fig. 8/3.

Table 8/2. Proportion (in percent) of velocity types in parts subserving central vision (0–5°
eccentricity)*

Velocity types	Areas		
	17 (n = 56)	18 (n = 30)	19 (n = 25)
Velocity low-pass	63	3	32
Velocity tuned	9	50	4
Velocity broad-band	21	37	64
Velocity high-pass	4	3	0

Lines below the proportions indicate significance level (χ^2 test) of the difference with the next
area: lines below the area 17 proportion indicate the significance level of the difference between
17 and 18; the lines below the area 19 proportion, the significance level of the 19–17 difference
⁻ Difference significant at 0.01 level
= Difference significant at 0.001 level
* A few cells had unclassified VR curves: hence the sum of percentages in a given area is not
necessarily 100%

cell. This probably explains why for most area 17 cells the spatial frequency
tuning hardly changes whether one uses constant velocity or constant
temporal frequency (see Chapter 7). On the contrary cells responding to
velocities over 50–60°/sec (most area 18 cells but also area 17 and 19 cells
subserving peripheral vision) change their response shape with velocity and
the duration of the response outlasts the stimulus duration at fast velocities.
Also, when stimulated with a grating the response peaks fuse over 200°/sec
(Orban and Callens, 1977 b). Therefore for these cells the firing of the cell no
longer represents the convolution of the stimulus and the spatial sensitivity
profile of the cells.

Velocity tuned cells *have optima ranging from 2 to 91°/sec.* The optimal
velocity of velocity tuned cells increases with visual eccentricity (Fig. 8/8A).
The median optimal velocity of velocity tuned cells in eccentricity class 0–5°
is 9°/sec compared to 41°/sec in eccentricity class 15–35°. Full width of
velocity tuning of velocity tuned cells significantly decreases with increasing
optimal velocity (Fig. 8/8 B). It is worth mentioning the parallel between
characteristics of spatial frequency tuning in area 17 and 18 cells (see Fig.
7/12) and of velocity tuning of those cells. As the optimal spatial frequency
decreases with eccentricity, optimal velocity increases. For both parameters
the range of optima decreases with eccentricity. As the bandwidth of tuning
decreases with optimal spatial frequency, the width of velocity tuning decreases with optimal velocity. The response strength of velocity tuned cells
increases with increasing optimal velocity. The correlation is stronger at
larger eccentricities.

While the characteristics of velocity-tuned cells changes with the eccentricity of their RF position, the characteristics of velocity high-pass cells
show no change with eccentricity nor with area. The threshold and satura-

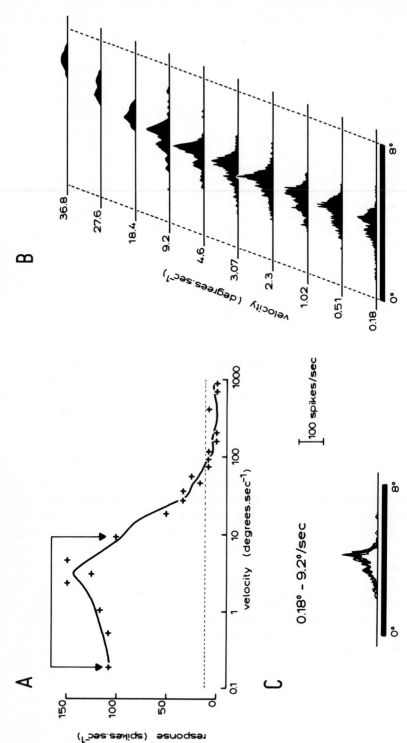

Fig. 8/7. Invariance of velocity low-pass (VLP) cells with velocity. A) Velocity-response (VR) curve of an area 17 C cell: horizontal stippled line significance level. B) PSTHs corresponding to the VR curve of A plotted as a function of position: horizontal bar indicates amplitude of movement (8°); within the plateau of the VR curve (velocities 0.1 to 9.2°/sec, arrows in A) the shape of the response is invariant with velocity. This is demonstrated by superposition of those responses in (C). The responses have been slightly shifted to account for the latency (85 msec).

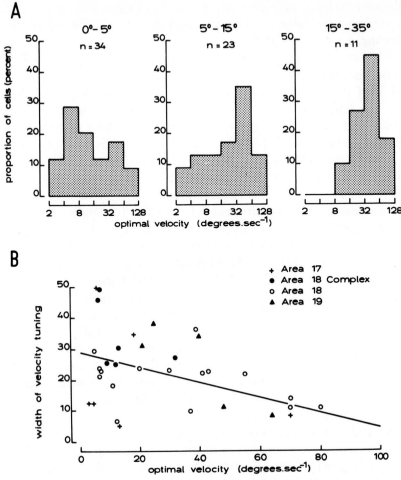

Fig. 8/8. Properties of velocity tuned (VT) cells: A) distribution of optimal velocities in 3 eccentricity classes: 0–5°; 5–15° and 5–35°. B) Full width of velocity tuning plotted as a function of optimal velocity. Crosses: area 17 cells; triangles: area 19 cells; dots: area 18 complex cells, circles: other area 18 cells. The differences in distribution of optimal velocities between the 0–5° class and each of the more eccentric classes were significant.

tion velocities of velocity high-pass cells were estimated by fitting a power function to the ascending part of the VR curve and flat lines to the plateaus below threshold and above saturation velocities. These threshold and saturation velocities do not change with eccentricity. Threshold velocities range from less than 0.36 to 45°/sec (median 4°/sec, first and third quartiles 1.5–17°/sec, n = 55). Saturation velocities range from 14 to 700°/sec (median 130°/sec, first and third quartiles 70 and 200°/sec, n = 55). The response of a single velocity high-pass cell increases on average only over a 25-fold change of velocity. The spread of threshold and saturation velocities among the population of velocity high-pass cells means that their activity as a group increases over a wider range of velocities than that of a single cell (single channel coding, see Chapter 5).

In area 17 velocity low-pass and velocity tuned cells are associated with S and B families while velocity broad-band and velocity high-pass cells are associated with A and C families. This association is highly significant ($\chi^2 = 26.7$, p < 0.00001) and is stronger when area 17 representing the central visual field is considered separately (Orban et al., 1981 a). In area 18 the correlation between velocity types and RF families is much weaker. Velocity broad-band cells in area 18 are associated with the S family ($\chi^2 = 5.8$, p < 0.025) while velocity high-pass cells are associated with A and C families ($\chi^2 = 9.8$, p < 0.005). Thus, in areas 17 and 18 velocity broad-band cells are associated with different RF families. In parallel with this difference, 68% of area 17 velocity broad-band cells were binocular, as compared to 32% in area 18. In area 19 the correlations between RF type and velocity type are weaker, although S and B families tended to be associated with velocity low-pass cells and velocity tuned cells and A and C families with velocity high-pass and velocity broad-band cells. While in area 17 almost all velocity tuned cells belong to the S family, velocity tuned cells in area 18 belong to any family. C family tuned cells have significantly (Mann-Whitney U test z = 3, p < 0.003) wider full width of velocity tuning than other velocity tuned cells in area 18 and their optimal velocities are all below 32°/sec. In area 17 subserving central vision, end-stopped cells are associated with velocity low-pass curves, while in the comparable part of area 18 most of the end-stopped cells are velocity tuned. In area 19 there is a weak association between end-stopped cells and velocity tuned cells.

Considering the overall population of areas 17, 18, and 19 we found a significant correlation ($\varrho = 0.6$, p < 0.005) between *RF width and half-height upper cut-off velocity*. Cells with higher half-height upper cut-off velocities have wider RFs. The correlation is partially due to the differences in RF width between the velocity types (Table 8/1). Velocity low-pass cells have the narrowest RFs and velocity high-pass cells the widest RFs. However a few velocity low-pass cells had wider RFs than some of the velocity high-pass cells. Within the different velocity types, there was a correlation between RF width and half-height upper cut-off for velocity tuned cells ($\varrho = 0.51$, p < 0.0005).

The correlation between half-height upper cut-off velocity and RF width could be related to a common factor: RF position in the visual field, since both upper cut-off and RF width increase with eccentricity. This is however only partially true: even within a given eccentricity class of areas 17 and 18 there is a correlation between RF width and velocity sensitivity (Fig. 8/9). Cells with wider RFs respond less to low velocities and better to fast velocities.

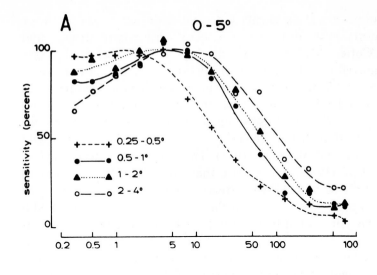

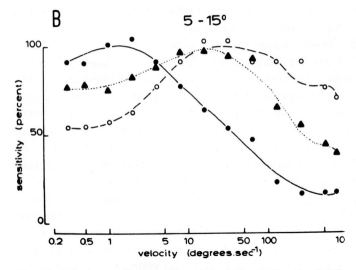

Fig. 8/9. Velocity-sensitivity profiles of area 17 and 18 cells of different RF widths. A) For eccentricity class 0−5°. B) For eccentricity class 5−15°. The RF widths are indicated in A. The four groups in A all had the same median eccentricity: 0.25−0.5° (11 cells), 2.8° eccentricity; 0.5−1° (28 cells), 2.7° eccentricity; 1−2° (24 cells), 2.8° eccentricity; and 2−4° (8 cells), 2° eccentricity. The three groups in B had approximatively the same median eccentricity: 0.5−1° (12 cells), 8.7° eccentricity; 1−2° (28 cells), 9.7° eccentricity; and 2−4° (15 cells), 10.7° eccentricity. Adapted with permission from Orban et al. (1981 a).

Our observations are in excellent agreement with earlier qualitative or more limited reports on the difference in velocity sensitivity of areas 17 and 18 (Dreher and Cottee, 1975; Stone and Dreher, 1973; Dreher et al., 1980; Riva Sanseverino et al., 1979; Tretter et al., 1975); on the difference between simple and complex cells in area 17 subserving central vision (Goodwin and Henry, 1978; Hess and Wolters, 1979; Leventhal and Hirsch, 1978; Movshon, 1975; Pettigrew et al., 1968 a; Wilson and Sherman, 1976), and on the increase in upper cut-off velocity with eccentricity in area 17 (Leventhal and Hirsch, 1980; Wilson and Sherman, 1976). There is disagreement with the data of Dreher et al. (1980) in the sense that in our data the changes in upper cut-off velocity with eccentricity are as striking in all three areas. Our results are also in good agreement with those of Berardi et al. (1982) who reported a negative correlation between upper cut-off velocity and optimal spatial frequency.

Temporal frequency (cycles/sec) is sometimes considered to be an alternative parameter to angular velocity (see Lennie, 1980) in providing information about rate of movement. Our results, in which most of the influence of temporal frequency was removed, demonstrate the strong influence of velocity on cortical cells. When stimulated with moving gratings, cortical cells display temporal frequency tuning (see Fig. 7/11).[2] It still has to be shown that temporal frequency is coded in the system by a set of filters in order to allow the system to use this parameter to evaluate to the rate of movement. Such a temporal frequency coding seems unlikely. An object (with an array of spatial frequencies) moving at a given velocity would produce an array of different temporal frequencies[3], so that coding of temporal frequency is not of any great interest to the organism. Moreover, as we have seen, cortical cells respond to both periodic and aperiodic stimuli. While both stimuli when moving can be characterized by a single velocity their temporal frequency composition will be very different. Finally, the changes in velocity sensitivity as a function of RF width or optimal spatial frequency easily explain psychophysical observations (Thompson, 1982; Breitmeyer, 1973), apparently suggesting a temporal frequency coding by the visual system.

---

[2] When using drifting gratings it may be more appropriate to consider temporal frequency as a parameter than angular velocity. Indeed velocity refers to an object moving over a given distance in some time. In a drifting grating there is not really a separate object moving from one point to another: each element in the grating is replaced by an identical one. Therefore, it may not be very surprising that Thompson (1982) observed that the rate of movement of drifting spatially periodic stimuli appears to be analyzed in terms of its temporal frequency (cycles/sec) rather than its velocity (deg/sec). In neuronal terms the same may be true, but one has to keep the limited RF size in mind. When the grating is relatively fine compared to RF size (i.e. when the spatial frequency is in the operating range of the neuron, see Chapter 7), then there is no distinct visual element moving through the RF and temporal frequency describes best the rate of stimulation by a drifting grating. However if the grating is rectangular and has wide bars compared to the RF size (i.e. outside the working range of the neuron) the individual edges move through the RF and one should rather consider the velocity of the edges.

[3] Temporal frequency (cycles/sec): spatial frequency (cycles/deg) × angular velocity (deg/sec).

In answer to the question of the range of velocities over which the cells operate, one can say that areas 17 and 19, especially the parts subserving central vision, are very responsive to low velocities, in the order of magnitude of slow drifts during fixation. Therefore these areas will probably be maximally active in the behaving animal *during fixation of stationary objects*[4] (or during pursuit). This of course fits in with the superiority of area 17 subserving central vision for the analysis of fine spatial detail. Area 18 subserving central vision does not respond well to the low velocities of the order of magnitude of slow drifts of the eyes and will in the behaving animal *only be activated by moving objects*. Since area 18 cells are able to some extent to analyze spatial parameters (spatial parameters as orientation, width or spatial frequency influence their activity, see Chapter 7), spatial analysis of visual objects can be performed either by area 17 or 18 depending on the velocity of the objects. The response to the question of velocity coding shows complementary evidence: the cells able to code for velocity, principally the velocity tuned cells as a set of bandpass filters and to a lesser extent velocity high-pass cells as a set of high-pass filters, occur chiefly in area 18, which thus seems to play a major role in the analysis of moving objects.

Our results are also in agreement with the observations of Noda et al. (1971) in the *awake* cat, although some of the neurons they reported to be in area 17 most likely belonged to area 18. Their cells, responding in the unanesthetized, unparalyzed cat to stationary stimuli (group 2), probably correspond to our velocity low-pass cells. Their motion-sensitive cells, responding little to stationary patterns, probably correspond to velocity tuned, velocity high-pass and some velocity broad-band cells (thus mostly area 18 cells): those responding best to velocities below 200°/sec (group 1) were probably velocity tuned or velocity broad-band cells and their fast-motion sensitive cells (group 3) correspond to velocity high-pass cells. We do not believe that the latter can signal saccadic eye movements since they also respond to lower velocities down to 10−20°/sec. Their group 4 cells were probably hypercomplex cells which must be very difficult to activate with a grating in an animal with freely moving eyes.

8.2 Influence of the Direction of Movement [5]

Direction of visual movement is a parameter ranging over 360°. When one investigates the influence of direction of movement over 360°, one studies

---

[4] One of the referees argued that human subjects can still process spatial structure without drift since we see the shape of objects under a low rate of stroboscopic illumination. We have recently shown (Cremieux et al., 1983) that most cortical velocity low-pass cells have long integration time constants whereby they are able to fuse even very low rate (2 Hz) stroboscopic flashes. For such cells, objects will still slowly drift over the retina during fixation.

[5] In this chapter we only consider direction in a frontal plane and direction in the Z axis will be considered in the next chapter.

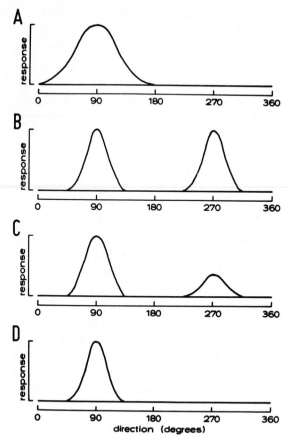

Fig. 8/10. Schematic example of directional tunings. Directional tunings (A) of a cell bandpass for direction, (B) of an orientation-selective cell without direction selectivity (stimulated with an elongated stimulus) (C) of an orientation-selective cell with a moderate direction selectivity (stimulated with an elongated stimulus), (D) of an orientation-selective cell with complete direction selectivity (stimulated with an elongated stimulus).

the directional tuning of the cell. In order to be a bandpass filter for direction of movement a cell has to respond over a limited range of directions (Fig. 8/10). Given their orientation selectivity, cortical cells when stimulated with elongated moving stimuli will show an axial selectivity whereby the optimal axis of motion is orthogonal to their optimal orientation.[6] In order to be a *bandpass filter for direction*, these cells then just need to suppress their response in one direction on the optimal axis. This additional property is referred to as direction selectivity. It is generally accepted (Hammond, 1978) that this direction selectivity is produced by a mechanism different from that producing orientation (and thus axial) selectivity and that the mechanism producing direction selectivity can be studied in "isolation" by using noise fields or spots provided the cell responds to these stimuli.

As for the influence of velocity, the investigation of *direction selectivity* (i.e. difference in response to opposite directions on the optimal axis) requires

---

[6] This supposes that the elongated stimuli move on paths orthogonal to their length. At least in the experimental studies this condition is verified.

1/4 to 1/3 of the cases (Orban et al., 1981 b). We have studied quantitatively the direction selectivity of areas 17, 18, and 19 neurons over a wide range of eccentricities and velocities (Duysens et al., 1982 a; Orban et al., 1981 b). Like other workers (Albus, 1980; Kato et al., 1978) we use the normalized difference between the responses to the two opposite directions on the optimal axis at a given velocity as a measure of direction selectivity:

$$DI = \frac{R_p - R_{NP}}{R_p} \times 100$$

Since we want to compare direction selectivity at different velocities and we have used maximum firing rate as a criterion in the VR curves, the responses R_p and R_{NP} are net maximum firing rates (i.e. maximum firing rate minus the mean spontaneous maximum firing rate). Most other studies (Albus, 1980; Gilbert, 1977; Kato et al., 1978; Leventhal and Hirsch, 1978) use the number of spikes as a response measure which will, for the same data, yield higher estimates of direction selectivity.

In more than half of the cortical cells, and especially in areas 18 and 19 cells, the *direction selectivity changes with velocity* (Table 8/3). The different types of direction selectivity velocity relationships are illustrated in Fig. 8/11. The most frequent change (2/3) being an increase in direction selectivity with increasing velocity, eventually followed by a decrease at very fast velocities (Table 8/3). Consequently in almost all cells the direction selectivity is maximum at the velocity yielding the largest response. This increase is not simply a reflection of the increase in response in the preferred direction (PD); in about 1/3 of the cortical cells the response in the non-preferred direction (NPD) decreases with velocity, changing symmetrically with the response in PD (Fig. 8/12). It is worth mentioning that velocity low-pass cells usually (70%) have a flat direction index (DI)-velocity relationship (Table 8/3), another example of the invariance of velocity low-pass cells with velocity.

Table 8/3. Association of velocity types with DI-velocity relationships*

Velocity types	No. of cells	DI-velocity relationship, %					
		Flat	In-crease	De-crease	Opti-mum	Re-versal	Ir-regular
Velocity low-pass	50	70	12	0	0	2	16
Velocity broad-band	98	31	32	1	9	12	15
Velocity tuned	36	30.5	30.5	3	33	3	0
Velocity high-pass	39	31.5	26.5	8	18	15	2
Total	274	39	26	2	13	9	11

* The different relationships are illustrated in Fig. 8/11

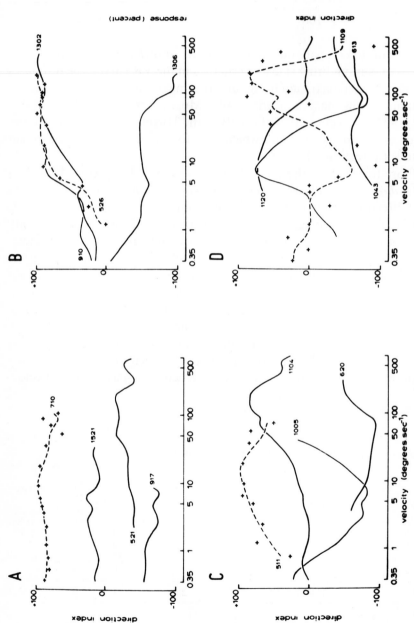

Fig. 8/11. Velocity-DI curves. A) Flat curves; B) increasing curves; C) curves with optimum; D) decreasing (cells 1120 and 1043) and reversing (cells 1109 and 613) curves. For one cell of each type data points are shown together with the interpolated curve (dashed line). Note that only changes in DI magnitude indicate changes in direction selectivity. Adapted with permission from Orban et al. (1981 b).

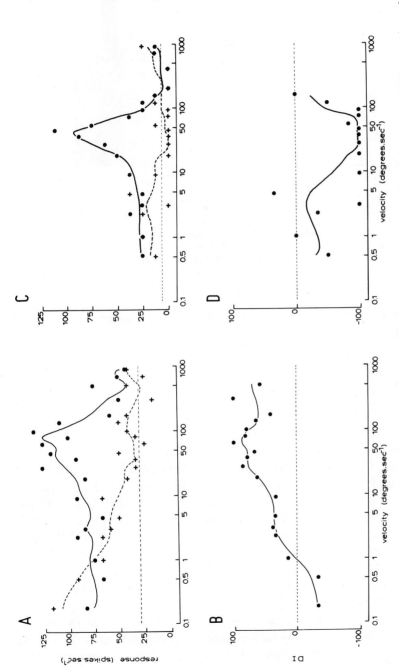

Fig. 8/12. Symmetry between response increase in the PD and response decrease in NPD. A and C: velocity-response (VR) curves in preferred direction (PD) (solid line) and non-preferred direction (NPD) (dashed line) of an area 17 velocity broad-band (VBB) cell (eccentricity 9.5°) (A) and an area 17 velocity tuned (VT) cell (eccentricity 1°) (C). Horizontal lines significance levels. B and D: DI-velocity relationships of the corresponding cells. The MDI of the cell in A and B was 52, and its DI increased with velocity. The MDI of the cell in C and D was −71, and its DI had an optimum (which corresponded to the optimum for the response in PD).

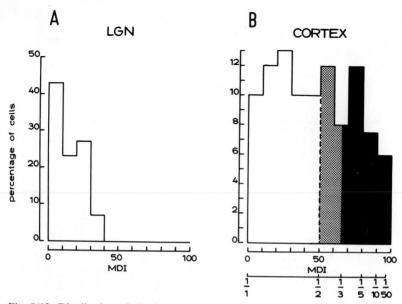

Fig. 8/13. Distribution of absolute mean DI (MDI) among LGN cells (n = 44) and among cortical cells (areas 17, 18 and 19 pooled) (n = 283). Ratios between preferred direction (PD) and non-preferred direction (NPD) are indicated below the corresponding MDIs. Open area: not direction selective (NDS) cells, hatching: direction asymmetric (DA) cells, dark area: direction selective cells.

Given the changes of DI with velocity we use a *weighted mean* as a measure of direction selectivity of the cell:

$$MDI = \frac{\sum\limits_{i=1}^{n} R_{Pi} DI_i}{\sum\limits_{i=1}^{n} R_{Pi}}$$

where R_{Pi} is the net response in PD at a given velocity, DI_i the DI at that velocity, and n = 20, the number of velocities ranging from 0.18 or 0.35 to 700–900°/sec. Cells having a *mean direction index* (MDI) less than 50 are considered as *not direction selective* (NDS), those having a MDI equal or larger than 66 are considered *direction selective* (DS), and those in between as *direction asymmetric* (DA) (Fig. 8/13). DS cells have a maximum firing rate three times larger in the PD than in the NPD averaged over all velocities. Comparing cortical cells to LGN cells shows that none of the LGN cells has a MDI larger than 40 and hence none qualifies as a DA or a DS cell. More cells are DS in area 18 than in area 17, which in turn has more DS cells than area 19 (Fig. 8/14).

Considering the different eccentricity classes separately, area 18 subserving central vision (0–5°) has by far the largest proportion of DS cells and the *proportion decreases steeply with eccentricity* (Fig. 8/15), as witnessed by the

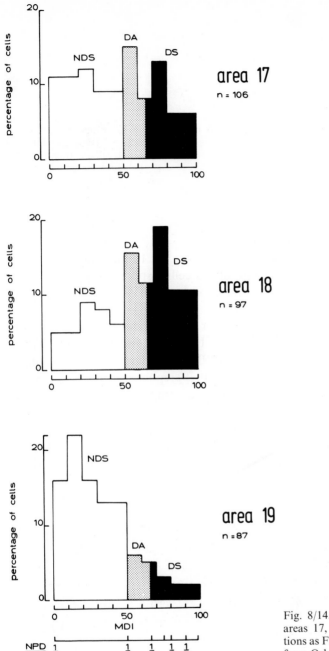

Fig. 8/14. Distribution of MDIs in areas 17, 18 and 19. Same conventions as Figure 8/13. With permission from Orban et al. (1982 b).

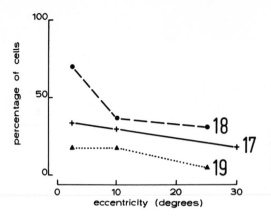

Fig. 8/15. Proportion of direction-selective (DS) cells plotted as a function of eccentricity in areas 17, 18 and 19. Number of cells, see Fig. 8/3.

negative correlation between MDI and eccentricity. In the other areas there is a slight decrease in the proportion of DS cells, especially in area 17, (see also Albus, 1980) but there is no correlation between MDI and eccentricity (Table 8/4).

Our estimation of 34% DS cells in area 17 subserving central vision is in agreement with that obtained by others. Leventhal and Hirsch (1978) observed 35% of area 17 cells with PD/NPD ratios larger than 3. Using a similar ratio to define DS cells Kato et al. (1978) reported about 28% DS cells among the simple family and 12% among the complex family. Albus (1980) reported about 40% of area 17 cells (0–10° eccentricity) to be direction selective when tested with a slit, the proportion dropping to 25% when testing both with a slit and dark bar. It is possible that some of our DS cells, presumably those with MDI just over 66, would have failed to pass Albus'

Table 8/4. Differences in direction selectivity between areas 17, 18 and 19

	17	18	19
Percent cells with DI dependent on velocity	39 (104)	74 (96)	71 (86)
Percent DS cells	30 (106)	45 (97)	14 (87)
Percent DA cells	24 (106)	21 (97)	7 (87)
Percent DS cells (0–5° eccentricity)	34 (56)	70 (30)	17 (25)
Correlation MDI-eccentricity	= 0.01	= −0.41	= 0.04

Numbers between brackets are numbers of neurons
Lines below the percentages: same conventions as in Table 8/2

more stringent criterion of contrast independence. Some of the older studies on area 17 mention higher proportions of DS cells: Pettigrew et al. (1968 a) 35% among simple and 44% among complex cells, Bishop et al. (1971 a) 76% among simple cells and Goodwin and Henry (1975) 49% among complex cells. Adequate precautions were not taken to ensure that cells were actually recorded from area 17, so the higher proportions of DS cells may be due to inclusion of area 18 cells.

Tretter et al. (1975) failed to find a difference between areas 17 and 18 with respect to direction selectivity, but these authors only used hand-held stimuli and few of their cells were within 5° of fixation point. Our results agree with those of Ferster (1981) who compared areas 17 and 18 over a range of 15° eccentricity: he observed 43% DS cells in area 17 compared to 62% in area 18.

In all areas but mostly in areas 17 and 18, DS cells were associated with S family RFs (see Chapter 4). *Direction selectivity is strongly associated with velocity tuning* (Table 8/5). Three fifths of velocity tuned cells were DS while

Table 8/5. Association of direction selectivity and velocity types (all 3 areas pooled)

	n	% NDS	% DA	% DS
Velocity low-pass	62	63	14	23
Velocity tuned	46	22*	17	61*
Velocity broad-band	120	58	18	24
Velocity high-pass	50	58	20	22

* The proportion of NDS cells among VT cells is significantly (p < 0.0005) lower than among any other velocity type. Conversely, the proportion of DS cells among VT cells is significantly (p < 0.0005) higher than among any other velocity type

for the other velocity types 3/5 of the cells were NDS. It is also noteworthy that velocity tuned cells have the least reversing or irregular DI-velocity relationships (Table 8/3). Consequently the velocity sensitivity of DS cells was much more tuned than that of NDS cells (Fig. 8/16).

Considering all DS cells in the different areas, all directions are about equally represented, although directions towards the fovea may be under-represented. Considering the different areas separately, area 18 DS and DA cells prefer direction away from the area centralis (Fig. 8/17) and area 17 DS cells directions on the principal axes (horizontal and vertical). In area 18 but not in areas 17 and 19, the NDS cells preferred the horizontal axis (Fig. 8/17).

If one considers the response of a cortical cell to a moving slit, the *directional tuning* (i.e. the response to all possible directions over a range of 360°) for such a stimulus is the result of the interaction of two selectivities: orientation selectivity specifying the optimal axis and direction selectivity

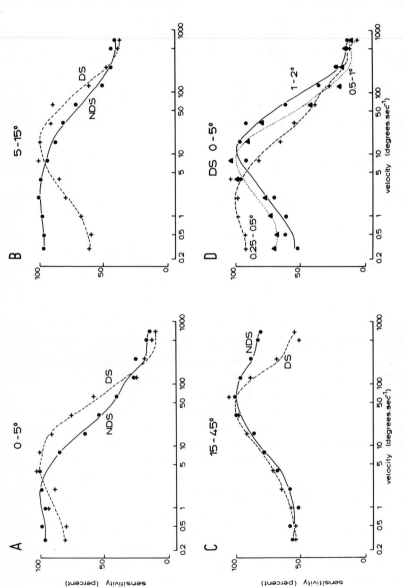

Fig. 8/16. Velocity sensitivity of DS cells. A, B, C: Velocity-sensitivity profile of DS and NDS cells of areas 17 and 18 for three different eccentricity classes. D) Velocity-sensitivity profiles of DS cells with RFs within 5° from the fixation point but different RF widths. All three groups of RF width had similar median eccentricities: 0.25–0.5° (7 cells), 2.8° eccentricity; 0.5–1° (17 cells), 2.95° eccentricity; and 1–2° (8 cells), 2.8° eccentricity. Adapted with permission from Orban et al. (1981 b).

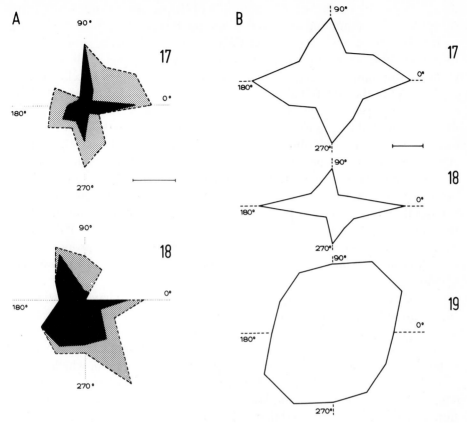

Fig. 8/17. Distribution of preferred direction and axes. A) Preferred directions of direction selective (DS) (dark area) and direction asymmetric (DA) cells (hatching) in areas 17 and 18. The proportion of DS and DA cells is too small in area 19 to estimate their preferences. B) Preferred axes of not direction selective (NDS) cells in areas 17, 18 and 19. 0° corresponds to horizontal movement into the ipsilateral field and 90° to upward movement. The neurons were recorded in the left cortex and all the RFs were in the lower right quadrant of the visual field. Thus directions between 0 and 90° correspond to movements towards the fovea. Horizontal bar represents 5 cells.

specifying the sense on that axis. The additional advantage of orientation selectivity is to decrease the width of directional tuning. Indeed, since complex family cells respond to moving noise fields and slits (Hammond and MacKay, 1977; Orban et al., 1975) one can investigate the directional tuning of those cells with and without the concomitant interaction of orientation selectivity. Hammond (1978) has clearly shown that for area 17 cells directional tuning is wider with a moving noise field than with a moving slit. Hammond also noted that many complex cells had different optimal directions for a moving slit and noise field, although some of the differences can be accounted for by the lack of smoothing of the curves. In about 1/3 of the complex cells, Hammond observed a bilobar directional tuning for noise, with a depression of sensitivity over the range of directions to which the cell responded best when stimulated with a moving bar (Fig. 8/18). Bishop et al. (1980) made similar observations in a weakly hypercomplex II cell and one of the lobes of the directional tuning for noise corresponded to the optimum for a moving spot. Hammond and Reck (1980) showed that the depression in the directional tuning for noise increases with increasing velocity of moving noise field. The latter observation strengthens the hypothesis of Movshon et al. (1980) that this depression is an effect of the velocity upper cut-off, since the moving noise has orientation components moving in different directions around the direction of movement, and the velocities in those directions are smaller than the velocity in the direction of movement of the pattern, being the cosines of that velocity (Movshon et al., 1980). Since about 30% of area 17 C cells have a low-pass function and the others do not, the proportion of complex cells with bilobar tuning fits with the proportion of velocity low-pass C cells.

Goodwin and Henry (1975) and Goodwin et al. (1975) have investigated the minimum traverse of stimulus movement required to maintain direction selectivity in area 17 simple and complex cells. Using a moving edge as stimulus they found a minimum amplitude of about 1 min of arc in unmasked conditions. With a mask the amplitude of movement required, which corresponds to the width of the mask, was larger (6 to 20 min of arc) (Fig. 8/19). This amplitude threshold in masking condition may well be an underestimation. Indeed we have observed that a mask of 0.3° width *completely abolishes the direction selectivity* of area 17 and 18 cortical cells (Orban et al., 1982 a). The difference between both observations is probably due to the method of testing direction selectivity. We evaluate the MDI over a range of velocities (0.5 to 900°/sec) while Goodwin et al. (1975) and Goodwin and Henry (1975) measure only the DI at one, low velocity (1°/sec or less). Indeed Goodwin et al. (1975) showed that the effect of masking on direction selectivity increases with stimulus velocity. According to Goodwin et al. (1975) the decrease in direction selectivity by masking is due to the removal of the steady illumination from the inhibitory region ahead of the discharge region in the NPD, demonstrated by these authors. If this is true, one wonders what would be the minimum amplitude required if one tests direction selectivity in the unmasked situation with a moving slit instead of a moving edge.

Payne et al. (1981) have suggested that there may be a columnar organization for direction preference in the visual cortex. However, these authors used hand-held stimuli and found only a few bidirectional cells in area 17, a finding very surprising in view of our data indicating that 45% of the area 17 cells are NDS. The much larger proportion of DS cells in area 18 suggests that this organization may be clearer in area 18 than in area 17.

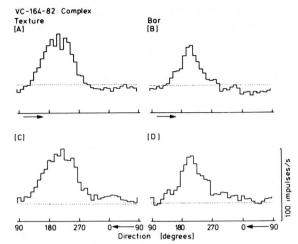

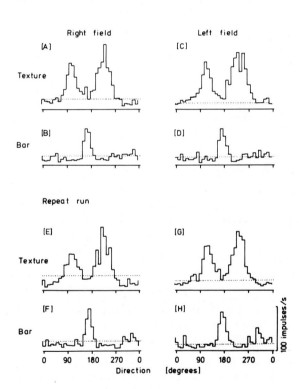

Fig. 8/18. Comparison of directional tunings for bars and texture. Upper part: Two pairs of directional tuning curves for texture and bar motion, respectively, in the same DS complex cell, to show the absence of sequence-dependent hysteresis for 10° increments of direction, stepped clockwise (A, B) and counter-clockwise (C,D). Sum of four responses per direction; resting discharge indicated by broken line. Note the broader, unimodal tuning for texture motion. Lower part: Four pairs of directional tuning for texture and bar motion interleaved, to show the interocular similarities and repeatability of tuning in a second complex cell (ocular dominance group 4). Runs taken in order A and B, C and D, E and F, and G and H; total analysis time: 51 min. Other conventions as above. Note the bimodal tuning for texture, with depressed sensitivity in directions optimal for bar motion. Adapted with permission from Hammond (1981 a).

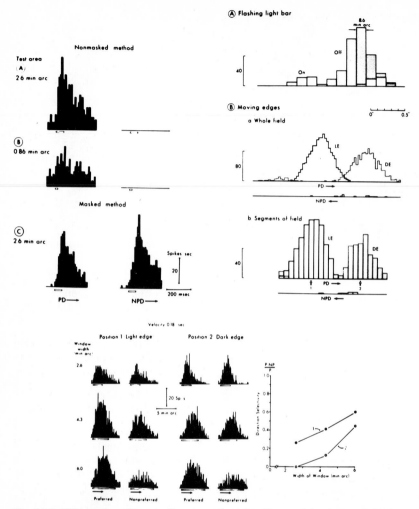

Fig. 8/19. Effects of masking on direction selectivity. Upper right: Aspects of RF organization and direction selectivity of a simple striate neuron (multihistogram method). Ordinate scale in spikes per second. A) Spatial distribution of ON and OFF areas as determined by flashing a stationary bar (4° × 0.14°) at successive locations across the RF. Each histogram column averages 10 responses sampled over the first 160 msec after the onset of each response. Flash rate 0.2 Hz. B) a: light-edge (LE) and dark-edge (DE) discharge centers determined by moving 4° long light and dark edges over the RF at 1.1°/sec. PD: preferred direction of edge motion; NPD: non-preferred direction. Each histogram averages 20 responses. B) b: direction selectivity of 4.3' segments of the LE and DE discharge centers. Each histogram column averages 10 responses. The vertical arrows indicate test segments used for upper left and lower parts. Upper left: Same unit as in upper right, showing responses to a dark edge moved in the preferred (PD) and non-preferred (NPD) directions at location 2 in upper right B, b over test areas of width as indicated. Each histogram averages 50 responses. Horizontal bars indicate onset and duration of edge motion. Lower: Same unit as in upper right using masked method of stimulation. Responses are to a constant edge velocity (0.18 deg/sec) with variable window widths, as indicated. Each histogram averages 50 responses. Direction selectivity plotted against window width: filled circles, light edge; open circles, dark edge. Adapted with permission from Goodwin et al. (1975).

8.3 Influence of Stimulus Movement Amplitude

Direction and velocity uniquely specify the motion of an object in visual space. However another description would be given by amplitude and direction of movement. A few cells in area 18 subserving peripheral vision have been shown to be selective to stimulus movement amplitude (Orban and Callens, 1977 b). By testing amplitude at different velocities Orban and Callens (1977 b) showed that cells were amplitude and not duration sensitive. A few cells had a bandpass amplitude-response function (Fig. 8/20). These cells had small fields and low spontaneous activity and thus had some similarity with the S family. A few other cells had a high-pass amplitude-response function. Those cells had larger RFs, responded to noise fields, and thus had some similarities with C family cells. All these cells were direction selective and some of them were velocity tuned.

8.4 Conclusion

Up to now we have used high contrast optimal slits for the study of spatio-temporal parameters coding by the visual cortex. We have preliminary evidence of the stability of velocity and direction tuning under those circumstances. Further work however is required to investigate the degree of invariance of this tuning. While we have evidence that slit width and orientation have little effect on velocity tuning, studies of velocity-spatial frequency interaction and of velocity-contrast interactions are required. Our present results however, allow us to conclude that there is *considerable specialization* among the 3 cortical areas with respect to the coding of spatio-temporal parameters. Areas 17 and 19, especially the parts subserving central vision, are suited for the analysis of stationary objects during fixation (or pursuit). It is especially interesting that area 17 S family cells, which have been shown to be of utmost importance for fine spatial vision, being all velocity low-pass, will be maximally active during fixation. Area 18 subserving central vision has a clear superiority for the coding of spatio-temporal parameters: direction and velocity of movement. There seems to be less superiority of S family cells over C family cells in this respect. This is in keeping with the observation that movement parameters are equally important for the analysis of visual objects (supposedly the function of S family cells) as for the analysis of the visual background [7], inducing subject versus surround perceptions (supposedly the

---

[7] Visual background is meant here in opposition to visual objects in a kind of figure-ground relationship. The visual background is the collection of visual objects not resolved as such by the visual system: this will occur mainly in the peripheral parts of the visual field (see Chapter 7).

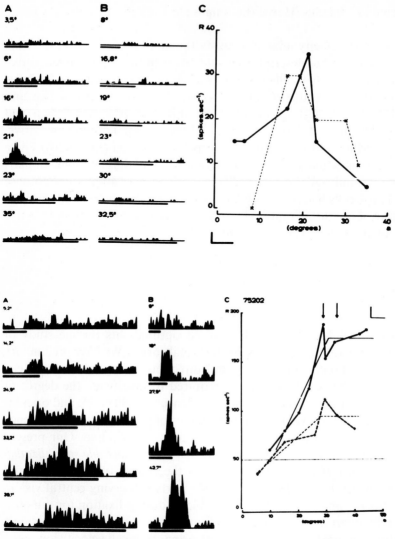

Fig. 8/20. Amplitude-response curves of cortical cells. Upper part: Response amplitude function of an amplitude specific cell. The average responses are to a 3.5 × 96° slit moving in the optimal direction (180°) over increasing amplitudes at two different velocities (10 (A) and 20 (B) degrees · sec^{-1}). Calibration marks indicate 20 spikes · sec^{-1} and 1 sec for left hand PSTHs and 40 spikes · sec^{-1} and 500 msec for middle PSTHs. In C, the maximum firing rate during response (R) is plotted as a function of amplitude (a) (full lines for movements at 10 degrees · sec^{-1} and dashed lines for movements at 20 degrees · sec^{-1}). Lower part: Response amplitude function of an amplitude sensitive complex cell. Average responses are to a two-dimensional noise pattern moving in the optimal direction (292°) over increasing distances at two different velocities (40 (A) and 180 (B) degrees · sec^{-1}). Vertical calibration mark indicates 30 spikes · sec^{-1} and horizontal mark 100 msec. In C, the maximum firing rate during response (R) is plotted in function of amplitude (a) (full lines for movements at 180 degrees · sec^{-1} and dashed lines for movements at 40 degrees · sec^{-1}). Thinner lines indicate possible theoretical functions. Horizontal line: spontaneous activity level. Adapted with permission from Orban and Callens (1977 b).

function of C family cells). It is also worth mentioning that the coding of spatio-temporal parameters, as the coding of spatial parameters, is more accurate in cortical parts subserving central vision.

Sensitivity of cortical cells to movement parameters, could conceivably contribute to more than motion perception. The direction selectivity of area 17 cells, especially of S family cells, can contribute to the outline of visual objects of which all parts will move in the same direction (see Marr and Ullman, 1981). In area 18 the velocity selectivity can also contribute to the outline of visual objects since all parts will not only move in the same direction but at the same speed. This is probably one of the reasons why, contrary to older views (Schneider, 1969; Trevarthen, 1968), spatio-temporal parameters are analyzed at the cortical level. Another reason may be that objects can be recognized not only by their spatial pattern (form) but also by their *pattern of movement* (e.g. the flight pattern of birds). In addition, under certain circumstances, *spatial structure can only be recovered from motion* (structure from motion, Ullman, 1979). This is demonstrated by a defocussed picture of a filmed visual scene: when the movie is held still it is unrecognizable, but as soon as the movie is put into motion the scene is recognized. A similar demonstration (Johansson, 1975) can be carried out by observing, in a dark room, human subjects wearing light sources attached at the joints. As soon as the subjects start to move they become recognizable.

Chapter 9. Binocular Interactions in Cat Visual Cortical Cells and Coding of Parameters Involved in Static and Dynamic Depth Perception

In the representation of the binocular visual field, *almost all cortical cells are binocular*. This is expressed to a certain extent by the *ocular dominance* of cortical cells. The binocularity of cortical cells does not necessarily imply that they show binocular interactions. Binocular interactions refer to neuronal responses to binocular stimulation different from the sum of responses to stimulation of each eye in isolation. Binocular interactions are far more important for the understanding of binocular vision than ocular dominance. In addition to binocular fusion and rivalry, binocular interactions underly the coding of a special class of visual parameters referred to as disparities i.e. differences between the eyes with respect to a given attribute. These disparities are important to binocular vision in two ways. On the one hand they have to be discarded by the visual system so as to allow fusion of the two slightly different retinal images to one cyclopean image. On the other hand they have to be used by the system in order to extract the information they contain on the *third dimension of space*. Students of stereopsis have mainly investigated the influence of position and orientation disparities, both cues for static depth perception (i.e. perception in depth of stationary objects). With respect to dynamic depth perception (i.e. the perception of objects moving in depth) both binocular cues (difference in velocity and direction between both eyes) and monocular cues (changing size) have been investigated. The binocularity of cortical cells will be described first.

9.1 The Binocularity of Cortical Cells and the Ocular Dominance Scheme

In their initial studies of areas 17, 18 and 19 of the cat, Hubel and Wiesel (1962, 1965) discovered a second major transformation of the geniculate input at the cortical level: in addition to orientation tuning they described the binocularity of cortical cells. Indeed unlike geniculate cells most cortical cells *had a receptive field (RF) in both eyes*. Although the RFs in both eyes were similar in RF organization, orientation and position, they could differ in the relative strength of the drive from either eye. To express this Hubel and Wiesel (1962) introduced a *7 point scale of ocular dominance groups* which they defined as follows: group 4, no obvious difference in the effects exerted by the two eyes; groups 1 and 7, exclusively contra- or ipsilateral respectively; groups 2 and 6, contralateral respectively ipsilateral eye much more effective and groups 3 and 5, contralateral respectively ipsilateral slightly more effective. Hubel and Wiesel (1962) not only tested each eye separately, but also studied binocular interaction in the sense that they looked for facilitation between the 2 eyes which they called synergy (although they also mention that "inhibitory inputs" from both eyes could be synergetic, probably referring to OFF regions). They included in classes 2 and 6 cells from which the non-dominant eye elicited no response on its own, but for which the non-dominant eye had a synergetic (i.e. facilitatory) influence on the response from the dominant eye. Apparently classes 1 and 7 were purely monocular cells. Hubel and Wiesel (1965) showed that in all three areas, but especially in area 19, most cells were binocular, that the different RF types (simple, complex and hypercomplex) had roughly the same ocular dominance distribution and that the contralateral input dominates the ipsilateral one, especially in area 18 (Fig. 9/1). It is noteworthy that Hubel and Wiesel (1965, p. 259) were surprised "that the functional separation of the two eyes should persist with so little change from one level to the next in the hierarchy, beginning with the simple and then complex cells in visual area I, and proceeding to complex and then to hypercomplex cells in visual area III". This is not just a formulation of the hierarchical theory, but it clearly shows that monocular cells in their view received input from only one eye.

Their ocular dominance scheme using hand-held stimuli has been used very extensively in studies of the normal cat (and also in a long series of papers on monocular deprivation). While the group 1, 7 and 4 were clearly defined, groups 2, 6, 3 and 5 were less well-defined and some authors consequently used only a five point scale (Wilson and Sherman, 1976).[1] Cells belonging to classes 1 and 7 are referred to as monocular cells, those of other classes as binocular cells. In another terminology which seems more fruitful (Poggio and Fischer, 1977) cells of classes 1, 2, 6 and 7 have an unbalanced ocular dominance and cells of classes 3, 4 and 5 a balanced ocular dominance. Figure 9/2 shows the ocular dominance distributions for two eccentricity classes of areas 17, 18 and 19. Our results confirm Hubel and Wiesel's (1965) observation that area 19 is much more binocular than areas 17 and 18. However Fig. 9/2 also shows that there are *clear changes in ocular distribution with eccentricity*: in areas 17 and 18, cells within 10° are more often monocular than cells with RFs further away from the area centralis. For area 19 the inverse is true. These observations run in parallel with those of Albus (1975 c)

---

[1] In our laboratory (Duysens et al., 1982 a; Orban and Kennedy, 1981) we have solved this problem by including in groups 2 and 6, cells with a response in the non-dominant eye, too weak to allow plotting of the RF in that eye, and in groups 3 and 5 cells giving reliable (i.e., allowing plotting) responses in both eyes, but with a clear superiority of one eye. Berman et al. (1982) seem to have adopted the same criteria.

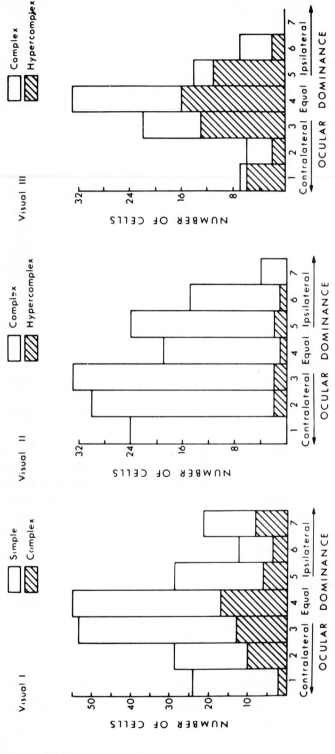

Fig. 9/1. Ocular distribution in the 3 cortical areas according to Hubel and Wiesel (1965). Distribution according to ocular dominance of (A), 223 cells in visual I, (B), 149 cells in visual II, and (C), 89 cells in visual III. Cells of group 1 are driven only by the contralateral eye; for cells of group 2 there is marked dominance of the contralateral eye; for group 3, slight dominance. For cells in group 4 there is no obvious difference between the two eyes. In group 5 the ipsilateral eye dominates slightly, in group 6, markedly; and in group 7 the cells are driven only by the ipsilateral eye. Adapted with permission from Hubel and Wiesel (1965).

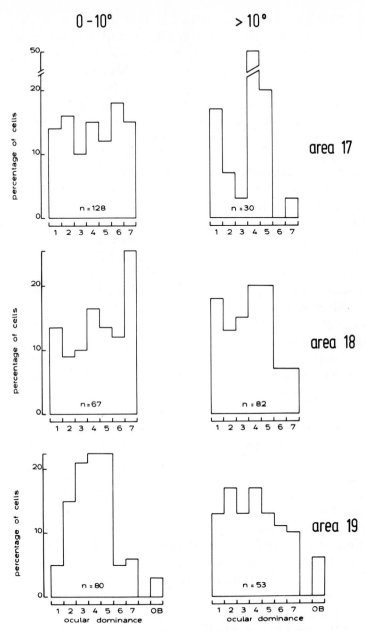

Fig. 9/2. Ocular dominance distributions in the 3 areas (17, 18 and 19) for 2 eccentricity classes 0–10° and >10° (10–50° in area 17 and 10–40° in areas 18 and 19).

who recorded from 640 cells with RFs within 12° from the area centralis: while about 55–60% of the cells with RFs within 4° from the fixation point were monocular only 26% of cells with RFs between 4 and 12° from the fixation point were monocular (Fig. 9/3). Wilson and Sherman (1976) recorded 150 cells in area 17 with RFs ranging in eccentricity from 0° to 45° and failed to see a change with eccentricity. Berman et al. (1982) recorded from 393 cells in area 17 and failed to see a change in binocularity with eccentricity up to 30°. They however report that cells are maximally binocular within a vertical strip extending up to 12° from the vertical meridian (VM), but curiously excluding the 4° around the area centralis. Over 12° from the VM, cells become strongly dominated by the contralateral eye. These authors try to link this 12° strip to the callosal input which, however, seems not to spare the projection of the area centralis.

At least part of these disagreements may be due to the use of hand-held stimuli and the difference in definition of monocular and binocular cells. Therefore a number of authors have used quantitative techniques to study the ocular dominance (Hammond, 1979, 1981 b; Kato et al., 1978; Leventhal and Hirsch, 1978). Macy et al. (1982) recently made a comparison between ocular dominance assessed by quantitative techniques and with hand-held stimuli. This comparison shows a reasonable agreement (1 class error) when the cell response is strong, but a much larger percent of error when the responses are weak. This calls for caution in the interpretation of developmental studies relying up to now exclusively on hand-held stimuli.

Many authors have reported a *difference in binocularity between area 17 simple and complex cells* (Albus, 1975 c; Berman et al., 1982; Hammond and MacKay, 1977; Leventhal and Hirsch, 1978), simple cells being more often monocular than complex cells. This is contrary to the findings of Hubel and Wiesel (1962) who found no difference in ocular dominance between simple and complex cells, and of Gilbert (1977) who found only a slight difference in binocularity between simple and standard complex cells. Our qualitative results show that difference in ocular dominance is a general feature of S and C families in all three areas (Table 3, Chapter 4). Hammond (1979, 1981 b) has studied quantitatively the ocular dominance of complex cells with bar and noise stimuli. In about half of the cells (14/31) the ocular dominance differed by 2 classes or more when bar and noise stimuli were compared. In view of this observation and of the difference in preferred directions for bar and noise stimuli (see Chapter 8) it is possible that complex cells (or C family cells in our terminology) carry different messages related to different stimuli, which could be decoded separately by different subcortical targets (Hoffmann, personal communication).

Hubel and Wiesel (1965) in their original contribution noted that in vertical penetrations most cells were dominated by the same eye, while in penetrations parallel to the cortex ocular dominance shifted from one eye to

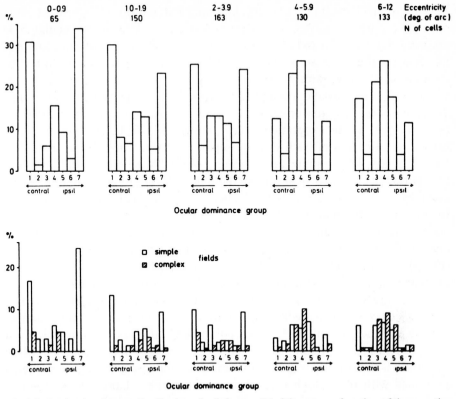

Fig. 9/3. Ocular dominance distribution of cells in area 17 of the cat as a function of the receptive field position of the cells. The response of the subdominant eye is given as a percentage of the response of the dominant eye; 0% are classified as ocular dominance groups 1 or 7, 1–20% as groups 2 or 6, 21–80% as groups 3 or 5, 80–100% as group 4. For each eccentricity class the range of eccentricity and the number of cells are given at the top of each diagram. The number of cells in each ocular dominance group is given as a percentage of the total number of cells in each eccentricity group. The cortical equivalent (mm cortex) for each eccentricity class is 2.3, 1.8, 2.0, 1.8, 2.4. Below: ocular dominance distribution of cells with simple and complex receptive fields. The number of cells in each ocular dominance group is given as a percentage of the total number of cells in each eccentricity group. A small proportion of cells in each eccentricity class has not been classified according to the receptive field properties. Adapted with permission from Albus (1975 c).

the other. These ocular dominance shifts were independent of changes in preferred orientation. Hubel and Wiesel suggested that cortical cells were grouped in *ocular dominance columns,* which constitute a set of columns or slabs running orthogonally (i.e., independently) to the orientation columns or slabs (Hubel and Wiesel, 1977). Hubel and Wiesel (1965) and Albus (1975 c) reported that ocular dominance columns are less well defined outside layer IV. According to Shatz and Stryker (1978) this corresponds to their own and Gilbert's (1977) observation that cells are more monocular in layer IV than in other layers. This observation has not been confirmed either by

Leventhal and Hirsch (1978) or by Berman et al. (1982). However, Mustari et al. (1982) have reported a very high incidence (64%) of monocular cells among layer IV monosynaptic S cells. In fact, the most striking laminar difference is the much larger number of binocular cells in layer V, linked to the dominance of C family cells in this layer.

Several authors have attempted to demonstrate the existence of ocular dominance columns anatomically by means of injections of labelled proline into one eye. These experiments have shown that in layer IV of the cat, geniculate afferents of each eye are separated in patches (Ito et al., 1977; LeVay et al., 1978; Shatz and Stryker, 1978; Shatz et al., 1977). When reconstructed on the cortical surface these patches, form slabs running orthogonal to the 17–18 border, the slabs being wider in area 18 than in area 17. In combining the injection of proline with microelectrode recordings in the same animal Shatz and Stryker (1978) have shown that cells dominated by one eye fit into the patches defined by the radioactive labelling of layer IV (Fig. 9/4), although they admit that the organization is less neat than in layer IV of the monkey. These experiments clearly show that the *geniculate afferents* are segregated in ocular dominance columns and that the physiological i.e. *cortical cell columns* are in register with those geniculate afferent columns, but the evidence for the cortical cell columns themselves remains at least in the cat exclusively physiological. As a brief report of Thompson et al. (1983) suggests it is likely that, as in the monkey, deoxyglucose labelling experiments combined with physiological recordings will in the cat provide anatomical evidence for ocular dominance columns extending over the whole cortical depth.

However the classicial concept of ocular dominance will probably have to be revised in view of the recent findings of Kato et al. (1981). These authors showed that in area 17 there are very few truly monocular cells and that monocularly driven cells are actually binocular cells, with an excitatory input from one eye and an inhibitory one from the other. Also the observation that some cells fire only upon combined stimulation of both eyes and not at all when stimulated through one eye (true binocular cells, Hubel and Wiesel, 1970) points to the inadequacy of the 7 point ocular dominance scale. Using moving slits as stimuli and different quantitative techniques to disclose interactions from the non-dominant eye (Fig. 9/5) Kato et al. (1981) found that in 16 cells exclusively driven by one eye (as tested quantitatively with a PSTH in each eye), only one cell was completely monocular. The effects of the non-dominant eye were distributed as follows: facilitation 2 cells, inhibition 6 cells, and inhibition flanked by a weak facilitation, 7 cells. Electrical stimulation experiments confirm this convergence of excitation from one eye and inhibition from the other eye in monocularly driven cells (Tsumoto, 1978). This convergence also fits with the finding that bicuculline, antagonizing GABA mediated inhibition, shifts ocular dominance towards class 4 (Sillito

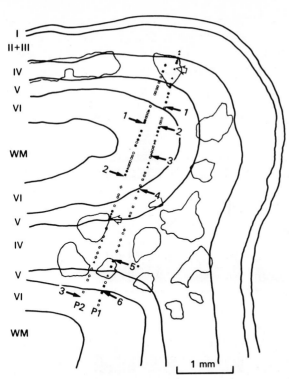

Fig. 9/4. Correspondence between anatomical and physiological demonstrations of ocular dominance columns. The ocular dominance columns in layer IV are marked by transneuronally transported radioactive proline injected in one eye. Single cells were recorded in the two penetrations (P1 and P2) into area 17 ipsilateral to the injected eye. The figure shows the histological reconstruction of the two penetrations based on Cresyl Violet stained sections. Layers are indicated by Roman numerals or WM (white matter). Numbered arrows indicate the positions of electrolytic marking lesions made along the electrode track. Filled symbols refer to the units preferring the injected (ipsilateral) eye (ocular dominance groups 5–7). Half-filled symbols indicate units equally driven by the two eyes (group 4). The dence patches of radioactive label seen in autoradiographs have been projected onto the reconstruction. Thus, in penetration 1, the electrode passed through two patches of label in layer IV, one at the upper right open arrow, the other just following lesion 5. In both cases, cells were dominated by the injected eye. Adapted with permission from Shatz and Stryker, 1978.

et al., 1980 a). It seems that binocular interactions studied with gratings spatially phase shifted in one eye with respect to the other eye yield less interactions in monocular cells than bar stimuli (Freeman and Robson, 1982). *Monocularly driven cells can better be described as EI* (excitatory input from one eye and inhibitory input from the other eye) *binocular cells and binocularly driven cells as EE* (excitatory-excitatory from both eyes) *binocular cells.* Ocular dominance columns would then be more accurately described as two EI slabs (one excitatory for each eye) in between two EE slabs, but the total width of these columns or slabs representing all combinations would be equal to the width of two classical ocular dominance columns (one for each eye). The finding of Kato et al. (1981) that with the exception of 1 out of 112 cells all cortical cells (including simple cells) have a binocular input, casts serious doubts on the statement of Gilbert (1977), based on ocular dominance distributions, that "the mixing of the input from the two eyes is progressive from geniculate cell to simple cell to complex cell". It rather seems that while C cells receiving almost an exclusively EE convergence, about 1/3 of the S cells have an EI convergence and 2/3 an EE convergence.

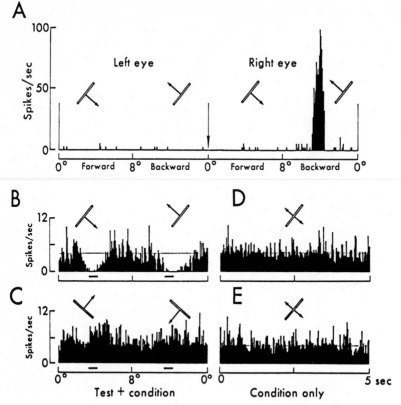

Fig. 9/5. Orientation-sensitive inhibitory receptive field (conditioning method) for the silent eye of a simple cell. A: average response histogram from the right (dominant) eye in response to an optimally-oriented light bar ($8° \times 0.23°$) moving at $3.2°$/sec. The left eye failed to fire to the same stimulus. B,C: binocular responses when the same stimulus as in A was moved in front of the left (silent) eye against a background discharge from the cell produced by repetitive stimulation of the excitatory region in the receptive field of the right eye. The orientation of the bar was optimal for B and at right angles to optimal for C. D, E: background discharge (condition only). The horizontal bars below the histograms in B and C indicate the 400 msec windows used to record the data for the orientation tuning of the inhibition (not shown). Adapted with permission from Kato et al. (1981).

9.2 Position Disparity Tuning Curves and the Coding of Static Depth

The obvious binocular cue for static depth is the difference in horizontal position of the images on the two retinae. In visual cortical physiology the difference in position of stimuli in the 2 eyes has been called the *position disparity*. Mainly the horizontal disparity, assessed by measuring the difference in position with respect to the VM, is of use for depth discrimination. In order to allow depth discrimination, the visual cortex should have neurons

(1) with a filter function for position disparity, preferably of the bandpass type *and* (2) with different disparity optima or thresholds depending on whether the filters are bandpass or not. Those two requirements seemed to be met by area 17 cells subserving central vision according to the two groups who initially reported on neuronal mechanisms for stereoscopic depth perception (Barlow et al., 1967; Nikara et al., 1968; Pettigrew et al., 1968 b). Both groups were mainly concerned with question (2), and they equated optimal position disparity[2] of a binocular cell with the position disparity, derived from the *RF locations in both eyes*. When the RFs in both eyes have the same position with respect to the fixation point (i.e., are located at corresponding retinal points), the cell has no or a zero disparity. When the RFs of the 2 eyes are in different positions, the cell has a (non-zero) disparity. Temporal offset of the RFs corresponds to a cortical cell receiving input from a small region behind the fixation point (crossed disparities), nasal offset of the RFs to a region in front of the fixation point (uncrossed disparities) (Fig. 9/6).

The determination of the position disparity of a binocular cell requires two problems to be solved: (1) to locate correctly the VM in each eye (2) to control *residual eye movements*. Both studies (Barlow et al., 1967; Pettigrew et al., 1968 b) used the same method to solve point (1): record as many neurons as possible in one animal and correct the disparities of the individual cells in such a way that the mean disparity of all binocular cells in the animal is zero. Barlow et al. (1967) fixed the eyes to rings and reported horizontal disparities ranging from 3 to +3°. Nikara et al. (1968) controlled the residual eye movement by plotting the retinal landmarks (retinal vessels) before and after recording each cell: with this correction they observed disparities ranging from −1° to +1°, while without correction they found disparities between −3 and +3°. Other authors (Ferster, 1981; Hubel and Wiesel, 1970) have used a simultaneously recorded binocular cell as control for residual eye movements. Barlow et al. (1967) showed some sketchy qualitative evidence that the binocular cells had a bandpass function for disparity, Pettigrew et al. (1968 b) gave quantitative evidence for this filter function. While these studies clearly outlined a possible mechanism for stereoscopic depth perception, it is not sure that adequate precautions were taken to ensure that the cells were recorded from area 17. The major criterion given by Barlow et al. (1967) is the absence of simple cells in area 18, a criterion of which the validity can be seriously doubted in view of recent reports on simple cells in area 18 (Ferster, 1981; Harvey, 1980 a; Orban and Callens, 1977 a; Orban and Kennedy, 1981). Subsequently these studies were extended to area 17 neurons with eccentric RFs by Joshua and Bishop (1970). According to these authors

---

[2] One could also measure optimal position disparity from a disparity-response curve, as has been done in later experiments.

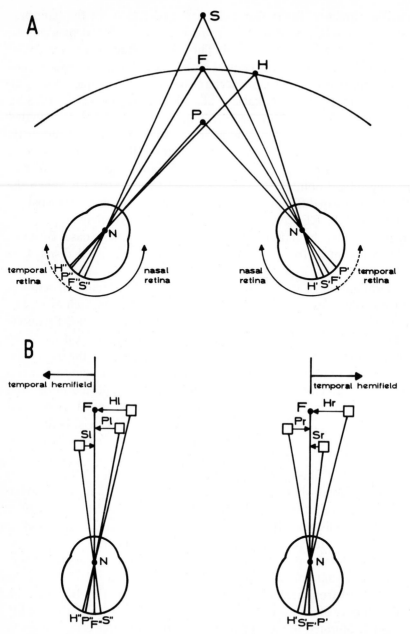

Fig. 9/6. Definition of RF disparities of cortical cells. A) Projection of different points in space onto the 2 retinae: F: fixation point, H: point of the horopter (collection in points, all at the same distance from the eyes as the fixation point), S: a point beyond the horopter and P: a point in front of it, N: nodal point of the eye. B) Position of RFs of cortical cells linked to corresponding retinal points (F' and F", H' and H") and of cells linked to non-corresponding points (S' and S", P' and P"). H_l, S_l, P_l, H_r, S_r and P_r indicate distances between the RFs and the vertical meridian in the left and right eye respectively. Temporally displaced fields indicate crossed disparities, nasally displaced fields uncrossed disparities.

Table 9/1. Changes in horizontal and vertical receptive field disparities with horizontal retinal eccentricity

Horizontal eccentricity	No. of units	Standard deviation of spread of receptive field disparities	
		Horizontal disparity	Vertical disparity
0°–4°	90	0.50°	0.52°
4°–8°	74	0.76°	0.57°
8°–12°	39	0.79°	0.34°
12°–16°	10	0.90°	0.37°

Adapted with permission from Joshua and Bishop (1970).

horizontal disparities increase with eccentricity (Table 9/1). Our own observations (Orban and Kennedy, unpublished) support this statement. The importance of the naso-temporal overlap for depth discrimination on the midline has already been pointed out (Chapter 2). The evidence in favor of this overlap has been reviewed in Chapter 2.

Bishop and his colleagues introduced two methods for the quantitative study of *disparity tuning* in the paralyzed animal: the use of a prism of variable diopter (Risley prism) (Bishop et al., 1971 c; Henry et al., 1969; Joshua and Bishop, 1970; Pettigrew et al., 1968 b) (see Fig. 9/8) and the variable delay method (Kato et al., 1981; Nelson et al., 1977) (see Fig. 9/7). The first method has also been used by others (Ferster, 1981; Fischer and Krüger, 1979; von der Heydt et al., 1978). From these studies the following consensus can be established. By far the most common type of disparity tuning is that of cells called *tuned excitatory cells* by Poggio and Fischer (1977) in their study of monkey visual cortex (see Chapter 14). These cells have a vigorous response for a near zero disparity and their response falls off very sharply at both sides of the optimal disparity (Fig. 9/7). Curves of this type were initially ascribed by Bishop et al. (1971 c) to binocular simple cells. Recent studies by Fischer and Krüger (1979) and by Ferster (1981) have shown that in the cat indeed 4/5 of these tuned excitatory cells have a balanced ocular dominance (class 3–4–5). Some of the tuned excitatory cells (1/5) have more unbalanced ocular dominance. It remains to be seen whether the latter include the gate neuron [3] (Henry et al., 1969) which is exclusively monocularly driven and has inhibitory regions surrounding a subliminally excitatory region (Fig. 9/8) (Bishop et al., 1971 c; Henry et al., 1969; Kato et al., 1981). The few simple cells with very weak monocular responses and strong (400%) sharp facilitation mentioned by Bishop et al. (1971 c) probably also belong to the tuned excitatory type (Fig. 9/8). According to Ferster (1981) tuned excitatory cells occur more often in area 17 than in area 18.

---

[3] The term gate neuron refers to the influence of the non-dominant eye which allows the dominant eye's response to get through only if the disparity is optimal.

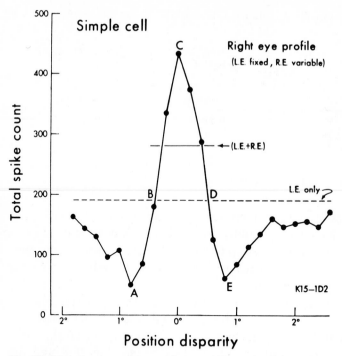

Fig. 9/7. Disparity-response curve of an area 17 tuned excitatory simple cell. Close-up look at the position disparity tuning curve in Figure 9/11B corresponding to the optimal stimulus orientation setting (86°) for the variable (right) eye. *Dashed line:* level of the monocular response from the left eye at the fixed (optimal) stimulus orientation of 93°. Short continuous line: summed monocular response from the two eyes with both stimulus orientations optimal (unit displays 54% facilitation). Adapted with permission from Nelson et al. (1977).

Ferster (1981) has disclosed the RF organization of tuned excitatory cells: they all have inhibitory sidebands in their monocular RFs. Thus all these cells would belong to the simple family as defined by Kato et al. (1978) or to the S family in our terminology (Orban and Kennedy, 1981). Ferster (1981) however maintains that some of them should be considered as complex in the Hubel and Wiesel sense, the main argument being that they have an exclusively ON or OFF excitatory RF. The latter cells however have 2 flanking inhibitory regions even for flashed stimuli and thus clearly fulfil the requirement of simple or S families (see also Palmer and Davis, 1981 a). The only valid objection to this seems to be Ferster's example of orientation dependence of the inhibitory sidebands in such cells, since Bishop et al. (1973) and Orban et al. (1979a) have reported examples of a simple cell and a hypercomplex I cell with orientation independent inhibitory sidebands. But neither study gives any indication as to whether orientation dependence or independence is a general property of inhibitory sidebands or not. It also remains to be seen whether or not orientation dependence of sidebands is different

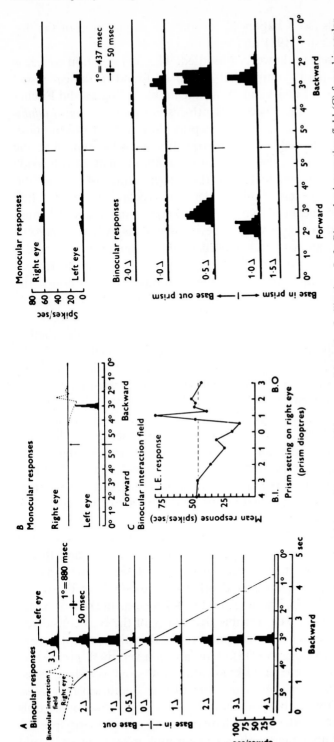

Fig. 9/8. Binocular interactions in a gate neuron and a neuron with extreme binocular facilitation. Left. Binocular interaction field (C) for a binocular gate neuron that discharged only to one eye (B: left eye) and then only on the backsweep of the stimulus. Binocular average response histograms (A) have been selected from the series used for the preparation of the plot in (C). Responses are to a slit of light (4° × 0.14°; orientation 0°) moved forwards and backwards over a 5.7° traverse at 1.14°/sec. Each histogram was compiled from 20 stimulus cycles using 200 analyser channels at 50 msec/bin. Horizontal dashed line in C: amplitude of monocular left eye response. Dashed lines represent a subliminal receptive field for the non-dominant (right) eye. Right. Average response histograms from a simple cell with very weak monocular responses but marked binocular facilitation. Responses are to a slit of light (5.7° × 0.28°; orientation 15°) moved forwards and backwards over a 5.7° traverse at 2.3°/sec. Each histogram was compiled from 20 stimulus cycles using 100 analyser channels at 50 msec/bin. Adapted with permission from Bishop et al. (1971 c).

among S1 and S2 cells (see Chapter 12 for another explanation of the disagreement between Ferster, 1981 and Bishop et al., 1973).

Four basic issues remain however unsettled. The first question concerns the other types of disparity tuning that are to be found in the cat visual cortex. In their study of V1 and V2 in the awake monkey, Poggio and Fischer (1977) reported on three other types of depth-response curves: *tuned inhibitory* cells, showing a sharp inhibition for depths close to the fixation point, and *far and near* cells, showing an asymmetric curve with facilitation at one side of the fixation point and a sharp transition to inhibition at the other side of the fixation point (see Fig. 14/12). In the interpretation of Poggio and Fischer tuned excitatory cells could underly binocular fusion and fine stereopsis, while far and near cells would underly coarse stereopsis and could also be used as a signal to trigger vergence eye movements. A few (10%) cells at the 17–18 border, all with unbalanced ocular dominance (i.e. ocular dominance classes 1, 2, 6 and 7) have been reported by Fischer and Krüger (1979) as fulfilling the requirements of tuned inhibitory cells although the inhibition in their Fig. 1 is not very pronounced. Kato et al. (1981) have reported a few cells (5%) among area 17 cells exclusively driven from one eye that could be tuned inhibitory. It is much more difficult to decide whether or not far and near cells are present in the cat. Ferster (1981) labelled 54 cells out of his sample of 280 area 17 and 18 cells as far and near (Fig. 9/9). While these cells had a wide inhibitory region asymmetrically located with respect to the reference point (disparity of another cell) only some of them showed a binocular facilitation (2 out of 6 cells in Fig. 9/9: cells in D and F). Moreover Ferster (1981) manipulated disparity in the dimension orthogonal to the optimal orientation: the horizontal disparities are smaller than those disparities and consequently he overestimates the extent of the inhibitory region. Furthermore, as pointed out by Kato et al. (1981) in order to consider a cell as far or near one has to show that the transition actually occurs close to the fixation point (i.e. the zero disparity in the absolute sense) and Ferster was in no position to do so. Finally, more than 3/4 of the so-called far and near cells recorded by Ferster (1981) were in area 18. Cynader and Regan (1978) studied dynamic binocular interactions in area 18 (see below) and have shown that their so-called direction in depth sensitive cells have mostly an unbalanced ocular dominance and wide inhibitory regions in their disparity tuning curve. It is thus very well possible that many of the cells considered by Ferster (1981) as far and near correspond to the direction in depth sensitive cells of Cynader and Regan (1978). And indeed a very high proportion "far and near" cells of Ferster (1981) are direction selective when tested monocularly, another property of many direction in depth sensitive cells. Fischer and Krüger (1979) observed that out of a population of 60 cells recorded near the 17–18 border 17 cells had an asymmetric disparity profile. However 7 of these 17 cells had an almost horizontal orientation and could

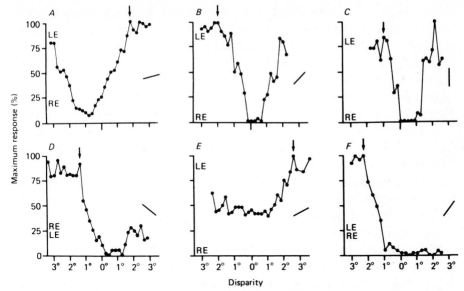

Fig. 9/9. Disparity-response curves of four far cells (B–D, F) and two near cells (A and E). 0° represents the reference point and uncrossed disparities are plotted to the left of zero. The short bar to the right of each curve is the orientation of each cell. LE and RE indicate the response of the cell to presenting the stimulus to left and right eyes alone. Arrows indicate optimal disparity, closest to the reference. The laminar position and receptive field type of each cell was: A, A17-layer VI, simple; B, A17-layer II, complex; C, A18-layer III, complex; D, A17-layer III, complex; E, A18-layer II, complex; F, A18-layer II complex. Adapted with permission from Ferster (1981).

thus not correspond to far and near cells; this leaves 10/60 cells as possible far and near cells. Considering all three studies, Ferster (1981); Fischer and Krüger (1979); Kato et al. (1981) it seems likely that there is a small proportion of far and near cells in the cat visual cortex and that they have ocular dominances of 2 or 6, since none of the disparity curves of class 1 and 7 cells obtained by Kato et al. (1981) really fit the definition of far and near cells. Whether far and near cells occur more frequently in area 18 than in area 17 remains to be seen.

A second unsettled issue concerns the proportion of cells in the visual cortex that are *disparity insensitive*. According to the Australian group the majority of area 17 cells is disparity sensitive: all simple cells according to Bishop et al. (1971 c) and at least some complex cells according to Pettigrew et al. (1968 b). Given the proportion of these types in area 17, disparity sensitive cells should amount to 60 or 80%. The observations of Fischer and Krüger (1979) agree with this figure: 60/71 cells at the 17–18 border were disparity sensitive. von der Heydt et al. (1978) take the opposite view, finding only 6 out of 46 cells to be disparity sensitive. Ferster (1981) reports a proportion in between the 2 extremes: 103 out of 280 area 17 and 18 cells were

disparity sensitive, although from his descriptions, it is clear that his definition of a disparity sensitive cell is very restricted, accepting only cells fitting
in what he defines as the tuned excitatory or far and near categories.

A third unsettled question is the *range of optimal disparities of tuned
excitatory* cells. Indeed Ferster (1981) who most recently studied the tuned
excitatory cells reports a very small range of optimal relative disparities (i.e.,
disparities measured with respect to the disparity of another cell) for these
cells. He is, however, in no position to give the optimal absolute disparities
(i.e. disparities measured with respect to the VM). If his data were correct (i.e.
if the relative disparities approximately corresponded to absolute disparities)
then the tuned excitatory cells of the cat, unlike those of the monkey, (Poggio
and Fischer, 1977) could *not* code for depth: they would all simultaneously
be either active or not, as Ferster himself points out. They could then only
be the substrate of binocular fusion. If the disparities given by Nikara et al.
(1968) (range of $-1°$ to $+1°$) could apply to the tuned excitatory cells which
have a range of interactions of about $0.5°$ to $1°$, then they could easily encode
depth (Fig. 9/10), although with an accuracy about $1/5$ to $1/20$ that of
monkey cortical cells. It is thus important to measure the optimal absolute
disparities in tuned excitatory cells of the cat and to compare them to their
width of disparity tuning. This is a difficult task since it requires an experiment combining the recording of many cells (to be able to assess correctly
absolute disparities) and a quantitative study of binocular interactions, but
with 4- or 5-day experiments this should be possible.

A fourth partially unsettled question is the *contribution of the different
areas* to static depth perception. The origin of this question is the report by
Hubel and Wiesel (1970) that in the *monkey* disparities are within the range
of measurement error in area 17 but are much larger in area 18. The data of
Ferster (1981) suggest that area 17 is more important than area 18 since it has
more tuned excitatory cells, although Ferster (1981) unfortunately only
mentions absolute numbers, not percentages. Since S family cells in area 18
have wider fields than their area 17 counterparts, their binocular interaction
range could be wider. It could well be that both areas 17 and 18 contribute
to static depth perceptions as they both can contribute to static pattern
analysis, but for different ranges of velocities of the objects (see Chapter 8).
Many of Ferster's (1981) tuned excitatory cells were end-stopped, and had
balanced ocular dominance. Therefore, area 19 HS cells (and possibly HB
cells if they have inhibitory sidebands) which have similar properties could
also contribute to static depth, but their proportion in area 19 is relatively
small, and their interaction range would be large due to their larger RF
width.

In conclusion the presently available results point towards the S cell
family, especially in area 17, as a possible substrate for static depth perception. Indeed due to their inhibitory sidebands, they produce sharp binocular

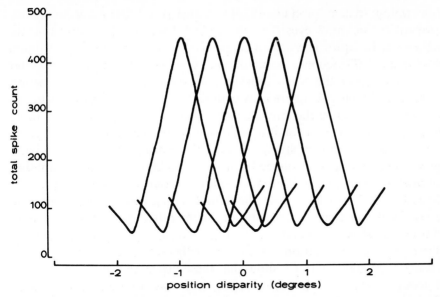

Fig. 9/10. Comparison of position disparity tunings with the range of disparity optima (admitting a range of -1 to $1°$ position disparity). Given the sharpness of position disparity tuning (same tuning as in Fig. 9/7) the response of a cell with optimal disparity $-1°$ is reduced to zero at zero disparity.

interaction curves required for fine depth discrimination. As for the two-dimensional spatial parameters (orientation and spatial frequency), there is a clear superiority of S family cells over C family cells for static depth discrimination (3rd dimension spatial parameter). As mentioned earlier, Ferster (1981) noted that half of the tuned excitatory cells were end-stopped compared to 25% or 30% of the other cells. It is then tempting to suggest that HS cells, the function of which has remained elusive up to now, play a major role in depth discrimination.

9.3 Orientation Disparity, Another Mechanism for Static Depth Discrimination?

Blakemore et al. (1972) made the remark that the retinal images of an object beyond or in front of the horopter[4] not only differ in position in the two eyes but also in *orientation, width, and length,* and when the object is moving also differ in *direction and velocity.* Since cortical cells are sensitive

---

[4] Horopter is the collection of points in space at the same distance of the eyes as the fixation point (see Fig. 9/6).

to orientation, Blakemore et al. (1972) investigated to what extent difference in orientation in the 2 eyes (i.e., *orientation disparity*) can contribute to signalling static depth. Their conclusion was that it could indeed contribute. Nelson et al. (1977) re-investigated the question and concluded that it could not. In this respect the two important questions are, just as for position disparity, (1) whether there are cells with different orientation disparities in the eyes and (2) whether the tuning curve for binocular orientation difference is bandpass and narrow enough to allow discriminations.

Both above-mentioned studies of area 17 neurons agreed on two basic observations: (1) there are indeed cells with different optimal orientation disparities and the range of optimal disparities extends from $-15°$ to $+15°$ difference and (2) the binocular orientation tuning (keeping orientation in one eye fixed and changing orientation in the other eye, which is really a tuning curve for orientation difference) has almost the same width of tuning as the monocular orientation tuning curve (Fig. 9/11).

While both studies clearly show that these orientation differences allow fusion of images of objects tilted in space, the answer to the question of their contribution to depth discrimination relies on the comparison of the range of optimal orientation differences with the width of binocular orientation tuning and thus in fact of monocular orientation tuning. Nelson et al. (1977) discard the orientation difference mechanism by a comparison with the position disparity mechanism showing that for a given example (a cat standing up looking 20 cm ahead) position disparities are a better cue (i.e. produce larger differences in neuronal response) than orientation disparity. However this is not a fundamental objection, since as Nelson et al. (1977) admit, the superiority may shift to the orientation disparity mechanism under other circumstances (e.g. more distant objects). One could even imagine that *both mechanisms are complementary:* the position disparity mechanism operating optimally for objects near the animal and the orientation difference mechanism operating optimally for objects further away from the animal.

Unfortunately the data of Blakemore et al. (1972) are not very adequate to compare the range of orientation disparities and the width of orientation tuning. Indeed their pooled histogram of orientation difference gives no indication of cell type and if one was to take the median orientation width of all cortical cells, the half-widths at half-height would be somewhere near $25°$ and one would have to conclude that the orientation tuning is too large to allow depth discrimination. Their figures showing data of a single animal can be of some help. They show that only 1 or 2 cells among the cells with a non-zero optimal orientation disparity have their response reduced to 50% or less at zero orientation disparity. From this data it seems that at best the orientation disparity mechanism could signal that objects are tilted away or towards the animal but not much more.

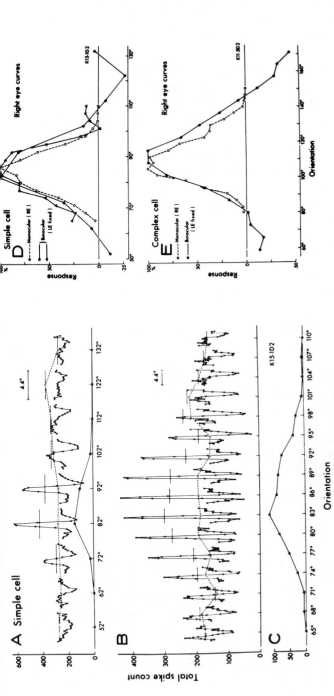

Fig. 9/11. Binocular and monocular orientation tunings compared. A and B: two independent matrix stimulation experiments on the same simple cell. Families of position disparity tuning curves are shown for two different ranges of orientation disparities. The left eye's stimulus was held at 93°; all orientation and position disparity changes occur in the right eye. Each position disparity curve has 22 increments of 12' arc disparity spanning 4.4°. Dashed lines (open circles): level of control monocular responses from the fixed orientation (left) eye. Short continuous lines: level of the summed monocular responses from the two eyes with the stimulus orientation for the variable (right) eye as indicated. A: nine position disparity tuning curves separated by coarse orientation disparity increments of 10° and spanning an orientation range of 80°. Continuous line (filled triangles): control monocular orientation tuning curve from variable orientation (right) eye. B: 16 position disparity tuning curves at finer orientation disparity increments of 3° to afford a close-up look at an orientation range of 45°. Fixed orientation control (i.e., monocular orientation control (i.e., monocular orientation tuning curve) obtained during collection of data for B. D and E: monocular and binocular stimulus orientation tuning curves match closely for both a simple cell (D) and a complex cell (E) following application of normalization procedures. For binocular curves only one stimulus varies in orientation and the resulting curve is labeled according to the eye receiving the variable stimulus. Results of two separate matrix stimulation experiments are shown for the same simple cell. The binocular curves have been drawn with respect to a zero base line taken as the level of control monocular response from the fixed orientation (left) eye in each case. The respective monocular stimulus orientation tuning curves have then been set on these zero base lines and their peaks normalized to peaks of their binocular curves. The simple cell is the same as in A, B and C. Adapted with permission from Nelson et al. (1977).

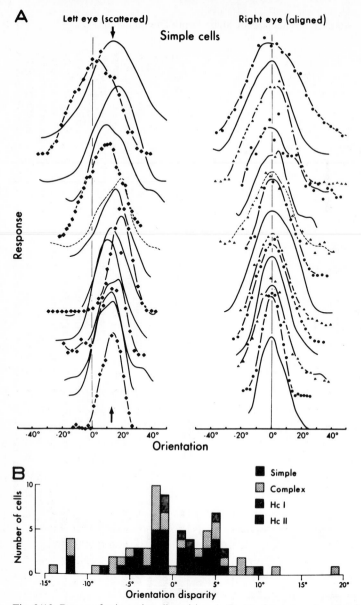

Fig. 9/12. Range of orientation disparities. A. Scatter in monocular stimulus orientation tuning curves for 14 binocular striate cells (13 simple, continuous lines; 1 hypercomplex I, dashed lines) in one cat. Optimal orientations of right eye curves are arbitrarily aligned at 0° and the total optimal stimulus orientation disparity for each cell is transferred to the left eye curve. Vertical arrows: mean displacement (13.1°) of left eye curves to the right, attributable to in-cyclorotation with paralysis. The scatter about this mean displacement gives the optimal stimulus orientation disparity distribution, describing the extent to which the binocular receptive-field pairs were matched in preferred stimulus orientations. All the tuning curves have been normalized to the same height, ordered according to half-width at half-height, and spaced vertically. Data points are shown for only one curve of each pair. B. Pooled distribution of the optimal stimulus orientation disparities for 74 striate cells (37 simple, 3 hypercomplex I, 31 complex, 3 hypercomplex II) from nine cats. Orientation disparities for each animal have been measured with respect to the mean orientation disparity in that animal. Disparity equivalent to that produced by in-cyclorotation of eyes is positive. Adapted with permission from Nelson et al. (1977).

The data of Nelson et al. (1977) are more adequate (see Fig. 9/12). Indeed they show that most simple cells (33/37), which have the narrowest orientation tuning, had their orientation disparity in the range -6 to $+6°$. The width of orientation tuning was comparatively relatively wide: median HW at HH 16.7° (range 7.2° to 43.2°). Therefore, even the most narrowly tuned cell with a 6° orientation disparity would give a response over 50% at zero orientation disparity. This is also apparent for the actual data of 14 simple cells (Fig. 9/12). Compare the coarseness of orientation disparity tuning with the sharpness of position disparity tuning in Fig. 9/11. The data at present available thus suggest that orientation difference is a *coarse mechanism* allowing discrimination of tilted toward and tilted away from the animal but not much more [5], and that it relies, as the position disparity mechanism, mainly on cells of the simple family.

9.4 Neuronal Mechanisms Underlying Dynamic Depth Perception (Motion in Depth)

Psychophysically two possible cues for motion in depth have been suggested: a binocular mechanism, *sensitivity to motion in depth*, using the difference in direction and velocity of motion in each eye (Beverley and Regan, 1973) and a monocular mechanism, *changing size* (looming) detection (Regan and Beverley, 1978 a, b). As shown in Fig. 9/13, directions in depth on axes between the eyes correspond to motion of opposite direction in both eyes (antiphase), while direction in depth on axes outside the eyes correspond to motion in the same direction in both eyes (in phase). Within each of these axial domains, the axes change with the velocity ratio in both eyes. With such a mechanism, axes close to the head are overrepresented. Cynader and Regan (1978) have reported cells sensitive to motion in depth which they recorded in area 18 of the cat. About 30% (29/101 cells) of the area 18 cells (eccentricities 3–10°) were direction in depth sensitive. The first type (20 cells) of direction sensitive units (Fig. 9/14A) was monocular and had in fact an inhibition in the non-dominant eye of which the preferred direction was opposite to the preferred direction of the excitation of the dominant eye. These units (opposed motion type) signal motion away or towards the animal on *axes hitting the head*. It is noteworthy that the inhibition persisted over a broad range of position disparities (Fig. 9/14A) reminiscent of some of the disparity curves of what Ferster (1981) called far and near cells. Some of the cells described as directional were really axially selective in depth. The second type of direction selective in depth cells (9 cells) were usually binocular and

---

[5] The orientation disparity mechanism would only be a coarse stereopsis mechanism as the far and near cells in the position domain.

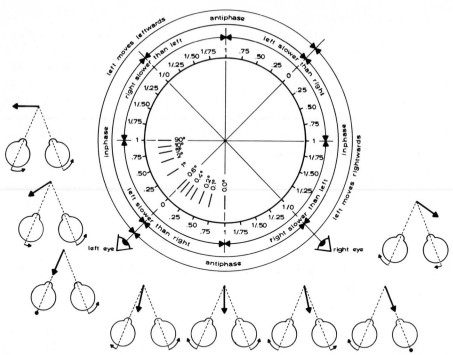

Fig. 9/13. Interocular differences in speed and direction corresponding to motion on different axes in space. Ratios of velocity in left eye and velocity in right eye (V_L/V_R) are marked round the circumference and are plotted linearly with azimuthal angle. These ratios were calculated geometrically by applying the method of Beverley and Regan (1975) to an interpupillary separation of 7 cm and a viewing distance of 145 cm. Note that a linear plot of V_L/V_R means that directions in real space are represented very non-linearly. Angles drawn inside the circle indicate that a 2.4° range of directions in real space is represented by the four central octants while the four octants represent the remaining 357.6° range of directions. The lettering outside the circle shows how each quadrant is related to the left and right image motions. These motions are illustrated for the four proximal quadrants. Modified from Cynader and Regan, 1978.

had a facilitatory interaction over a more restricted range of disparities. These cells were selective for directions on *axes missing the head* (Fig. 9/14B). In addition to direction selective in depth cells Cynader and Regan (1978) described "positional disparity units" or better sideways direction selective units. These cells responded only over a limited range of disparities and preferred a direction in a *fronto-parallel plane* (Fig. 9/14C): about 20% (17/101 cells) of the sample recorded by Cynader and Regan belonged to this category.

It is particularly striking that responses measured by Cynader and Regan (1978) are *usually less than 5 spikes/sweep*, although area 18 neurons are very responsive in terms of peak firing rate (Chapter 8). One wonders what would have been the direction in depth tuning if firing rate would have been used instead of number of spikes. Since the velocity changes in one eye, the duration of stimulation also changes and *firing rate seems more appropriate*

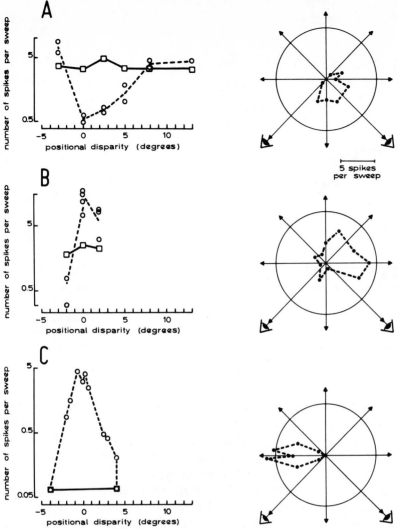

Fig. 9/14. Different types of direction selectivity in depth: selectivity for direction hitting the head (A), for directions missing the head (B) and for directions in a fronto-parallel plane (C). For each cell, the numbers of spikes per sweep is plotted logarithmically as ordinate versus the positional disparity (plotted linearly) in the graphs on the left-hand side. In these plots the zero disparity is arbitrary. The continuous lines plot the linear sum of responses to separate stimulations of the left and the right eyes. The heavy dashed lines plot the actual responses to identical stimulation of both eyes simultaneously (i.e., binocularly viewed sideways motion). The cell in A was strongly inhibited over a larger range of disparities, the cells in B and C were facilitated. For each cell, the plot on the right side shows the binocular selectivity for direction of motion plotted in polar coordinates looking down onto the left and right eyes. The number of spikes per sweep is plotted radially on a linear scale (dashed lines, dots). The ratio between the speeds of the left and right retinal image is plotted linearly round the circumference of the circle. This angular scale is very non-linear and emphasizes the 2.4° range of directions that pass between the eyes at the expense of the remaining 357.6° range of directions that misses the head (see Fig. 9/13). The cell in A had appreciable responses only to a narrow (2°) range of directions of motion for which the target would either hit or narrowly miss the head. The cell in B had best responses to directions away from the head along a line wide of the head. The cell in C leftward motion in a fronto-parallel plane. The stimulus settings were as follows, velocity: 37°/sec for the cell in A and 78°/sec in C, orientation: 30° anticlockwise from vertical for cells in B and C. Number of sweeps 20 in A and B, 30 in C. Modified from Cynader and Regan (1978).

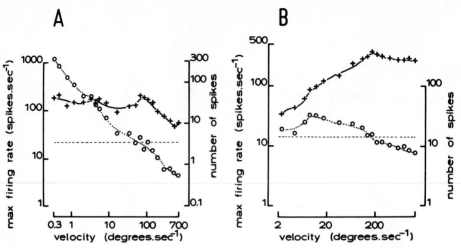

Fig. 9/15. Comparison of VR curves with maximum firing rate (crosses) and number of spikes (circles) as response measure for a velocity broad-band cell (A) and a velocity high-pass cell (B). Horizontal stippled lines: significance levels for maximum firing rate. For the cells illustrated in Fig. 9/14 Cynader and Regan (1978) used velocities between 35 and 80°/sec in the dominant eye.

as response measure. As shown in Fig. 9/15 both measures change differently with stimulus velocity and therefore the direction in depth tuning will be different with (maximum) firing rate as criterion. There are also other problems with the conclusions of Cynader and Regan (1978). Even admitting that cells with inhibition in the non-dominant eye (as in Fig. 9/14) are tuned to directions on axes hitting the head, it is difficult to conclude that they are specific for that direction. Indeed, since the binocular interaction is purely inhibitory, the response to the optimal direction in depth never exceeds the monocular response (e.g. evoked by a stimulus moving, in any direction, in front or behind the binocular interaction zone). Furthermore, the cells reported to be specific for axes missing the head (Fig. 9/14B) have a rather broad tuning. According to Van Essen and Maunsell (personal communication) such a tuning is observed when the position disparity, at which the different directions in depth are tested, is not optimal. The coarseness of the steps (2°) with which position disparity was actually investigated, for the cell of Fig. 9/14B, leaves this possibility open. And indeed in a later study Cynader and Regan (1982) found that the majority of selective cells changed their direction in depth tuning with position disparity. In a third study Regan and Cynader (1981), studied the velocity dependence of the direction in depth tuning. Their claim that velocity tuning of the inhibition in the non-dominant eye cannot explain the selectivity for axes hitting the head is even more dependent on their choice of number of spikes as response measure. Clearly the question of direction selectivity in depth requires further investigation.

Regan and Cynader (1979) also explored area 18 of the cat in search of cells *sensitive to changes in size*. They tested this with 2 edges of opposite polarity moving in or out of phase and found no conclusive evidence for such cells in area 18. Almost all of 56 area 18 cells studied by Regan and Cynader (1979) responded to change in size (49/56), but the bias favoring contraction or expansion switched, either when the contrast polarity (light bar or dark bar) was reversed (in 19/56 cells, mostly S1 cells), or when the change in size occurred in a different position in the RF (29/56 cells). Again their analysis is done using the number of spikes and it remains to be seen what results would have been produced by an analysis of peak firing rate.

9.5 Conclusion

Ocular dominance reflects only partially the binocularity of visual cortical cells. Binocular interactions are far more important than ocular dominance for the understanding of binocular vision. Although it is clear that these binocular interactions use the many differences between the attributes of the retinal image in both eyes, the neuronal mechanisms of static and dynamic stereopsis in the cat are still in dispute. There are indications that the tuned excitatory S cells of area 17 could play a major role in static fine stereopsis. It seems that the involvement of area 18 in dynamic stereopsis needs reinvestigation, with appropriate response measures.

Chapter 10. The Output of the Cat Visual Cortex

Important *laminar differences* in cortical output have been established: the deep layers (V and VI) project subcortically, while the superficial layers give rise to commissural (mainly layer III) and associative (layers II and III) projections (Gilbert and Kelly, 1975; Toyama et al., 1969 a). While this distinction is quite clear in area 17, the picture is less clear for areas 18 and 19 of which the deep and superficial layers project to area 17 (Bullier and Kennedy, personal communication). The *subcortical targets* include the pons, the superior colliculus, and the pretectum, the claustrum, the LGN, the pulvinar, and the lateralis posterior. The main *cortical targets* are other visual cortical areas: the lateral suprasylvian areas and areas 20 and 21. Relatively few projections to non-visual areas have been demonstrated. The subcortical projections of the visual cortex have been well studied and their function begins to be understood: most of them are related to the control of body motion and oculomotor function by vision. Relatively little is known of the corticocortical projections, which probably are important for further processing of the visual images and hence for visual perception.

10.1 The Projections of Layer V to the Superior Colliculus, Pons, Pretectum, and Pulvinar-LP Complex

It is now well established, both anatomically and physiologically, that *layer V of areas 17, 18, and 19 project to the superficial layers of the superior colliculus* (SC) (Gilbert and Kelly, 1975; Harvey, 1980 b; Hoffmann, 1973; Holländer, 1974; Lund et al., 1975; Magãlhaes-Castro et al., 1975; McIlwain, 1973; Palmer and Rosenquist, 1974). The projection is topographically organized (Kawamura et al., 1974; Updyke, 1977) and there is convergence on the same collicular cell of inputs from topographically related regions of all three areas (McIlwain, 1973, 1977). The projection is mainly ipsilateral, but a small contralateral projection has been claimed by Powell (1976) and Galletti et al. (1981). The visual cortical projection is part of a larger corticotectal projection arising from the whole cerebral cortex (Kawamura and Konno, 1979).

The corticotectal cells are *pyramidal cells* of layer V (Fig. 10/1) (Gilbert and Kelly, 1975; Lund et al., 1979). Gilbert and Kelly found about 1/3 of the

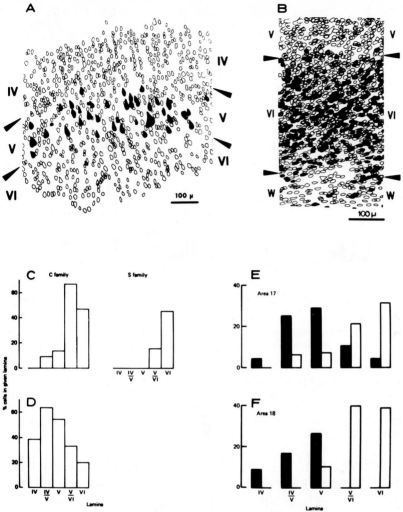

Fig. 10/1. Lamination of corticotectal and corticogeniculate efferents. A. A camera lucida drawing of the soma outlines of labeled and unlabeled cells in area 19 after injection of peroxydase in the SC. It is evident that the labeled cells represented a distinct class, the largest in layer V, and that they comprised a relatively high proportion of all the cells in the layer. Layers IV and VI were free of labeling. B. Camera lucida drawing of the outlines of labeled and unlabeled cell somata taken from a section of the postlateral gyrus, after counterstaining. Peroxydase injection in layer A of the LGN. The blackened outlines represent labeled cells, the clear outlines unlabeled cells. The labeled cells were confined to layer VI. Approximatively half of the total number of cells in the layer were labeled. A few labeled cells were found in the white matter, but neurons considered to be part of layer VI are commonly found in the white matter near the apex of a gyrus. C-D. Relative proportions of cells in the S and C families in each lamina which send axons to the dLGN (C) or superior colliculus (D). Data pooled from areas 17 and 18. E-F. Proportions of units in each of the deeper cortical laminae with axons efferent to the superior colliculus (filled blocks) or thalamus (open blocks). E: area 17; F: area 18. Units encountered at the boundaries between laminae have been placed in separate border groups (Henry et al., 1979; cf. Harvey, 1980 b). Adapted with permission from Gilbert and Kelly (1975) and from Harvey (1980 b).

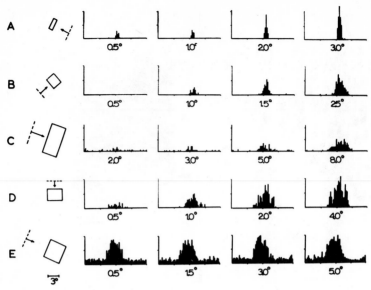

Fig. 10/2. Selected PST histograms illustrating summation with stimulus length (or its absence) several cortical cell types. Fields drawn to scale at the left of each series of histograms. In each case, stimuli are of constant width but length (given in degrees below each histogram) increases from a fraction of the field length up to the total field length in each case. Stimuli of various lengths presented in random order. Other parameters as follows. A: simple cell. Field 1.0 × 3.0°, abscissa 10.0°, 5.0 sec, ordinate 120 spikes/sec, slit width 10 min, 16 passes each. B: complex cell. Field 2.5 × 3.0°, abscissa 10.0°, 5.0 sec, ordinate 120 spikes/sec, slit width 7.5 min, 14 passes each. C: complex cell. Field 4.0 × 8.0°, abscissa 13.5°, 1.0 sec, ordinate 96 spikes/sec, slit width 1.0°, 16 passes each. D: complex cell. Field 3.0 × 4.0°, abscissa 7.0°, 1.0 sec, ordinate 128 spikes/sec, slit width 12 min, 20 passes each. E: complex corticotectal cell. Field 4.5 × 5.0°, abscissa 17.0°, 1.0 sec, ordinate 96 spikes/sec, slit width 0.5°, 24 passes each. Adapted with permission from Palmer and Rosenquist (1974).

layer V pyramidal cells to be retrogradely labelled after injection of HRP in the superior colliculus. Lund et al. (1979) insist that the cells labelled after tectal injections are in layer VB (lower part of layer V), while cells in layer VA project intracortically to the superficial layers. Inactivation of the visual cortex results in a loss of binocularity and direction selectivity of collicular cells (Mize and Murphy, 1976; Rizzolatti et al., 1970; Rosenquist and Palmer, 1971; Wickelgren and Sterling, 1969).

The corticotectal cells have been *identified physiologically* by antidromic stimulation of the SC. Palmer and Rosenquist (1974) reported that area 17 corticotectal cells were complex cells characterized by large RFs, little length summation (Fig. 10/2), almost equal input from both eyes (ocular dominance class 3, 4, 5), and in many instances direction selectivity and responses to fast stimuli (over 80°/sec). Gilbert (1977) took area 17 corticotectal cells as prototypes of his special complex cells (see Chapter 4). Harvey (1980 b) used the A, B, C, S classification scheme to study area 17 and 18 corticotectal cells. According to Harvey, all corticotectal cells belonged to the C family and were binocular (classes 3, 4 and 5). This is in keeping with the strong peak of C family distribution in layer V (Harvey, 1980 b; see also Chapter 4). Harvey (1980 b) further reports that almost all corticotectal cells were recorded in layer V and its border with layers IV and VI, although occasionally one was recorded in layer IV or VI (Fig. 10/1). Since it is fairly well established that all corticotectal cells are layer V pyramids, this can be seen as an indication that one can record at some distance from the cell soma, at least of pyramidal cells. The corticotectal cells have fast-conducting axons (Harvey, 1980 b; Hoffmann, 1973). The corticotectal cells can be further subdivided (Harvey, 1980 b) into HC cells (4/22), C cells showing no length summation (i.e. the Palmer and Rosenquist (1974) type, Fig. 10/2 or spot cells) (10/22) and C cells showing length summation (8/22). The first two types were mostly direction selective, the latter not. Corticotectal C family cells usually have high spontaneous activity, wide orientation tuning and respond to fast movements even in area 17 (Harvey, 1980 b). Harvey (1980 b) estimated that about 60% of C family cells of layer V project to the SC (Fig. 10/1).

It is also anatomically (Albus et al., 1981; Kawamura and Chiba, 1979) and physiologically (Albus and Donate-Oliver, 1977; Gibson et al., 1978) established that *layer V of areas 17, 18 and 19 projects to the rostral parts of the pons*. The projection is denser from areas 18 and 19 than from area 17 (Albus et al., 1981; Sanides et al., 1978), although Brodal (1972 a, b) found projections in equal strength from areas 17 and 18. Albus et al. (1981) note that in terms of number of cells per visual degree the difference between areas 17 and 18 or 19 may be quite small given the larger magnification in area 17. Exactly as with the corticotectal projection, the visual corticopontine projection is part of a larger corticopontine projection arising from the whole cortex (Kawamura and Konno, 1979). More important is that the corticopontine projections arise mainly, if not exclusively, from cortical regions subserving the peripheral visual field (over 10° eccentricity) (Albus and Donate-Oliver, 1977; Albus et al., 1981; Gibson et al., 1978; Sanides et al., 1978). This suggests that there is a demagnification of central visual field regions in this projection, which is monosynaptically linked to the cerebellar vermis (Fries and Albus, 1980), so that in the cortico-pontino-cerebellar pathway the peripheral visual field is represented as largely as the central visual field.

Although the corticopontine cells have not been studied in the A, B, C, S scheme, all their properties, large RFs, equal excitatory input from both eyes, and response to diffuse flash and to multispot patterns (Albus and Donate-Oliver, 1977; Gibson et al., 1978), suggest that they are C family cells as are the corticotectal cells and in fact Albus and Donate-Oliver (1977) found a few cells projecting both to the pons and the SC. According to Gibson et al. (1978), area 18 corticopontine cells were often direction selective (preferring downwards movements) and preferred fast stimulus speeds (some of VR curves shown by Gibson et al., 1978 suggest that they may be VHP cells). Gibson et al. (1978) reported that corticopontine cells preferred faster movements than other area 18 cells. [1]

Areas 17, 18 and 19 have been shown to *project topographically to the pretectum*, more precisely to the nucleus of the optic tract (Kawamura et al., 1974; Updyke, 1977). This projection also probably arises from layer V pyramidal cells (Schoppmann, 1981). In addition there is a projection from area 19 (and possibly area 18) to the anterior pretectal nucleus (Updyke, 1977). The properties of the corticopretectal cells suggest that they also belong to the C family (Schoppmann, 1981). Some of the corticopretectal cells also project to the SC. According to Schoppmann (1981) areas 17 and 18 give rise to a stronger projection to NOT than does area 19.

Finally areas 17, 18 and 19 project topographically (Kawamura et al., 1974; Updyke, 1977) to the *lateral part of the lateralis posterior* (cortico-recipient zone, see Chapter 3). Area 19 also projects topographically to the pulvinar (Updyke, 1977). At least for area 17, Lund et al. (1979) have shown that the projection to lLP arises from layer V pyramidal cells (layer VB). Lund et al. (1979) suggest that the large layer V pyramidal cells send axon collaterals to both the SC and lLP, which would then suggest that corticolateralis posterior cells also belong to the C family.

It seems thus that layer V C family cells have extensive projections to neuronal centers involved in visuomotor function and that eventually the same layer V pyramidal can send axons to all 4 major subcortical targets. Since corticotectal cells belong to the Y system (Hoffmann, 1973), this is a further example of branching in the Y system. Depending on the subcortical target, the sensitivity of C family cells to movement of large patterns (multi-spot or noise) or to movement of small spots will be important. Spot sensitivity could be important for the projection to the SC possibly involved in foveation (visual grasping). Sensitivity to movements of large patterns may be important for the projection to the pretectum which is involved in oculo-motor stabilization reflexes such as the OKN (Hoffmann, 1982), and possibly for the projection to the pons which may signal the movement of the animal with respect to the terrain and contribute to visual guidance of movements (Gibson et al., 1978).

10.2 The Projections of Layer VI to the dLGN and the Claustrum

The 3 visual areas 17, 18 and 19 *project back to dLGN* in a topographical order (Kawamura et al., 1974; Updyke, 1977). This projection has been

---

[1] It remains to be seen to what extent this results from the large bin widths (over 200 msec) used by Gibson et al. (1978). Indeed corticopontine cells have wide RFs and cells with smaller RFs give shorter responses at fast velocities, which will be underestimated by the use of large bin widths (Orban et al., 1981 a Fig. 2).

shown, both anatomically (Gilbert and Kelly, 1975; Lund et al., 1979; Tömböl et al., 1975) and physiologically (Harvey, 1980 b; Tsumoto and Suda, 1980; Tsumoto et al., 1978), to arise from layer VI of areas 17, 18 and 19 (Fig. 10/1). The termination of the corticogeniculate projection differs according to the area of origin (Updyke, 1975). Area 17 projects heavily to all geniculate layers giving rise to a column of labelled cells orthogonal to the geniculate layers. The area 18 projection is less heavy but extends throughout all layers although the interlaminar plexi and the magnocellular C lamina are more densely labelled after HRP injection into area 18. Area 19 projects mainly to the parvocellular C layers. Thus the corticothalamic projections mirror the thalamocortical projections (see Chapter 3). Anatomically, topographical projections have been demonstrated from areas 17, 18 and 19 to the MIN and the ventral LGN although the projections of area 17 to this latter nucleus is scant (Updyke, 1977).

The cells of origin of corticothalamic projections are mostly pyramidal cells according to Gilbert and Kelly (1975). Tömböl et al. (1975) distinguished three types of corticothalamic cells: the majority were pyramidal cells in the upper part of layer VI, some of them had a smaller ovoid soma and some, still smaller, had a fusiform aspect. The corticothalamic projection has both excitatory and inhibitory effects on LGN cells, mostly on X cells (Tsumoto et al., 1978). The excitatory effects were seen between pairs of LGN and cortical cells having RFs up to 2.3° apart and inhibitory effects between pairs having RFs up to 3.1° apart (Tsumoto et al., 1978).

There is now evidence that there are *3 projection systems from layer VI to the dLGN:* a fast projecting system arising from C (Harvey, 1980 b) or complex (Gilbert, 1977; Tsumoto and Suda, 1980) cells in the upper part of layer VI, an intermediate projection system arising from S (Harvey, 1980 b) or simple (Tsumoto and Suda, 1980) cells in the lower part of layer VI, and finally a slow projecting system arising from visually unresponsive cells in lower layer VI (Tsumoto and Suda, 1980). It is tempting to correlate these 3 physiologically identified systems to the 3 types of efferent cells described by Tömböl et al. (1975): the pyramidal cells in the upper part of VI to the C cells, the cells with an ovoid soma to the S cells and the very small fusiform cells to the unresponsive cells. The corticothalamic C cells were mostly binocular (ocular dominance classes 3, 4 and 5) and half of them showed length summation the other half did not (Harvey, 1980 b). Corticothalamic C cells further resembled corticotectal cells in having high spontaneous activity, broad orientation tuning, responses to fast movements, and often direction selectivity (Harvey, 1980 b). The corticothalamic S cells were often direction selective, but in opposition to C cells, often monocular (class 1 and 7). Many of these corticothalamic S cells were monosynaptically driven from the LGN, in oppositon to corticotectal cells which were usually disynaptically activated (Harvey, 1980 b). This has been confirmed by the intracellular study of

Ferster (1981). According to Harvey (1980b) about 60% of the lamina VI C family cells and 45% of the layer VI S family cells are efferent to the dLGN (Fig. 10/1).

The intermediate projection arising from layer VI S cells has been implicated by Harvey (1980 b) and Tsumoto and Suda (1980) in the control of binocular interactions in the dLGN following the suggestion of Schmielau and Singer (1977) and Singer (1977). These latter authors suggested that cortical disparity sensitive cells when optimally activated would excite the appropriate LGN cells, both by direct facilitation and by removal of the geniculate binocular inhibition, and would let the geniculate binocular inhibition come into play when not activated. This requires the corticothalamic cells to be very disparity sensitive as are S cells (see Chapter 9). This hypothesis receives strong support from the finding of Tsumoto and Suda (1980) that the intermediate projection is absent in the monocular segment of area 17. The fast projection from C cells would have a more diffuse effect through perigeniculate cells (Harvey, 1980 b) or be involved in a local amplification through a positive feedback loop (Tsumoto et al., 1978). Finally, Tsumoto and Suda (1980) suggested that the slow projecting cells may play a role in the development of the reciprocal geniculocortical connections.

The visual areas 17, 18, and 19 together with other visual areas such as the lateral suprasylvian area, project ipsi- and contralaterally *to the dorsal caudal parts of the claustrum* (Jayaraman and Updyke, 1979; Sanides and Buchholtz, 1979; Squatrito et al., 1980 a, b). Anatomically no retinotopic organization was found (Jayaraman and Updyke, 1979; Squatrito et al., 1980 a, b). LeVay and Sherk (1981) demonstrated that the corticoclaustral projection arises from layer VI and has a retinotopic organization. According to Sherk and LeVay (1981 a, b) claustral cells display important length summation as do layer VI simple cells according to Gilbert (1977). They therefore concluded that corticoclaustral projections arise from layer VI simple cells. Little is known of the function of the reciprocal corticoclaustral connections. Sherk and LeVay (1982) have suggested that claustral input to area 17 may contribute to the end-stopping of area 17 cells.

10.3 The Commissural Projections

Although the commissural projections through the corpus callosum form a complex system of fibers linking different visual areas in both hemispheres (see Table 3/6) only the projection of the 17–18 border has been studied *physiologically*. It is clear from recent studies (Harvey, 1980 b; Innocenti, 1980) that the RF types of the efferent neurons are more diverse than those of recipient neurons. According to Harvey (1980 b) any RF type of the 4

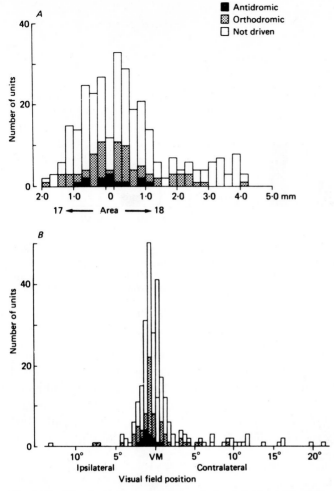

Fig. 10/3. Histological location (A) and visual field position (B) of cells tested by electrical stimulation of the corpus callosum (c.c.) and contralateral visual cortex (c.v.). A: position with respect to the 17–18 border, B: position with respect to the vertical midline (VM). *Filled blocks*, antidromically activated cells, stippled *blocks*, orthodromically activated cells, open blocks, cells not excited from c.c. or c.v. Adapted with permission from Harvey (1980 b).

families of the A, B, C, S scheme projects through the corpus callosum, while the recipient cells are more often B or C cells. While the projecting neurons are monocular as well as binocular, recipient neurons are more often binocular although some were monocular (Harvey, 1980 b). The RF position of efferent and afferent neurons (Fig. 10/3) is clearly concentrated on the vertical meridian (VM) with an extension in the ipsilateral visual field (up to 5°). This confirms that at the 17–18 border level, the corpus callosum is really an expansion of intracortical connections linking retinotopically adjoining regions on the VM exactly as the intracortical fibers link neighbouring regions

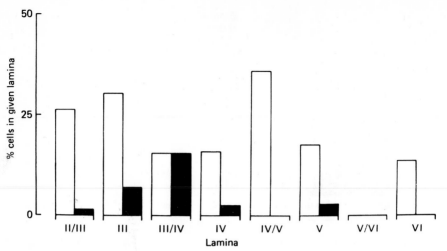

Fig. 10/4. Proportion of cells in each cortical lamina antidromically (filled blocks) or orthodromically (open blocks) activated after electrical stimulation of the corpus callosum and/or contralateral visual cortex. Data pooled from areas 17, 17–18 and 18. Cells encountered at the
boundaries between laminae have been placed in separate border groups. Adapted with permission from Harvey (1980 b).

further away from the VM [2]. The efferent neurons were recorded mainly from
deep lamina III (Fig. 10/4) while the recipient neurons were more scattered
through all layers (Harvey, 1980 b). While all recipient cells were indirectly
driven from the optic radiation some of the projecting cells were monosynaptically linked to the LGN (Harvey, 1980 b). This is in agreement with Hornung and Garey's (1980) observation that spiny stellate callosal neurons bear
geniculocortical synapses.

10.4 The Associative Corticocortical Projections

The 3 cortical areas 17, 18, and 19 are *reciprocally connected* (Gilbert and
Kelly, 1975; Kawamura, 1973; Squatrito et al., 1981 a, b). Most of these
connections arise from lamina II and III (Gilbert and Kelly, 1975; Lund et
al., 1979) although the projection from area 19 to area 17 arises from layer
VI (Gilbert and Kelly, 1975) and spiny stellate cells of area 17 layer IV project
to area 18 (Meyer and Albus, 1981 a). Using fluorescent tracers, Bullier and
Kennedy (personal communication) observed that both superficial and deep

---

[2] Recently the corpus callosum have been implicated by Elberger (1982) in the development of
maximal visual acuity. It may well be that this development depends on intracortical connections
at the level of the area centralis representation.

layers of area 19 project back to area 17. Connections between areas 17 and 19 seem especially dense and to occur in patches (Gilbert and Wiesel, 1980). Given the parallel operation in these 3 areas these intracortical connections could have mainly "coupling" functions, linking the activity in topographically related parts of the 3 areas (see Chapter 2). This "coupling" function may be important if the 3 cortical regions analyse different aspects of the same visual object or analyse the same object under different circumstances (e.g. when it moves or remains stationary).

The cortical output of the three cortical areas 17, 18 and 19 as a whole is mainly *to other visual areas*, most notably to the lateral suprasylvian (LS) areas (Gilbert and Kelly, 1975; Hubel and Wiesel, 1965; Lund et al., 1979; Squatrito et al., 1981 a, b; Toyama et al., 1969 a). The lateral suprasylvian areas send reciprocal connections back to areas 17, 18 and 19. Areas 17 and 18 also project to areas 20 and 21 while area 19 only projects to area 21 (Squatrito et al., 1981 a, b). The only non-visual targets are areas 5 and 7[3] to which both areas 18 and 19 project (Squatrito et al., 1981 a, b) and area 6 to which area 19 (Squatrito et al., 1981 b) and possibly areas 17 and 18 project (Garey et al., 1968). The visual cortex projections to the lateral suprasylvian areas (LS) arises from lamina III (Gilbert and Kelly, 1975; Lund et al., 1979) and terminates mainly in layer III and V (Sugiyama, 1979). It seems that LS areas are the necessary, or at least the main, relay through which information processed by the visual cortex can reach non-visual areas such as the limbic areas (see Fig. 10/5). If this were true, then there may be an analogy with the monkey where according to Mishkin (1980) and Macko et al. (1982) the visual information flow divides between areas processing the *"where"* (areas 5 and 7) and the *"what"* (inferotemporal areas), the latter information finally

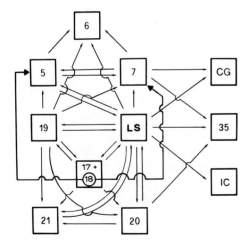

Fig. 10/5. Flow diagram of corticocortical connections. Block diagram derived from Squatrito et al.'s (1981 a, b) data and previous data (Heath and Jones, 1970, 1971; Kawamura, 1973; Shoumura, 1972; Shoumura and Itoh, 1972), summarizing the known interconnections of cortical visual areas and the spreading of the visual input to other cortical areas. LS = lateral suprasylvian visual area limited to PMLS + PLLS subdivisions. CG = cingulate gyrus; IC = insular cortex. Adapted with permission from Squatrito et al. (1981 b). Compare with Fig. 2/11C.

---

[3] Dow and Dubner (1971) have described visual responses in area 7 under chloralose anesthesia.

reaching the amygdala and limbic areas. In this analogy, LS areas may represent a further stage in the visual processing leading to recognition of visual objects ("what") and hence play an important role in cat visual perception as witnessed by the large deficit of lesions in this region (Sprague et al., 1977).

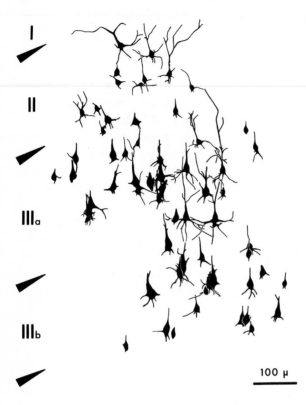

I

II

IIIₐ

IIIᵦ

100 μ

Fig. 10/6. A camera lucida drawing of the cells in layers II and III of area 18 after a peroxidase injection in the Clare-Bishop area (part of the LS areas). The labeled cells were all pyramids. The boundaries of the layers were drawn after the section was counterstained. They are indicated by Roman numerals. Adapted with permission from Gilbert and Kelly (1975).

The physiological properties of cortically projecting neurons are almost unknown. One of the reasons is that in a given cortical area very few cells are antidromically driven from other cortical areas (Henry, personal communication). This is no wonder given the observation of Gilbert and Kelly (1975) that very few area 17 or 18 cells (Fig. 10/6) were retrogradely labelled after HRP injection in other cortical areas (no more than 5% in each layer). Henry et al. (1978 b) have shown that indeed only 6.5% of cells in laminae II and III of area 17 could be driven by antidromic stimulation from PMLS, despite the use of 6 stimulation electrodes. The majority of these cells (8/11) belonged to the B family, 2 others belonging to the S family. On the contrary, area 17 cells receiving afferents from LS were more numerous and belonged to any family.

10.5 Conclusion

The subcortical projections of areas 17, 18 and 19 are relatively well understood. They project to brainstem structures involved in motor and oculomotor control and to the thalamic nuclei afferent to the visual cortex. The corticocortical projections of area 17, 18 and 19 are poorly understood. The major output seems to be to the LS areas. It seems that further study of this output is essential for understanding the cat visual system.

Chapter 11. Correlation Between Geniculate Afferents and Visual Cortical Response Properties in the Cat

The properties of cortical cells depend to a certain extent on *the type of their geniculate afferents*. Since the first description of cortical RF organization (Hubel and Wiesel, 1962), attempts have been made to explain RF structure by the type of geniculate afferents (ON or OFF center). More recently, the discovery of different functional streams in the retino-geniculo-cortical pathway (X, Y, W) has promoted the view that many properties of cortical cells are the reflection of the X, Y or W type of geniculate afferents (see Stone et al., 1979 for review). In the extreme, labels of subcortical functional types have been used to categorize cortical cells (De Valois et al., 1982 b). More commonly, it has been believed that spatial frequency sensitivity or velocity sensitivity depend on the X, Y or W type of afferents. Recent evidence however suggests that velocity sensitivity depends mainly on intra-cortical mechanisms, leaving only spatial frequency sensitivity dependent on the type of LGN input. Only electrical stimulation of the visual pathways allows, within certain limits, *direct identification* of the type of geniculate afferents (X, Y, or W) of a cortical cell. This type of experiments relies on the different conduction velocities of the different types of afferents (see Chapter 3). All other attempts to identify the type of geniculate input to cortical cells provide only *indirect* evidence and should be interpreted with the greatest caution.

11.1 Electrical Stimulation of the Visual Pathways

The first report in which electrical stimulation of the visual pathways was used to identify the type of afferents to cortical cells, was a short note by Hoffmann and Stone (1971) showing that 40% of the complex cells of area 17 could be driven monosynaptically by fast conducting afferents, while simple and hypercomplex cells were not discharged by fast afferents, although some of them could be activated by slow afferents. These results, which have often been misquoted by saying that complex cells receive Y afferents and simple cells X afferents, showed that electrical stimulation experiments, in which optic radiation (OR) *and* optic chiasm (OX) are stimulated, can answer two questions: (1) by which type of afferents (X, Y or W) are the different RF types driven (2) which RF types are monosynaptically or polysynaptically connected to LGN afferents. It should be noted that answering the second question implies that the first question has been answered. And as mentioned in Chapter 3, this supposes the measurement of OX and OR latencies. The state of the literature only allows us to consider LGN inputs of the different RF types in areas 17 and 18, as the only paper correlating LGN afferents with properties of area 19 neurons (Kimura et al., 1980), erroneously considered all area 19 cells as complex.

It should be noted that a substantial number of cortical cells can apparently *not be driven* by electrical stimulation of the afferent visual pathways. Singer et al. (1975) and Tretter et al. (1975) reported that 75% of area 17 cells and 81% of area 18 cells responded to LGN stimulation compared to 36% of area 17 cells and 75% of area 18 cells responding to OX stimulation. The larger proportion of cells driven from the chiasm in area 18 compared to area 17, is compatible with the larger proportion of Y afferents to area 18. Indeed it has been reported that LGN cells responding to OX stimulation with short latencies (as Y cells do) tend to respond more reliably than cells responding with long latencies (as X cells do) (Hoffmann et al., 1972; Stone and Dreher, 1973). According to Bullier and Henry (1979 a) 92/258 (36%) of area 17 cells cannot be driven by electrical stimulation of the OR and according to Harvey (1980 a) 29% of area 18 cells cannot be driven either from the OX or from the OR. In both areas the cells not driven by electrical stimulation occur mainly in layer II–III and VI (Bullier and Henry, 1979 c, Harvey, 1980 a). On the contrary, most cells in layer IV and deep layer III could be driven.

Another difficulty with the electrical stimulation experiments is the possible convergence of 2 types of afferents onto the same cortical cell. This may be further complicated by the convergence of excitatory and inhibitory inputs onto the same cell, since the latter inputs could mask longer latency excitatory responses. Intracellular recordings have indeed shown that areas 17 and 18 cells driven monosynaptically from the LGN are also disynaptically inhibited by electrical stimulation of the LGN (Toyama et al., 1977 a). Similarly cells driven disynaptically from the LGN, show trisynaptic inhibitory postsynaptic potentials. However the relative separation of X and Y afferents within layer IV (see Chapter 3) suggests that at least stellate cells with their restricted dendritic tree, must receive predominantly one type of input.

All studies (Bullier and Henry, 1979 a; Harvey, 1980 a; Henry et al., 1979; Singer et al., 1975; Toyama et al., 1977 a; Tretter et al., 1975) agree that *most RF types, including complex types, can be monosynaptically driven from the LGN* (Fig. 11/1). A notable exception seems to be the B family, although the numbers studied up to now are small: Henry et al. (1979) reported on 4 B cells and Bullier and Henry (1979 a) on 9 B cells in area 17: none of them was driven monosynaptically. Similarly in area 18 Harvey (1980 a) found only one out of 9 B family cells to be monosynaptically driven from the OR. All

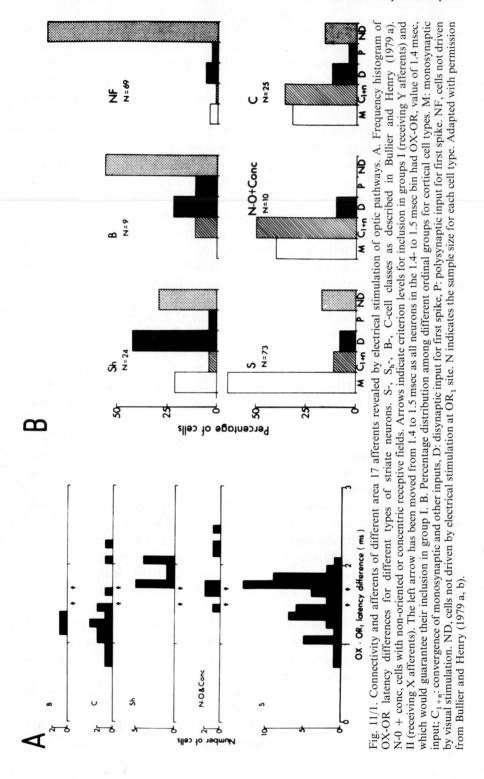

Fig. 11/1. Connectivity and afferents of different area 17 afferents revealed by electrical stimulation of optic pathways. A. Frequency histogram of OX-OR latency differences for different types of striate neurons. S-, S_h-, B-, C-cell classes as described in Bullier and Henry (1979 a). N-0 + conc, cells with non-oriented or concentric receptive fields. Arrows indicate criterion levels for inclusion in groups I (receiving Y afferents) and II (receiving X afferents). The left arrow has been moved from 1.4 to 1.5 msec as all neurons in the 1.4- to 1.5 msec bin had OX-OR, value of 1.4 msec, which would guarantee their inclusion in group I. B. Percentage distribution among different ordinal groups for cortical cell types. M: monosynaptic input; C_{1+n}: convergence of monosynaptic and other inputs, D: disynaptic input for first spike, P: polysynaptic input for first spike. NF, cells not driven by visual stimulation. ND, cells not driven by electrical stimulation at OR_1 site. N indicates the sample size for each cell type. Adapted with permission from Bullier and Henry (1979 a, b).

Table 11/1. The afferent connectivity of parastriate receptive field classes

	Latency group						
	1	2	3	OR only	Ox only	N.e.s.	Total
S	43	8	3	10	4	13	81
S$_H$	7	2	0	0	0	2	11
C	7	19	8	3	0	2	39
C$_H$	1	7	2	1	0	1	12
B	1	3	2	0	0	0	6
B$_H$	0	1	0	1	0	1	3
A	1	0	0	0	0	0	1
N.o.	2	0	0	0	0	1	3
N.v.c.	16	12	6	28	2	62	126

N.e.s., not driven by electrical stimulation
N.v.c. not visually classified
N.o. non-oriented
Latency group 1 OR latency between 1 and 2 ms and OX latency between 2 and 3 ms, probably
monosynaptically driven
2 OR latency between 2 and 3 ms and OX latency between 3 and 4 ms, probably
disynaptically driven
3 remaining cells of which OR and OX latencies do not fall into either of the
above groups
Adapted from Harvey (1980 a)

studies further agree that simple cells or S cells are more often monosynaptically driven (60–80%) than complex cells or C family cells (20–40%) (Table 11/1). These results fit with the recent intracellular study of Ferster (1981), showing that most area 17 cells, except those in layer II and deep V, receive monosynaptic LGN input. Bullier and Henry (1979 a) noted that among the C cells, those monosynaptically driven are more often direction selective. In area 17 at least, less end-stopped S cells seem to be monosynaptically linked to the LGN than end-free S cells. While Singer et al. (1975) reported that *all* their area 17 class I cells (having exclusively ON or OFF subregions) were monosyaptically driven compared to only 60% of their simple cells, other reports (Bullier and Henry, 1979 a; Harvey, 1980 a) including that of Tretter et al. (1975) on area 18, do not support the idea that S1 cells (see Chapter 4) are more often monosynaptically driven than S2 cells. All these reports are difficult to reconcile with the serial hypothesis of Hubel and Wiesel (1965), and rather suggest that the different RF types are first order elements of different streams running in parallel within the cortex (Bullier and Henry, 1979 a). The latter hypothesis is strongly supported by the recent experiments of Malpeli (1981) showing that layer IV simple cell activity is not necessary to support the visually driven activity of complex cells in layers II and V (see Chapter 4 for further arguments in favor of a parallel operation of the different RF types).

The question of the correlation between RF type and type of LGN afferents is trivial in area 18, since almost all direct LGN afferents are Y

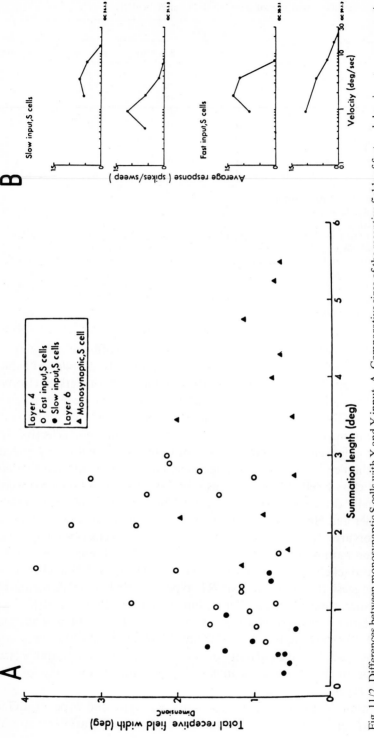

Fig. 11/2. Differences between monosynaptic S cells with X and Y input. A. Comparative sizes of the receptive fields of fast and slow input monosynaptic S cells of lamina 4 and all monosynaptic S cells of lamina 6 portrayed by plotting the total width of the receptive field, against its summation length measured in a length-response curve. B. Velocity tuning curves of four monosynaptic S cells in lamina 4. Top two curves are from slow input S cells (i.e. X-recipient); lower two curves from fast input S cells (i.e. Y-recipient). Adapted with permission from Mustari et al. (1982).

afferents. This clearly underlines that Y afferents can be connected to any cortical RF type. For area 17 there seems to be some disagreement between Singer et al. (1975) and later work. According to Singer et al. (1975) there seems to be no difference in proportion of simple and complex cells driven by Y, X or W afferents. Indeed in their Fig. 4 the number of cells showing a OX-OR latency difference below 1.55 msec (receiving Y afferents) between 1.55 and 2.2 ms (receiving X afferents) and over 2.2 msec (receiving W afferents) is almost equal for simple or complex cells. Later work (Bullier and Henry, 1979 b; Henry et al., 1979), however, clearly suggests that *while X and Y afferents are about equally represented among afferents to S cells, B and C cells are mostly fed by Y afferents*[1] *and strongly end-stopped S cells chiefly by X afferents* (Fig. 11/1). Bullier and Henry (1979 b) found few differences between S cells fed by X and Y afferents, at least when using hand-held stimuli. This point was taken up further in a quantitative study of mono-synaptically driven S cells of area 17 by Mustari et al. (1982). These authors showed that among monosynaptically driven S cells, those driven by Y afferents, as a population, have larger RFs (both in length and width) than those fed by X afferents. These authors further report that there may be less difference in end-stopping between S family cells driven by X or Y afferents than initially (Henry et al., 1979) reported. There was much less difference in velocity tuning than in RF dimensions between S cells driven by X and Y afferents (Fig. 11/2), both types of S cells being mostly of the velocity low-pass type as far as the data, which unfortunately plot the response in number of spikes, allow us to conclude. However Mustari et al. (1982) noted that almost all S cells having cut-off velocities over 20 deg/sec, which probably correspond to our (Orban et al., 1981 a) area 17 velocity tuned and broad-band S cells, and to Kulikowski et al. (1981) fast simple cells, had Y afferents. These results clearly show that Y afferents project upon area 17 S cells, including a large proportion of velocity low-pass cells, and are therefore as X afferents probably involved in the spatial analysis of retinal image, although in a lower spatial frequency range.

As an alternative to electrical stimulation experiments, the study of the correlation between firing of cortical cells and retinal ganglion cells (Lee et al., 1977 b) or geniculate cells (Tsumoto et al., 1978) has been used. Although the experiments seem feasible the number of pairs recorded until now is still too small to allow any firm conclusions.

11.2 The Question of ON or OFF Cell Input to Cortical S Cells

Originally Hubel and Wiesel (1962) hypothesized that a simple cell receives input from a single row of geniculate cells, ON *or* OFF center cells.

---

[1] Recent data of Henry, Mustari and Bullier (personal communication) however suggest that B cells could be the X driven complex cells and C cells, the Y driven complex cells.

Bishop et al. (1973) proposed a model for simple cells, derived mainly from responses to moving stimuli, in which area 17 simple cells receive input from both ON *and* OFF LGN cells. Recently three different approaches have been used to tackle this question. Bullier et al. (1982) compared the responses of first order S cells and of LGN cells to stationary flashed light bars and to moving light and dark bars. From the observations of responses of ON and OFF center LGN cells, they concluded that when responses to a moving stimulus are put in accurate register with the stationary response, taking into account the latency, then a moving bar with its contrast appropriate to the RF center evokes a response on the near side of the center response to the stationary slit and a moving bar of opposite contrast a response on the far side (Fig. 11/3). Occasionally the moving bar of appropriate contrast evokes a secondary peak at the far side of the RF center. Bullier et al. (1982) also noted that geniculate responses to moving bars of contrast appropriate to the RF center had shorter latencies (60–95 msec) than those evoked by moving bars of opposite contrast (140 to 185 msec). We have made similar observations in the LGN (Orban et al., 1981). Transferring these rules to the responses of first order S cells, Bullier et al. (1982) considered that *one quarter of these cells received input from a single type of ON or OFF LGN* cell (Fig. 11/4). All these cells had a response to stationary flashed slits consisting of a single ON or OFF region and correspond to what we call S1 cells. Most first order S cells however, *receive a dual input (ON and OFF center)* according to Bullier et al. (1982). That the response to stationary flashed stimuli has a second (OFF in Fig. 11/4) component and that the responses to moving light and dark bars correspond to the ON and OFF regions of the flashing bar responses is seen by Bullier et al. (1982) as evidence for a dual input (Fig. 11/4).

Lee et al. (1981 a) have taken another approach: they measured the phase of retinal and geniculate cell responses to moving sinusoidal gratings. They obtained a bimodal distribution clustering at phases −0.1 and 0.4 cycles, corresponding respectively to ON and OFF center ganglion or geniculate cells. Lee et al. (1981 b) have applied the same methods to cortical cells, which they claim were simple cells, although the response to moving light and dark bars of some of the cells suggest that they were not simple cells. Those authors conclude that simple cells also show a bimodal phase distribution with two modes separated by 0.5 cycles and are thus predominantly driven by 1 type of input (ON or OFF center) (Fig. 11/5).

The two previous studies consider only excitatory inputs from ON or OFF center LGN cells onto cortical cells. Cortical S cells could also receive an excitatory and an inhibitory input from the same type of LGN afferents (ON or OFF). This conclusion was reached by Heggelund (1981 a) who tested the interactions between two stationary flashed stimuli. Heggelund (1981 a) showed that when one of the slits was in the dominating part of the field (ON or OFF), then simultaneous presentation of a second slit in phase

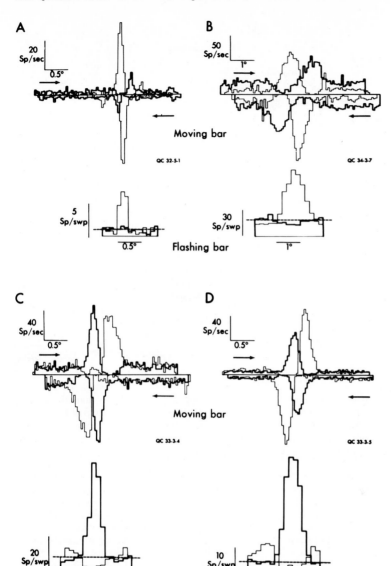

Fig. 11/3. Correspondence between flashing light field and moving bar response patterns for ON-center (A and B) and OFF-center (C and D) neurons in the LGN. The average response histograms for light and dark bars have been shifted by a number of bins corresponding to the cell's response latency and the resulting patterns positioned in spatial correspondence with the flashing bar response field. The flashing bar response field is made up of the strength of the ON-response (thin line) and OFF-response (thick line) at different positions. The unit of response is the spike per sweep and each sweep is made up of an 0.8 sec presentation (ON or OFF) with 1 to 2 sec hold times between presentations. The interrupted lines in the flashing bar histogram record the level of spontaneous activity. A: $0.1° \times 0.2°$ moving bar, 20 sweeps at $0.46°$/sec. B: $0.2° \times 0.6°$ moving bar, 20 sweeps at $1.83°$/sec. C: $0.1° \times 0.5°$ moving bar, 20 sweeps at $0.46°$/sec. D: $0.1° \times 0.7°$ moving bar, 20 sweeps at $0.46°$/sec. Adapted with permission from Bullier et al. (1982).

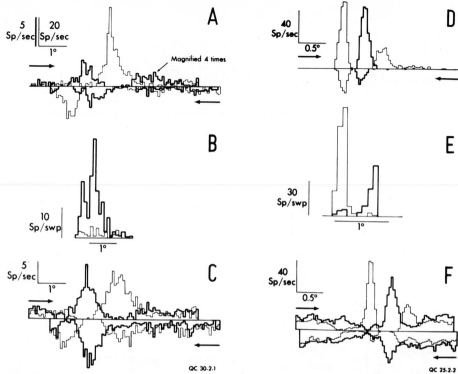

Fig. 11/4. Response patterns of monosynaptic S cells with single and dual (ON and OFF center) input. A-C: Response patterns of a monosynaptic S cell receiving from one group of LGN input neurons (OFF-center brisk transient). A: shows the cell's response to light and dark moving bars (LB and DB). The response to the dark bar is magnified 4 times to reveal small discharge peaks, B: the flashing light response field, C: the cell's response to light and dark moving bar under the influence of monocular conditioning. The average response histograms in A and C have been shifted to compensate for the cell's response latency. A: $0.1° \times 1.8°$, 55 (LB) and 100 (DB) sweeps at $1.83°$/sec. B: $0.1° \times 1.8°$, 5 presentations. C: $0.1° \times 1.8°$, 182 (LB) and 160 (DB) sweeps at $3.66°$/sec. D-F: Response patterns of a monosynaptic S cell receiving from two groups of LGN brisk sustained neurons. D: shows the histograms to light and dark moving bars (shifted to compensate for response latencies). E: illustrates the flashing light response pattern and F: the response histogram to moving light and dark bars in the presence of a monocular conditioning stimulus. D: $0.1° \times 0.3°$ moving bars, 20 sweeps at $0.46°$/sec. E: $0.1° \times 0.5°$ flashing bar, 5 presentations. F: $0.1° \times 0.5°$ moving bar, 40 sweeps at $0.46°$/sec. Adapted with permission from Bullier et al. (1982).

with the first one (e.g., ON with ON) produced strong suppression on 1 side of the RF center and a weaker one on the other side. Presentation of a second slit in opposite phase (e.g., OFF with ON) had weaker, opposite effects (Fig. 11/6). Heggelund (1981 a) concluded that simple cells receive an *excitatory input* from one type of LGN cells (ON or OFF) and a *spatially offset inhibition* from the *same type* of LGN cells. Heggelund (1981 a) completed his demonstration by a computer simulation of a RF receiving this type of double input and found good agreement between the simulated and the

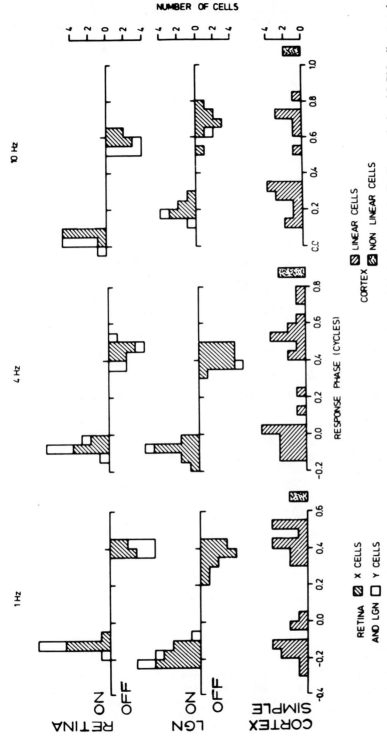

Fig. 11/5. Distribution of response phase P_r in 21 retinal ganglion cells, 27 LGN cells, and 31 simple cortical cells. For cortical and LGN cells, at each temporal frequency different numbers of cells are represented due to selectivity for temporal frequency in some cells. Cells were on- and off-center, sustained and transient, as indicated for retinal and LGN cells; non-linear cortical cells have non-linear phase-spatial frequency relationship and probably correspond to non-linear simple cells in Fig. 7/16. For each cell abscissa values are calculated as averages of the two directions of movement. Integer values indicate that the cell responds in phase with maximum grating luminance passing over the response locus; at half-values the cell responds in phase with minimum grating luminance passing over the field. Adapted with permission from Lee et al. (1981 b).

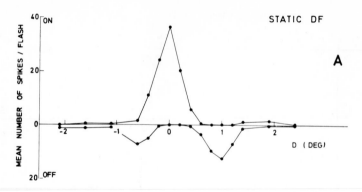

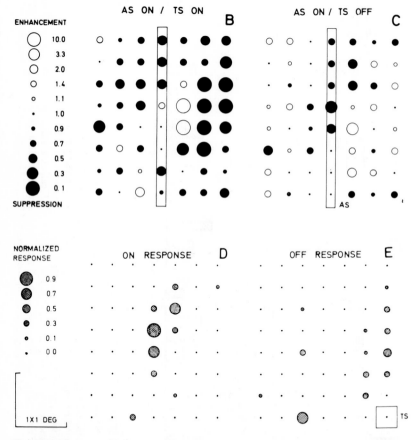

Fig. 11/6. The type of LGN unit (ON or OFF center) providing inhibitory input to a simple cell. A. Static discharge field plot made with an optimally oriented light slit (0.17 x 3.3 deg). B. Effects of test stimulus (TS) ON on the ON-response to activation stimulus (AS). Mean response to AS alone 14.2 spikes/presentation. C. Effects of test stimulus OFF on the ON-response to activation stimulus. D–E. Two-dimensional plot of the ON- and OFF-zones determined from the response to the test stimulus alone. Maximal mean response −4.8 spikes/presentation. For enhancement and suppression scale see Fig. 11/7. Adapted with permission from Heggelund (1981 a).

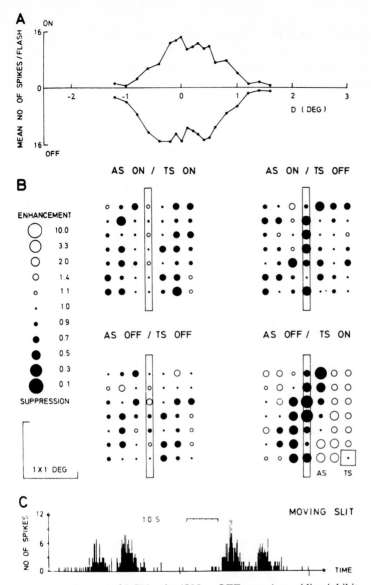

Fig. 11/7. The type of LGN units (ON or OFF center) providing inhibitory input to a complex cell. A. Plot of the discharge field (DF) with an optimally oriented light slit (0.1 × 2.1 deg) at different broadside distances (D) from DF-center. B. Effects of test stimulus (TS) in four different combinations with the activation stimulus (AS). The effects were expressed by the ratio between the responses to combined presentation of the two stimuli, and to AS alone. The magnitude of the effects are indicated by the size of the spots according to the scale on the left. The scale expresses the factor by which TS modified the AS response. The enhancement scale categories (open spots) represent the inverse value of the suppression categories (filled spots). Mean ON-response to AS alone −11.1 spikes/presentation. Mean OFF-response −6.8 spikes/ presentation. The rectangle in the center of the maps indicates AS size and position and the square in the lower right corner the size of TS. C. Response to a 2.1 x 2.1 deg light square moving forward and backward over the receptive field in directions perpendicular to the optimal stimulus orientation (N = 10 sweeps, velocity 3 deg/sec, bin width 12.8 msec). The first half of the histogram (cf. marks below the abscissa) shows response to forward sweep and the second half to backward sweep. In both movement directions the first response peak was produced by leading edge and the second by trailing edge. Adapted with permission from Heggelund (1981 b).

actually recorded responses. It remains however to be seen how general Heggelund's conclusions are, i.e. whether they applied to the whole S cell population or only to those S cells giving predominantly either ON or OFF responses, as his data suggest.

Using the same methods-Heggelund (1981 b) tested area 17 complex cells and found them to have suppressive zones, demonstrated by the simultaneous presentation of in phase flashed slits, both for OFF *and* ON stimuli (Fig. 11/7). These observations are in agreement with those of Movshon et al. (1978 b) who reported on subunits in the RF of area 17 complex cells. Heggelund (1981 b) concludes that complex cells receive an excitatory input both from ON and OFF LGN cells and a spatially offset inhibitory input from both types.

The question of ON and OFF center input to the S family cells certainly requires further investigation, especially in view of the wide variety of RF types in this family (S1 versus S2, even and odd symmetric, see Chapter 4). The results at present available however suggest that in part of the S or simple cell stream ON and OFF information is kept separate, while their informations are merged in another part of the S of simple cell stream and in the complex of C cell stream.

11.3 Other Attempts to Identify the LGN Input to Cortical Cells

Ikeda and Wright (1975a) described *transient and sustained* cells in area 17 of the cat, which they considered as recipient of X and Y afferents respectively. Yamane et al. (1977) described a larger proportion of transient cells in area 18 than in area 17. However it is now recognized that even at the retinal and LGN level, the transient or sustained time course of the response to a stationary flashed stimulus is a poor criterion to separate X from Y cells. Therefore it can be of *little use* in the identification of the type of afferents of cortical cells. Mustari et al. (1982) in their study of first order S cells of area 17 found little correlation between the sustained-transient character of the cells and their type of input. It seems rather, that the ratio between the transient and sustained part of the response to a flashed stimulus correlates with the behavior of the cortical cell in the velocity domain (Duysens et al., 1982 c). Cortical cells with low velocity upper cut-offs are much more tonic than those with high velocity upper cut-offs. One wonders whether tonicity may not be the reflection of the cortical transformation in the velocity domain (a temporal low-pass filtering) rather than a reflection of the geniculate afferents.

Leventhal and Hirsch (1980) distinguished in area 17 among SAS (small area slow) cells with low upper cut-off velocities and small RFs, LAS (large area slow) cells with a large RF and low upper cut-off velocity and F cells which have high upper cut-off velocities (see Chapter 4). These authors used the correlation of velocity sensitivity and RF width of cortical cells with their type of afferents identified by electrical stimulation (Dreher et al., 1980; Stone and Dreher, 1973; Stone and Hoffmann, 1971) as the main argument supporting their hypothesis that *SAS, LAS and F cells receive X, Y and W afferents respectively*. Furthermore they use as supporting evidence the increase in proportion of F cells with eccentricity which matches the retinal distribution of X, Y and W ganglion cells and the layering of their cortical cell types which matches the termination of afferents (but see Chapter 3 for this latter point). It is likely that cells with a high velocity upper cut-off (especially the velocity high-pass cells) receive Y input. This is in keeping with the observation of Dreher et al. (1980) and ours (Orban et al., 1981 a) that those cells are more numerous in area 18 and increase in proportion with eccentricity in areas 17 and 19. However, cells with lower velocity upper cut-offs may also receive input from Y afferents. And indeed from the observation of Mustari et al. (1982) it is clear that some of area 17 S cells fed monosynaptically by Y afferents have velocity low-pass curves. From the comparison of velocity-response curves in the LGN (Orban et al., 1981 c) and in the cortex it is quite clear that the velocity tuning of cortical cells is not the passive reflection of that of their geniculate afferents. Indeed the difference in velocity characteristics of X and Y cells is much too small to account for the differences between areas 17 and 18 in those respects (Fig. 11/8). On the contrary there seems to be a considerable modification of the velocity characteristics, at the cortical level most notably a low-pass filtering (also noted by Lee et al., 1981 b in temporal frequency terms). Similarly for the RF width, cortical cells with very narrow widths (e.g. below 0.5°) very likely receive their input from X cells. This is in keeping with both Dreher et al. (1980) and our (Duysens et al., 1982 b) observation that very narrow RFs only occur in area 17. However, this is not to say that cells with a wider RF cannot be X recipient. Indeed C or A family cells with afferents from 2 or 3 rows of LGN cells could produce wider RFs despite their X input. It seems thus that RF width and velocity sensitivity give some indication of the type of LGN afferents to cortical cells belonging to the lower end of the RF width distribution and to the upper end of the velocity upper cut-off distribution, *but that for most cortical cells these characteristics do not allow a definite identification of their afferents.*

Another approach to identifying the type of afferents to cortical cells is the construction of response planes and their derivation, the contour plane (Citron et al., 1981). The response plane is produced by stacking average responses to stationary slits flashed in different closely spaced positions throughout the RF (see Chapter 4). The contour plane is a cut through the response plane at the level of the spontaneous activity. The starting point of

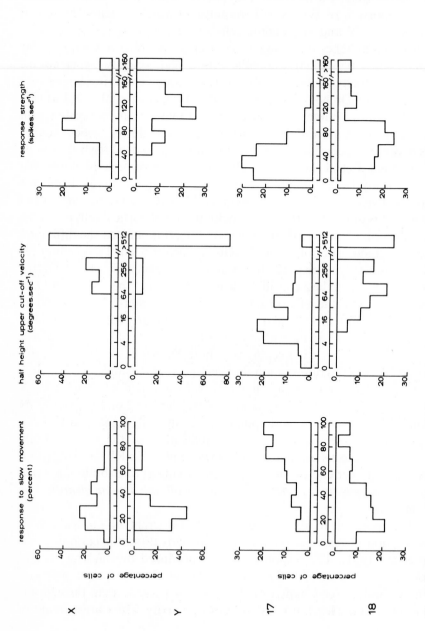

Fig. 11/8. Response to slow movement, half-height upper cut-off velocity and response strength distribution of X (n = 19), Y (n = 16) dLGN cells and area 17 (n = 89) and 18 (n = 71) cells (all cells had RFs within 15° from fixation point). For definitions see Chapter 8. The differences between X and Y cells are too small to account for the difference between area 17 and 18 cells.

this approach are the observations of Stevens and Gerstein (1976) and Bullier and Norton (1979) that X cells have an heterogeneous plane and Y cells an homogeneous one. In the latter case ON and OFF responses (taken as activity larger than spontaneous activity) are present over the whole extent of the RF and have a similar latency over the whole extent. From the comparison of these LGN planes with those of area 17 and 18 cells (unfortunately only 46 cells in total) Citron et al. (1981) conclude that area 17 simple cells are driven by X afferents while complex cells (both in areas 17 and 18) and a simple-like cell type in area 18 (which they call segregate cells) receive input from Y cells. This response plane approach has been taken up again by Mullikin et al. (1981), who suggested that the response domains of area 17 Y like simple cells had "arms" on either side of the central excitatory response and X like simple cells had not. These results however *have to be validated by* measurements of conduction velocity. Another indirect approach is the linearity of spatial summation: linear simple cells (see Chapter 7) are thought to receive input from linear X cells and non-linear simple cells (Fig. 7/16) from non-linear Y cells.

11.4 Conclusion

Except for the electrical stimulation experiments, all the methods reviewed here are indirect and have to take into account possible transformations at the cortical level. However a certain picture is starting to emerge. In area 18, all RF types seem to receive Y afferents [2]. In area 17, C family cells receive predominantly Y input while the S family receives either input, although the X input seems to be more common, especially among the end-stopped members of the family. In keeping with this, HS cells of area 17 were found to have narrower RFs than S cells (Orban and Kennedy, unpublished). With respect to ON and OFF center afferents, some S family cells seem to keep these afferents separate while other S family cells and C family cells mix them.

---

[2] Recently however Sawyer and Palmer (1982) have reported that the RF organization of about 15% of the area 18 cells could reflect a mixture of Y input and area 17 (X-like) input .

Chapter 12. Intracortical Mechanisms Underlying Properties of Cat Visual Cortical Cells

The spontaneous activity of visual cortical cells is much lower than that of LGN cells (Fig. 12/1). This leads us to suspect[1] that cortical cells are subject to important inhibitory influences. Indeed many cortical properties rely on intracortical inhibitions and not just on excitatory connections. Evidence for the involvement of intracortical inhibition in functional properties of cortical cells will first be reviewed. In the second and third part of this chapter, possible sources of this inhibition will be examined, both from physiological and anatomical points of view.

12.1 The Role of Intracortical Inhibition

12.1.1 Orientation Selectivity

In their original model of simple RFs Hubel and Wiesel (1962) proposed that a simple RF was built from the *excitatory convergence of a row of LGN cells*. Although Hubel and Wiesel (1962) did not rule out inhibitory connections, they did suggest that the flanks of the simple fields arose from the surrounds of LGN receptive fields eventually supplemented by excitatory afferents from LGN cells with centers of opposite polarity (i.e. ON center or OFF center). The orientation specificity arose according to them from the layout of the subregions, the response being maximal when the stimulus fell entirely within the central activating region. From this description it has been deduced that the main mechanism of orientation selectivity in simple RFs is summation along the length of the RFs resulting from geniculocortical convergence. Since complex orientation specificity was supposed to be a reflection of simple cell orientation specificity (Hubel and Wiesel, 1962) orientation tuning in the visual cortex relied essentially on excitatory processes. While such a mechanism can qualitatively explain orientation selectivity, it does not account for the absence of response to orientations 90° apart from the optimal orientation since LGN cells respond, sometimes unequally

---

[1] A lower synaptic efficiency could also contribute to the decreased spontaneous activity of cortical cells.

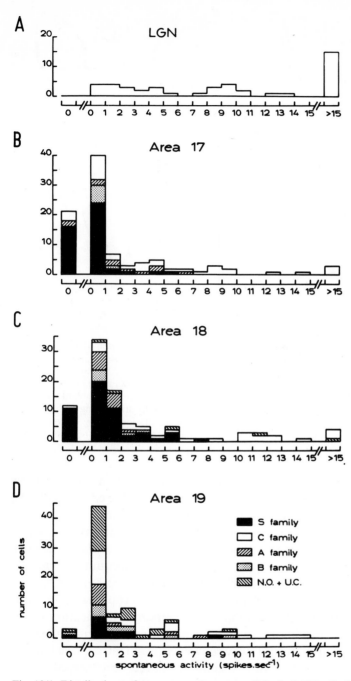

Fig. 12/1. Distributions of average spontaneous activity in LGN cells (A, n = 44) areas 17 (B, n = 95), 18 (C, n = 97), and 19 (D, n = 85) cells. Cortical RF types are indicated. N.O. = non-oriented cells; U.C. = unclassified cells. While in the LGN 9% of the cells had a spontaneous activity below 1 spike/sec, 64%, 47% and 55% of cells in areas 17, 18 and 19 respectively did.

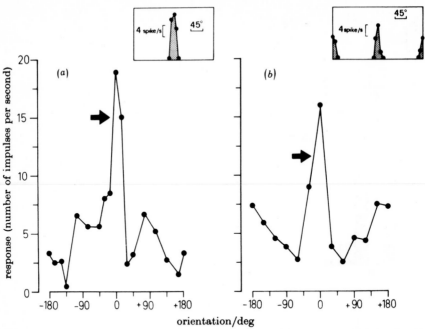

Fig. 12/2. Orientation tuning of cross-orientation inhibition for two representative simple cells, one uni- and one bidirectional. The response was elicited by a sinusoidal grating (spatial frequency 0.8 and 1.2 cycle/deg; velocity 2.8 and 1.5 deg/sec; contrast 20%) and inhibited by 37% contrast 1-D visual noise, free to vary in orientation. The arrows indicate the response (mean discharge) to the grating alone, obtained by replacing the noise with a blank field. The insets show the orientation-selectivity band of the cells, obtained by stimulating with the noise alone. Note that the inhibition arises over a wide range of orientations, being of comparable strength at all orientations outside the cells' selectivity bands. Adapted with permission from Morrone et al. (1982).

(Vidyasagar and Urbas, 1982), to all orientations. Thus at least a tonic inhibition, eventually operating at all orientations, is required. Actually the results of Morrone et al. (1982) suggest that cortical cells are inhibited only for orientations outside the range of their perferred orientations (Fig. 12/2). The same authors also report that this *"cross orientation" inhibition* is much stronger for simple than for complex cells. This could account for the narrower orientation tuning of simple cells (see Chapter 7).

Sillito (1975) investigated the changes in functional properties induced by removal of GABA mediated inhibition by iontophoretic application of the GABA antagonist bicuculline. His initial observations were in agreement with the hypothesis that both excitatory convergence and intracortical inhibition were implicated in orientation selectivity. Indeed he observed only a reduction in orientation selectivity of simple cells after bicuculline application, in marked and surprising contrast to complex cell orientation selectivity which was lost completely in many cases. Tsumoto et al. (1979) supplemented the iontophoretically applied bicuculline with 3 mercaptoproprionic acid

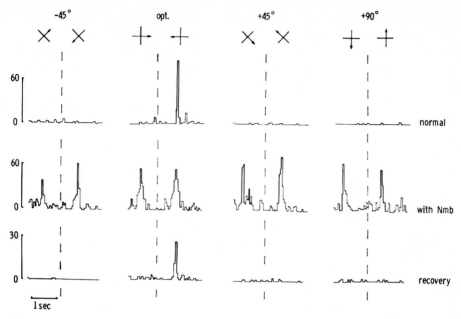

Fig. 12/3. Action of N-methyl bicuculline (Nmb) on simple cell orientation selectivity. Testing orientation and direction of stimulus motion is indicated above each set of PSTHs. Dotted line subdivides records into zones corresponding to the two directions of motion. Optimal orientation is arbitrarily referred to as zero, −, indicates anti-clockwise rotation from optima, +, clockwise rotation. Each PSTH constructed from 25 trials. Bin size 50 msec. Vertical calibration indicates number of counts per bin. Adapted with permission from Sillito et al. (1980 b).

(MP) given intravenously, and observed a complete abolishment of orientation selectivity in 2 out of 4 simple cells. Sillito et al. (1980 b) re-investigated the question with N-methyl bicuculline (Nmb), a more potent antagonist of GABA. With iontophoresis of this drug they observed a *total loss of orientation selectivity in all 13 simple cells* studied (Fig. 12/3). Moreover Sillito et al. (1980 b) noted that the width of the discharge peaks evoked during Nmb application by slits oriented orthogonally to the optimal orientation were not wider than those evoked by a slit of optimal orientation, as one would expect if the simple cell received input from a row of LGN cells. They conclude that very few LGN cells, possibly only one, drive a simple cell, a feature also incorporated in the Heggelund (1981 a) model for simple cells (see Chapter 11). On the other hand, the results of Hoffmann et al. (1980) suggest that the extreme sensitivity of simple cells to a slit embedded in noise is due to convergent input from several LGN cells, since a single LGN cell does not respond much more to the slit than to the dots of the noise. As stressed in Chapter 4, the S family has both end-stopped and end-free members. Distinction of these two types of S cells may well solve the contradictions with respect to the number of LGN cells converging into a simple cell.

In his 1979 report Sillito distinguished between *two types of complex cells:* those (52%) in which orientation selectivity was abolished by bicuculline and those (48%) in which it was only reduced. This great effect of bicuculline on orientation selectivity of complex cells was surprising in view of the fact that at least 50% of the complex cells are second order cells.[2] To account for his observations (Sillito, 1979) put forward the hypothesis that complex cells pool excitation from (simple) cells with different optimal orientations and are inhibited by an interneuron of which the optimal orientation is 90° out of phase with that of the complex cell under consideration. Actually Lee et al. (1977 a) observed in their vertical penetrations a few cells of which the preferred orientation was out of phase compared to that of the other cells and these cells were usually broadly tuned complex cells. However, in a brief note on the effect of GABA applied iontophoretically Rose (1977) reports that the inhibition acting on a corticotectal complex cell, a type excluded from Sillito's (1979) study, is maximal at the optimal orientation. It should be noted that Heggelund's model for complex cells can also account for a loss of orientation selectivity in at least first order complex cells.

Studying the effect of bicuculline on the orientation selectivity of *superficial layer hypercomplex cells* (including simple-like hypercomplex cells), Sillito and Versiani (1977) made the even more surprising observation[3] that bicuculline abolished the orientation tuning of these cells. These authors explained their finding by supposing that the superficial layer hypercomplex cells receive input from layer V complex cells with weak end-stopping resembling corticotectal cells described by Palmer and Rosenquist (1974). The orientation tuning of corticotectal cells is indeed broad compared to that of other cortical cells, but is much narrower than what is left of tuning of superficial layer hypercomplex cells with bicuculline application. While some of these iontophoresis experiments remain difficult to interpret, they do clearly show that orientation selectivity critically depends on intracortical inhibition.

12.1.2 Direction Selectivity

Hubel and Wiesel (1962) noticed that some of the simple cells were direction selective and suggested that direction preferences of a simple cell could be predicted from the static RF plot, in that a stronger response in the preferred direction arises *from the simultaneous effect of leaving an inhibitory*

---

[2] i.e. are driven disynaptically from the LGN and are likely to receive an input which is already orientation selective.
[3] The surprise srems from the fact that most superficial layer cells are likely to be second order cortical cells.

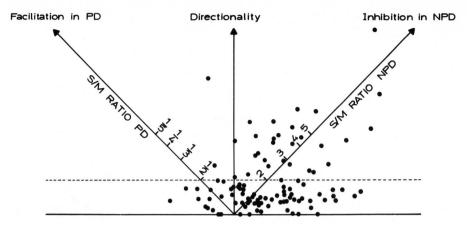

Fig. 12/4. S/M ratio (ratio of responses to stationary flashed and to moving slit) in PD plotted as a function of SM ratio in NPD for 104 cortical cells (areas 17, 18 and 19 pooled). Axes turned 45°; vertical up represents the directionality (i.e. PD/NPD ratio), stippled horizontal line PD/NPD ratio = 2. Note the clustering of datapoints around axis indicating inhibition in NPD.

region and entering an excitatory region. While such a mechanism can explain a stronger response in one direction than in the other, it cannot explain a total absence in the non-preferred direction and in addition it is difficult to see how it can account for contrast independent direction preference (i.e. preferences identical for light and dark bars). This latter point explains why some authors (Albus, 1980; Emerson and Gerstein, 1977 b) include contrast independence in their definition of direction selectivity. In addition to the RF asymmetry proposed by Hubel and Wiesel (1962), two other mechanisms have been proposed to account for direction selectivity: *forward facilitation in the preferred direction* (Emerson and Gerstein, 1977b; Movshon et al., 1978 b) and *forward inhibition in the non-preferred direction* (Goodwin et al., 1975). The relative importance of these two mechanisms can be evaluated from the comparison of S/M ratios[4] in the preferred (PD) and non-preferred (NPD) direction (Duysens and Orban, 1981). These two ratios have been plotted on two orthogonal axes in Fig. 12/4. The two axes have been turned 45° so that the vertical axis now represents directionality (i.e. PD/NPD ratio) at the optimal velocity. The intersection of the axes corresponds to the point where both S/M ratios are 1 and where the directionality is zero since responses in both directions are equal. Depending on whether forward facilitation in the PD or inhibition in the NPD contribute to direction selectivity the datapoints of direction selective cells should cluster around the end of the left-hand and right-hand oblique axes respectively. Considering the cells with directionality

---

[4] Ratio of responses to stationary (S) and moving (M) slit, see Chapter 4.

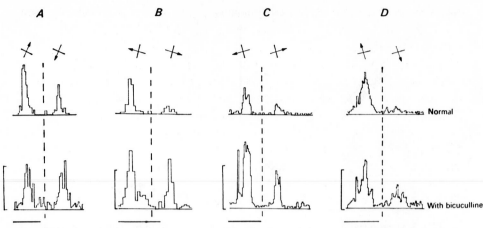

Fig. 12/5. Action of iontophoretically applied bicuculline on complex cell directional specificity. A, type '1' complex cell. Vertical calibration bar indicates range corresponding to 0–100 counts/ 50 msec bin (0–80 impulses/sec) for the upper record (normal) and 0–200 (0–160 impulses/sec) for the lower record (during bicuculline application) No. of trials, twenty-five. Horizontal bar corresponds to 1.0 sec. Bicuculline applied with 40 nA ejecting current. B, further example of type '1' complex cell. Vertical bar indicates range corresponding to 0–100 counts/50 msec bin (0–80 impulses/sec); calibration same for upper and lower record. Horizontal bar indicates 1.0 sec. No. of trials, twenty-five. Bicuculline applied with 100 nA ejecting current. C, type '2' complex cell. All other details as for B except that bin size is 20 msec (vertical calibration 0–100 counts/bin, 0–200 impulses/sec) and bicuculline ejecting current 140 nA. D, type '2' complex cell. All details as for B except that bin size is 20 msec (vertical calibration 0–100 counts/bin, 0–156 impulses/sec). No. of trials, thirty-two and bicuculline ejecting current 90 nA. See Chapter 4 for details of type '1' and '2' complex cells. Adapted with permission from Sillito (1977a).

over 2/1 (response in PD at least double of that in NPD), it is plain that most of them cluster around the right-hand oblique axis indicating that *inhibition in the NPD is the main mechanism* for direction selectivity. Actually the forward facilitation in PD only made a clear contribution to direction selectivity in one cell.

The nature of the inhibitory mechanism in the non-preferred direction of simple cells is still unclear: Emerson and Gerstein (1977 b) supposed a lateral inhibition between sequence-detecting subunits, while Goodwin et al. (1975) supposed a blanking out inhibition operating on radial direction asymmetry of LGN cells caused by gradient detection. Both studies however agree that the lateral spread of the inhibition is about 1/4 of a degree, the inhibition falling off rapidly at larger values.

The importance of intracortical inhibition in simple cell direction selectivity was clearly demonstrated by iontophoresis experiments of Sillito (1975, 1977) and of Tsumoto et al. (1979). They showed that almost all simple cells lost their direction selectivity with bicuculline application. With respect to direction selectivity of complex cells Sillito (1977 a) distinguished between 3 types of complex cells (Fig. 12/5) of which only type (1), corresponding probably to B cells (see Chapter 4), lost its direction selectivity with bicuculline application. Types 2 and 3, resembling those C and HC cells, did not. In agreement with this, Goodwin and Henry (1975) noticed that the spontaneous activity of complex cells was not inhibited in the NPD, an observation which could be taken as evidence that complex cells received an already direction selective input. However Bishop et al. (1980) have clearly shown that the spontaneous activity of complex cells can be inhibited in the NPD. *Negative results* in bicuculline experiments are hard to interpret[5]. It is possible that a neuro-transmitter other than GABA is involved in complex cell direction selectivity, or possibly use of the more potent Nmb will cause the loss of direction selectivity in complex cells. It is, however, beyond doubt that intracortical inhibition is a major mechanism for direction selectivity of simple cells and at least some complex cells.

12.1.3 End-Stopping

The origin of length preference or end-stopping of cortical cells is in dispute. Hubel and Wiesel (1965) proposed an *intracortical inhibitory input.* Many authors (Heggelund, 1981 a; Rose, 1977; Schiller et al., 1976) have suggested however that end-stopping is just a *reflection of LGN surround antagonism.* One of the main arguments is that geniculate cells also show a reduction in response when stimulated with long bars, although the effect is clearer in ON-center cells (50% reduction on average) than in OFF-center cells (40% reduction on average for X cells). This of course could not account for the hypercomplex cells with complete inhibition at long lengths. The other argument is that cortical length-response curves can be modelled by summing outputs of geniculate cells. Rose (1979) described a model (Fig. 12/6) in which simple and complex cells receive input from LGN units with their centers scattered (perhaps aligned in a row) while their hypercomplex counterparts receive input from LGN cells with closely superimposed fields (also possibly in a short row). Rose (1979) further assumed that between those two extremes there is a continuity in the degree of overlap of LGN fields. While the last part of Rose's proposal is untenable in view of the bimodal distribution of end-zone inhibition (Kato et al., 1978), the first part could be acceptable, although difficult to reconcile with Sillito's et al. (1980 b) recent observations (see above). It could however be that the inputs from the end of the row of LGN fields are much weaker or even subliminal (e.g by ending on more distant parts of the dendrites). From his model Rose (1979) predicted

---

[5] Technical difficulties can also account for some of the negative findings in bicuculline iontophoresis experiments: one has to record from the cellbody (and not from the axon or a dendrite) and the drug has to be injected near the synapses which affect the property of the cell under study.

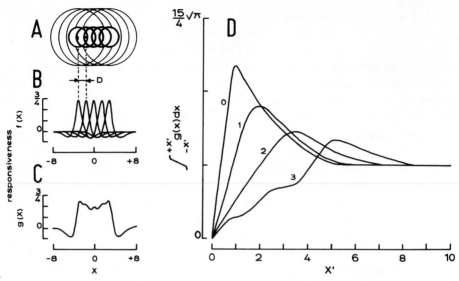

Fig. 12/6. Lengthwise RF organization of simple cells according to Rose (1979). At the top (A) is a plan view of 5 LGN receptive fields aligned in a row (thick lines show field centers, thin lines, the surrounds). In B, the profiles of the 5 LGN fields are shown superimposed in alignment with the plan view in A. In A, the center and surround radii are drawn at a distance of 2.5 x the standard deviation of their respective Gaussian functions from the exact middle of the receptive field. The offset of each receptive field from its neighbor is D, which equals $2/\sqrt{2}$ in this figure. C. The algebraic sum of the 5 LGN receptive field profiles in B is shown. This is the cortical receptive field profile g(x). It is shown in alignment with A and B, so the x-axis (distance across the receptive field) applies to all parts of the figure (If D were equal to $1/\sqrt{2}$, then g(x) would have a single central peak with a rounded top, and if $D = 3/\sqrt{2}$, 5 distinct peaks would be visible.) D. The curves obtained by integrating the cortical field profile shown in C between $x = -x'$ and $x = +x'$, are plotted here as functions of x'. The four curves in each panel are for different offsets between the LGN fields (D in A); this was $n/\sqrt{2}$, and the value of n is displayed alongside each curve. Adapted with permission from Rose (1979).

that cells with scattered LGN input would have a lower response at optimal length than those with overlapping input (Fig. 12/6). This prediction is clearly not verified for simple and hypercomplex I cells (see Kato et al., 1978, Table II).

Therefore others (Cleland et al., 1983) have suggested that end-stopping seen in hypercomplex cells is *partially a cortical phenomenon* (39%), but also *partially a subcortical phenomenon* (37% geniculate and 25% retinal). The main argument of Cleland et al. (1983), in addition to modelling cortical length-response curves (see objections above), is the comparison of the reduction of responses for long bar lengths in retinal, geniculate and hypercomplex I cortical cells. In calculating the cortical contribution (39%) Cleland et al. are unfair in comparing only ON-center geniculate cells with the cortical cells of Kato et al. (1978), while they insist that the cortical sample included both ON and OFF dominated cells and their data show that the response reduc-

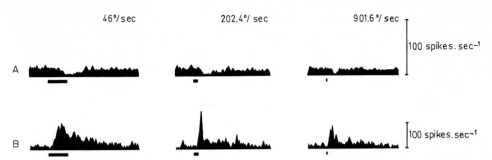

Fig. 12/7. Suppression of spontaneous activity by end-zone inhibition. PSTHs representing average responses to a moving slit of an area 19 VHP, HC cell at 3 different velocities. A: long slit (30°), B: short slit (2°). Horizontal bar indicates movement duration.

tion at long lengths is smaller in OFF center cells. Furthermore the relative contributions given by Cleland et al. are only valid under one set of experimental conditions. It could well be that by lowering the background illumination (which was 4 cd/m² in their experiments) the subcortical contributions to end-stopping would decrease. We use lower background levels in our set-up and while our proportion of cortical end-stopped cells is about similar to that obtained by Kato et al. (1978) with high background levels, geniculate cells with very few exceptions, seem quite happy to respond to long bars. One of the main characteristics of the cortical contribution to end-stopping could well be its *generality* (i.e. that it operates in a very large range of stimulus conditions). Cleland et al. (1983) further doubt whether a localized inhibitory end-zone region is necessary to explain the cortical contribution to end-stopping, but it is difficult to see how the firing threshold (Henry et al., 1978 a) they indicate as an alternative, could bring about a reduction in response at long stimulus lengths.

There are a number of experimental findings that are difficult to account for, if end-stopping were to a large extent to result from inhibitory actions onto the excitatory geniculate input to cortical cells. Orban et al. (1979 b) have shown that inhibitory end-regions, both weak and strong ones, are orientation selective and much wider than the discharge region of hypercomplex I cells, two observations difficult to reconcile with a substantial subcortical contribution to the end-stopping. Furthermore, in some instances the spontaneous activity of end-stopped cells can be inhibited by stimuli of long lengths (Orban and Duysens, unpublished; Rose, 1977; see Fig. 12/7). Both results taken together *suggest intracortical inhibitory inputs as the major origin of end-stopping* (Orban et al., 1979 b). Finally, Sillito and Versiani (1977) observed a reduction but not an abolishment of length preferences in superficial layer hypercomplex cells in area 17 after bicuculline application. Since this was accompanied by a loss in orientation selectivity but not of direction selectivity, Sillito and Versiani (1977) proposed that the non-oriented directional input with length preference originated in layer V cells, similar to corticotectal cells, sending collaterals to the superficial layers. While this possibility is not excluded, one could also consider that the input to these hypercomplex cells arises from LGN afferents (no orientation tuning and some length preference) and that their direction selectivity, as for some complex cells (see above), is mediated by another transmitter.

12.1.4 Ocular Dominance

Sillito et al. (1980 a) recently presented evidence that intracortical inhibition also contributes to the ocular dominance of area 17 cells. Considering only area 17 cells clearly dominated by one eye (mostly ocular dominance classes 1, 7, 2 and 6 of Hubel and Wiesel, 1962), these authors observed a *clear shift in ocular dominance towards class 4* (i.e. equal drive from both eyes) after bicuculline application in about 50% of the cells, independently from their RF type (simple or complex). Sillito et al. (1980 b) concluded that more cortical cells are binocular than indicated by their ocular dominance, but that nevertheless, there are truly monocular cells, namely those not affected by bicuculline application. As mentioned above, negative results are difficult to interpret in these experiments and there may be an alternative explanation to their negative finding. Kato et al. (1981) observed in almost all (15/16) monocularly driven cells a binocular input. However the input from the non-dominant eye could either be purely inhibitory or both inhibitory and subliminally excitatory. While one would expect a shift of ocular dominance under bicuculline in the latter case, this need not be the case in the former (see below). Both experiments however underscore the importance of intracortical inhibitions in binocular interactions. In this respect the observation of Ferster (1981) that all tuned excitatory cells, whether in area 17 or 18, have inhibitory sidebands, is also of considerable interest since these sidebands are of intracortical origin (Innocenti and Fiore, 1974).

12.1.5 Velocity Upper Cut-Off

In the same report, Sillito et al. (1980 a) also mentioned the influence of bicuculline iontophoresis on velocity tuning of area 17 cells. They showed that after bicuculline application, area 17 cells become responsive to fast velocities (100 deg.sec^{-1}), to which they normally do not respond. This is in agreement with our observation (Orban et al., 1981 a) that the spontaneous activity of some velocity low-pass (VLP) cells can be inhibited by fast moving stimuli. Goodwin and Henry (1978) postulated the existence of a *retroactive inhibition* arising at fast velocities from a region past the discharge region.

While we (Orban, Duysens and Cremieux, unpublished) have confirmed their data showing that velocity upper cut-offs appear only for larger amplitudes of movement, it is by no means sure that this is an indication of an inhibitory interaction. Furthermore, we (Duysens et al., 1982 c, 1983) have evidence that velocity upper cut-off of many VLP cells is caused by a *temporal threshold* (too short a duration of activation), due either to failure of excitation or to inhibition. While intracortical inhibition probably is a cortical factor determining velocity tuning it may not be the only one.

12.1.6 Absence of Response to Two-Dimensional Noise

Recently Hammond and MacKay (1981) have shown that the absence of responses in area 17 simple cells to moving textures of static two-dimensional noise is not just a *lack of activation* but actually a *reflection of a strong inhibitory input*. Using a moving bar as a conditioning stimulus and noise fields as test stimuli, they found that 3/4 of the simple cells were depressed by moving fields of static noise. These data confirm earlier observations by Hoffmann and von Seelen (1978) that when the noise field moves relative to the slit (on the same axis), it inhibits the response of area 17 simple cells to the slit, while when both patterns move together this inhibitory influence is removed at least for area 17 cells (Hoffmann et al., 1980), but not for area 18 cells (Dinse and von Seelen, 1981 b). Whether the inhibition demonstrated in the Hoffmann and von Seelen (1978) and Hammond and MacKay (1981) experiments, actually explains the absence of response of simple cells to the noise fields moving on their own, remains to be seen. An alternative explanation is certainly length summation, since simple cells respond to unidimensional noise (Burr et al., 1981) (see Chapter 7 for discussion). It should also be noted that the inhibitory input demonstrated by Hoffmann and von Seelen (1978) and Hammond and MacKay (1981), has *the same preferred axis* as the simple cell and is therefore different from the cross orientation inhibition demonstrated by Morrone et al. (1982) which has an optimal axis orthogonal to the preferred axis of the simple cell. By using small patches of moving noise fields of variable dimensions and location, Hammond and MacKay (1981) showed that the inhibitory input shows length summation more than width summation and extends lengthwise further than the length of the excitatory discharge region. Often they observed a weak facilitation at the end of the receptive field. This latter point shows that the inhibition from noise fields is different from end-zone inhibition. Hammond and MacKay (1981) interpreted this inhibition as coming through complex cells. This "sea of complex cell inhibition" covering simple cells, as demonstrated by Hammond and MacKay (1981) as well as by other experiments discussed later, may explain some of the effects from "outside the RF" seen by Maffei and Fiorentini (1977), Nelson and Frost (1978) and Blakemore and Tobin (1972).

In conclusion one can say that intracortical inhibition is an important if not critical factor in most functional properties of the cortical cells. The only property which has escaped attention in this respect is spatial frequency tuning. Since however cortical cells have a clear low frequency attenuation, which LGN cells lack and which is due to antagonistic flanks, it seems likely that intracortical inhibition is also involved in this tuning.

12.2 Properties of the Intracortical Inhibitions

Originally Bishop et al. (1973) proposed that *intracortical inhibitory inter-neurons were non-oriented cells*. Their argument was that *inhibitory sidebands of simple RFs seemed to be non-oriented*. Indeed raising the activity with a conditioning slit and turning the test slit orthogonal to the optimal orientation yielded a large inhibitory response instead of the two inhibitory valleys flanking the excitatory peak evoked by an optimally oriented test slit (Fig. 12/8). In contradiction with this Ferster (1981) observed that tuned excitatory "complex" cells have *oriented inhibitory sidebands* (Fig. 12/8). As mentioned in Chapter 4 those particular complex cells would be considered as S cells by us (Kato et al., 1978; Orban and Kennedy, 1981). The discrepancy between both observations may simply be due to the difference in *level of activity* induced by the conditioning slit. In the experiments of Bishop et al. (1973), the level was around 8–10 spikes/sec, much higher than in Ferster's (1981) experiment where it was 1 spike/sec (Fig. 12/8). Recently Burr et al. (1981) and Morrone et al. (1982) have also provided evidence for an inhibition of simple cells caused by a test pattern moving at right angles to the optimal axis. Again the conditioning stimulus (1 dimensional noise) induced a high level of activity (over 10 spikes/sec). Sillito (1979) has shown that by raising the resting discharge of complex cells to a high level (either visually by a conditioning stimulus or chemically with iontophoresis of DL homo-cysteate), one can turn the activation of complex cells (as defined by Kato et al., 1978) into an inhibition by using an optimal stimulus and that non-optimal stimuli under those circumstances also generate inhibition, both inhibitions being cancelled by bicuculline application. It could well be that the appearance of inhibition at non-optimal orientations in simple cells is due to a similar mechanism coming into play when the conditioning slit induces too high an activity level, and is not related to inhibitory sidebands, since complex cells (as defined by Kato et al., 1978) have no inhibitory sidebands.

It thus seems thus that great care is required *in the use of conditioning stimuli* to disclose inhibitory sidebands. A weak conditioning stimulus (pro-ducing < 5 spikes/sec) will only disclose the inhibitory sidebands at optimal

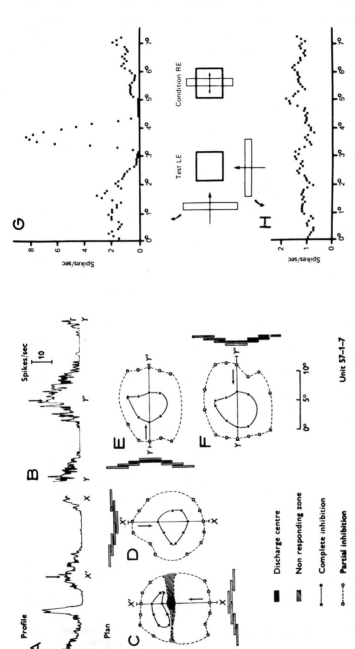

Fig. 12/8. Are simple cell inhibitory sidebands orientation dependent or not? A–F. Selected activity profiles (A, B) and plan representations (C, D, E, F) of the organization of a unimodal simple cell in response to a narrow slit (3.4° × 0.29°) moved forward and backward across the field at the optimal orientation (A, C, D–75°) and at 90° to the optimal orientation (B, E, F–165°). Profiles and plans are drawn to the same scale but slits are not to scale and are only diagrammatically located in relation to the plans. Monocular conditioning was used and the testing slit moved over a 14.0° traverse at 11.3°/sec. The two activity profiles (A, B) were obtained over the traverse X–X′–X and Y–Y′–Y respectively as shown in C, D, E, and F. Receptive field 5° from visual axis. Adapted with permission from Bishop et al. (1973). G–H. Two activity profiles of the same receptive field of a tuned excitatory complex cell. G: as shown in the diagram, the test slit and the conditioning slit had the optimal orientation and, as was usually observed, the receptive field consisted of a central excitatory region and two flanking inhibitory regions. H: the test slit was turned 90° to the receptive field orientation. Both the excitatory and inhibitory regions were orientation-selective. Note that a cell as shown in G and H would be considered by the author as S cell. Adapted with permission from Ferster (1981).

orientation in S cells but requires of course many sweeps to make them apparent. A stronger stimulus (10–20 spikes/sec) will still allow the test slit to disclose inhibitory sidebands of S cells but some inhibition will also be induced by the test slit at non-optimal orientations. Combined with stronger conditioning stimuli test stimuli will even induce inhibition at optimal orientation, which could create the impression of sidebands even in C or complex cells (as defined by Kato et al., 1978); however the latter inhibition will be accompanied by a strong reduction of the excitatory response (see e.g. Fig. 8 B of Sillito, 1979). Even further increase in the conditioning stimulus strength (30–50 spikes/sec resting discharge) will cause the test stimulus to induce only inhibition in complex cells (Sillito, 1979). This suggests an important control for experiments in which one wants to disclose inhibitory sidebands typical of S or simple family (in the Kato et al., 1978 and Sherman et al., 1976 sense), namely, the excitatory peak should be about as large (or larger) with as without conditioning stimulus.

The origin of this inhibition at higher resting levels is unclear, although for complex cells Sillito (1979) suggested that it is due to the interneuron (with optimal axis orthogonal to the cell considered) bringing about orientation specificity in complex cells (see above). The same may be true for simple cells, as the results of Burr et al. (1981) and Morrone et al. (1982) suggest. It could even be that in addition to inhibition by complex cells with optimal orientation at right angles to that of the cell considered, simple cells also receive inhibitory input from complex cells with the same optimal orientation as the cell considered, as suggested by Hammond and MacKay (1981). Indeed even optimal stimuli generate inhibition (Creutzfeldt et al., 1974; Toyama et al., 1974).

If *the pool of complex cells acting on the simple cells* produces a divisive inhibition as the results of Morrone et al. (1982) suggest, the effect of the strength of the conditioning stimulus is readily explained (Fig. 12/9). When the conditioning stimulus of optimal orientation is weak (arrow 1 in Fig. 12/9) the effect of the divisive inhibition is minimal and one will not see much influence from the test stimulus at right angles to the optimal orientation. When the conditioning stimulus is stronger (arrows 2 and 3) the effect of the divisive inhibition will be clear and the test stimulus at right angles to the optimal orientation will produce a substantial inhibition. The difference between strengths indicated by 2 and 3 is that when the test stimulus has the optimal orientation, it will raise the contrast of the conditioning stimulus and this will increase the response, provided the conditioning stimulus is not too strong (arrow 2), but will have little effect if the conditioning stimulus is already saturating the cell (arrow 3). Hence one can derive the optimal contrast of the conditioning stimulus to disclose inhibitory sidebands: the contrast should correspond to the middle of the dynamic range (about arrow 2 in Fig. 12/9).

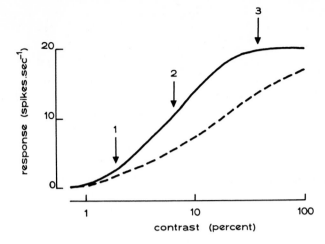

Fig. 12/9. Contrast-response curves for an optimally oriented stimulus (conditioning stimulus) on its own (full line) and combined with a non-optimally oriented test stimulus, supposing that the inhibition is divise. Arrows indicate 3 contrast levels corresponding to a weak, medium, and strong inhibition by the conditioning stimulus (see text).

Before returning to the question of inhibitory interneurons, it is worth noting that if inhibitory sidebands, which by definition (Bishop et al., 1973), are disclosed with moving stimuli (Fig. 4/9), are orientation dependent, then their relationship with the suppressive flanks seen with stationary stimuli (Heggelund 1981 a, b) becomes clearer. In simple cells they may be the expression of the same inhibitory input. It seems that non-oriented inhibitory interneurons are not really required by the available data and anyway non-oriented cells are rare in the visual cortex (see Chapter 4). On the contrary the properties of intracortical inhibitions suggest that *the inhibitory interneurons have the properties of ordinary cortical cells* (e.g. orientation selectivity). This leads us to the interesting possibility that interneurons should appear to the physiologist just as "ordinary" cortical cells. Evidence for this suggestion rests on experiments making extensive use of double stimulus techniques. These experiments done in collaboration with P.O. Bishop and H. Kato will now be reviewed.

Let us first consider the *inhibition from the non-dominant eye* of monocularly driven cells. Kato et al. (1981) showed (1) that it was orientation selective (Fig. 12/10) and that its width of orientation tuning decreased with the length of the stimulus and (2) that in some cases (30%) it was direction selective. Both properties clearly suggest that the inhibition is of intracortical origin. These authors further noted that the optimal orientation of the inhibition in the weak eye was always in close agreement with that of the excitation of the dominant eye. For direction selectivity the match was not as clear. Some of the results reported by Sillito et al. (1980 a) could be interpreted by saying that monocular cell inhibition from the weak eye is velocity dependent (e.g. their Fig. 8).

Kato et al. (1981) further observed that in about half of the cells only inhibition could be evoked through the non-dominant eye. Any RF type

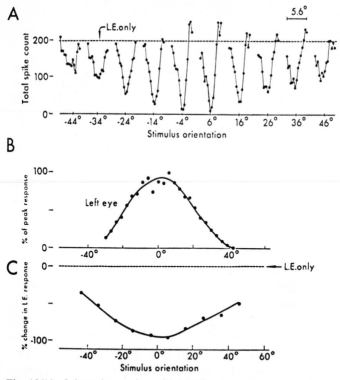

Fig. 12/10. Orientation tuning of inhibition from the non-dominant eye of monocular cells. Orientation tuning curves for the dominant (B) and silent (A, C) eyes of the same simple cell. A: family of position disparity tuning curves for the silent eye using the variable delay method. Each curve is for a different stimulus orientation setting for the silent eye (10° steps) keeping the orientation for the dominant eye fixed at its optimal value throughout. For each curve, disparity increments of 24 min arc were used over a total range of 5.6°. Binocular facilitation (25%) is more narrowly tuned than binocular inhibition (95%) but both have the same preferred orientation (6°). B: monocular orientation tuning curve for the dominant eye. Half-width at half-height = 18°. C: binocular inhibitory tuning curve for the silent eye given by the values of the inhibitory peaks of the tuning curves in A. Inhibitory curve: half-width at half-strength = 41°. Adapted with permission from Kato et al. (1981).

driven by the weak eye could cause this inhibition and those monocular cells may correspond to the monocular cells in which bicuculline induces no change in ocular dominance (see above). In the other half of the cells, subliminal facilitation in addition to inhibition could be elicited through the weak eye. For some of these cells, Kato et al. (1981) could further show that the plan of the RF was similar in both eyes, except for strength of excitation, and that a moving noise field was as effective in producing the inhibition as a moving slit. This suggests that this second type of monocular cells receives a similarly organized input from both eyes but that in the non-dominant eye a strong inhibitory input from a complex cell is superimposed. This explains the fact that noise fields can induce inhibition from the non-dominant eye and that the orientation tuning of the inhibition is broad. The removal of the inhibitory input from the complex cell would then reveal the excitatory input from the weak eye and hence the ocular dominance would shift, as observed by Sillito et al. (1980 a) for certain monocular cells.

For *end-zone inhibition* of hypercomplex cells we (Orban et al., 1979 b) were also able to show that it was orientation dependent (Fig. 12/11) and in some instances direction selective. Again the optimal orientation of the end-zone inhibition corresponded to that of the excitatory region. Furthermore, the end-zone was in close register with the discharge region both being maximally sensitive at the same level in the width profile. This again shows that end-zone inhibition is at least partially of intracortical origin and arises through "ordinary" cortical cells with matched properties. Our experiments (Orban et al., 1981 a) on velocity tuning of cortical cells suggest that at least in velocity tuned cells, the end-zone influence is also velocity dependent, increasing in parallel with the excitation from the discharge region (Fig. 2 Orban et al., 1981 a).

Direction selective inhibition has been shown to be parameter dependent (Bishop et al., 1980). From the observation of the inhibition of spontaneous activity in complex family cells, Bishop et al. (1980) could demonstrate a certain orientation and length dependence of direction-selective inhibition. Again the same orientation and length were optimal for both excitation in preferred direction and inhibition in non-preferred direction. The results of Orban et al. (1981 b) on direction selectivity of cortical cells, show that, especially in area 18 cells, direction selective inhibition becomes more efficient with increasing velocities in parallel with the increase in response in the prefered direction (Fig. 8/12). This shows that direction selective inhibition in area 18 is velocity dependent, exactly as the excitatory responses of cortical cells of that region.

Morrone et al. (1982) have recently provided evidence that yet another inhibition, *cross-orientation inhibition* is parameter dependent (Fig. 12/2). Since they used drifting gratings the parameters they investigated were spatial and temporal frequency. As shown in Fig. 12/12, cross-orientation inhibition is spatial frequency tuned. The tuning is broader than that of the excitatory drive of the cell but both are matched in optimal spatial frequency.

All this evidence clearly suggests that cortical inhibitory interneurons have the properties reported for ordinary cortical cells and that S or C cells could well be interneurons for each other. *Many of the inhibitions may arise from C* cells: the noise field inhibition, possibly the end-zone inhibition (because of their width, Orban et al., 1979 b), some of the monocular cell inhibition (Kato et al., 1981 and above), direction selective inhibition (because of its large extent, Bishop et al., 1980) and the cross-orientation inhibition (Morrone et al., 1982). But the inhibitory sidebands and suppressive flanks in the stationary interaction profiles of Heggelund (1981 a) suggest

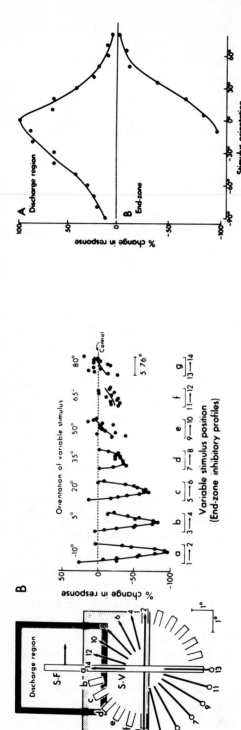

Fig. 12/11. Orientation tuning of end-zone inhibition. Left. End-zone activity (inhibitory) profiles prepared by the variable delay method for seven different stimulus orientations on a hypercomplex II cell. The configurations used for the fixed (S−F) and variable (S−V) stimuli are shown at A in relation to the discharge region and end-zone. The lower-case letters indicate orientations of the variable stimulus and end-zone. The lower-case letters indicate orientations of the variable stimulus and the numerals, 1 → 2, 3 → 4 …, etc. show the corresponding direction of movement at each orientation. Right. Stimulus orientation tuning curve (A) for the discharge region and inhibitory orientation tuning curve (B) for an end-zone from the same hypercomplex II cell as shown on the left side. The abscissa and ordinate scales are common to both curves. The optimal stimulus orientation for the discharge region has been arbitrarily set at 0°. Data for curve B come from the end-zone inhibitory profiles on left side. Adapted with permission from Orban et al. (1979 b).

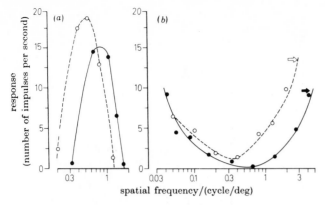

Fig. 12/12. Spatial frequency tuning of the cross-orientation inhibition for two simple cells. (a) The spatial frequency tuning curve of the discharge region of the two cells (mean discharge), obtained by stimulating with a sinusoidal grating (temporal frequency 2 Hz; contrast 30%) of varying spatial frequency (b). The spatial tuning for the cross-orientation inhibition, obtained with a noise conditioning stimulus of 37% contrast, together with an orthogonally oriented grating (temporal frequency 4 Hz; contrast 30%) of variable spatial frequency. The arrows indicate the response to the conditioning noise alone. The inhibitory 'tuning curves' have nothing like the sharp bandpass characteristics of the excitation curves, suggesting that the inhibition arises from a wide range of spatial frequencies. Adapted with permission from Morrone et al. (1982).

that S cells receive inhibitory input from other S cells. I propose therefore to modify the wiring diagrams introduced by Heggelund for simple and complex cells (Chapter 11), just by stating that in the simple cell model, the inhibitory interneuron is another simple cell, while in the complex cell model, the inhibitory interneuron is another complex cell (Fig. 12/13). We would have, *right at the input of the cortex (in layers IV and VI), 3 types of cell pairs generating inhibition:* a pair of ON center S1 cells each connected to LGN cells with slightly offset centers in the same eye and reciprocally inhibiting each other, a pair of OFF center S1 cells, with offset centers inhibiting each other, and a pair of C cells with slightly offset excitatory input and reciprocal inhibitory connections. The recent observation of Palmer and Davis (1981 a) of two S cells recorded simultaneously and having RFs with complementary subregions is very suggestive of the existence of such pairs of S cells. Figure 12/14 shows the modelling of spatial frequency and orientation tunings of a pair of S cells, each receiving input from only one ON center LGN neuron and inhibiting each other (Daugman, personal communication). The modelling was done with two-dimensional Fourier analysis and shows that both tunings are, to a first approximation, independent of each other. The orientation tuning is too wide compared to the actual selectivity (see Chapter 5). Sharpening could probably be provided either by taking elongated inputs (both excitatory and inhibitory) and or by supposing inhibitory inputs from cells with different orientation preferences (see below).

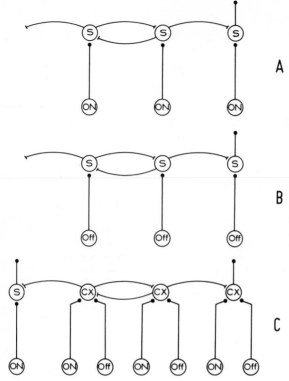

A

B

C

Fig. 12/13. Model of interneurons generating intracortical inhibitions. A: pair of ON-center S cells, B: pair of OFF-center S cells, and C: pair of C cells. The RFs of the ON LGN cells in A are slightly offset as are those of the OFF LGN cells in B. In C the ON and OFF LGN cells converging into 1 cell have overlapping RFs but the RFs of the LGN cells projecting to the other member of the pair are slightly offset. Interneurons of each pair can inhibit cells not belonging to the pair (one of such cells is indicated in A and B, two of them in C). Dots indicate excitatory inputs, short lines inhibitory inputs.

Figure 12/15 summarizes the possible *wiring diagrams* of different members of the area 17 S family, at least for inputs from the dominant eye. The basic input of an S1 cell (here an ON center S1 cell) is *two rows of LGN cells* (here both ON center), one projecting directly and excitatorily onto the S1 cell and the other exerting an indirect inhibition through an S1 interneuron. The latter contribution produces the oriented sidebands and suppressive flanks of S1 cells. In addition to those inputs, the S1 cell receives inhibitory input from *a pool of complex cells* of which the RFs cover the excitatory ON center row and which respond to all orientations including the one of the S1 cell they feed into. The input from complex cells with orientation different from the S1 cell is strongly suggested by the results of Morrone et al. (1982) and input from a complex with the same optimal orientation as the S1 cell is suggested by the Hammond and MacKay (1981) results. It is possible that the latter input is not always as strong as that from complex cells generating the cross-orientation inhibition, and this would explain why some S cells respond weakly to 2D noise fields (Morrone, 1982 and Chapter 4). The orientation selectivity of the cell would result from three factors: the length summation in the excitatory drive, the inhibition from the suppressive flank and the tonic inhibition from the pool of complex cells. The direction selectiv-

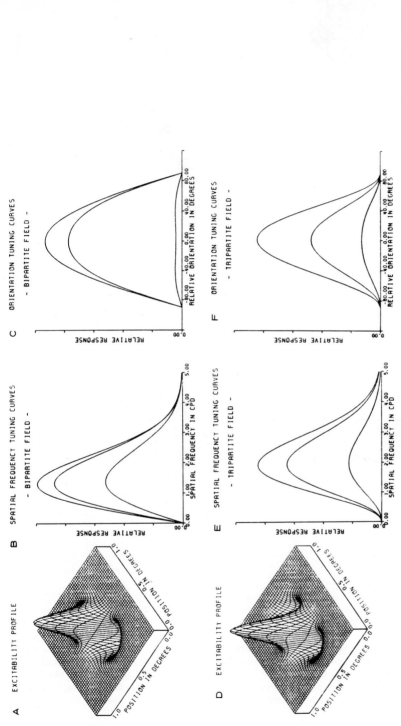

Fig. 12/14. Simulation of spatial frequency and orientation tuning of S cells with excitatory and inhibitory input of same polarity (ON or OFF): A, B, C model with one excitatory and one inhibitory input as explained in the text, D, E, F more evolved model with two inhibitory inputs. The dimension of the RF lobes (half-width at half-height) and the distance between centers has been arbitrarily set to 0.1°. Spatial frequency tunings (B, E linear scales) and orientation tunings have been calculated from the two-dimensionel Fourier transforms (not shown) of the excitability profiles (A, D). Spatial frequency tunings are shown for the optimal orientation and orientations 30° and 60° away from the optimal. Orientation tunings are shown for the optimal spatial frequency and for half and twice this frequency. While the spatial frequency tuning approximately fits the actual values, the orientation tuning is too wide. For additional mechanisms see text (Daugman, personal communication).

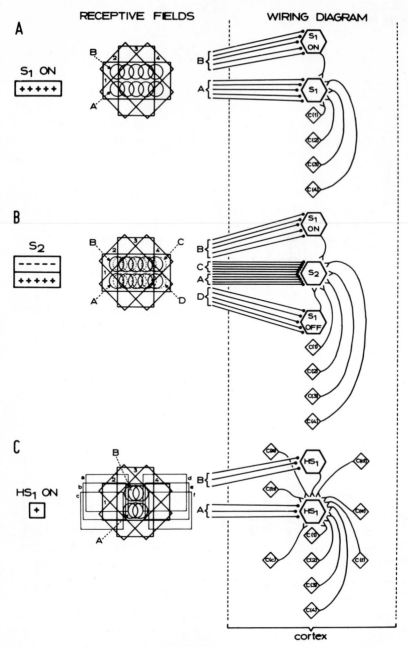

Fig. 12/15. Wiring diagram of different members of the S family: a S1 ON-center cell (A), a S2 cell (B) and a HS1 ON-center cell (C). For each cell the schematic RF outline (as revealed by stationary flashed slits), the RFs of the different input to cell and the wiring diagram are shown. A, B rows of ON-center LGN cells, C, D rows of OFF-center LGN cells, 1, 2, 3, 4 RFs of complex cells C(1) to C(4) and a, b, c, d, e and f RFs of complex cells C (a) to C (f). In the wiring diagrams, dots indicate excitatory inputs and Vs inhibitory inputs. Note that the pool of inhibitory complex cell inputs could account for the firing threshold of simple cells postulated by Henry et al. (1978 a). This firing threshold could also explain why cortical simple cells, contrary to geniculate cells, do not respond to the body of a wide slit, but only to its edges (Bishop et al., 1971 a).

ity could arise from the asymmetric inhibition by the suppressive flank combined with the inhibition from the pool of complex cells. The latter will be mostly driven by Y afferents and could operate as the transient inhibition required by the Marr (1982) model of direction selectivity. Furthermore the pool of Y-driven complex cells could intervene in the temporal low-pass filtering occurring in area 17 S cells, as the complex cells would cause a very brief, phasic inhibition. Finally, by their tonic inhibitory influence these complex cells could account for the firing threshold of simple cells postulated by Henry et al. (1978 a). The S2 cell would have very similar inputs, except that on top of the row of inhibitory ON center LGN afferents, there would be a row of OFF center LGN afferents providing an excitatory drive to the cell. This is suggested by the results of Bullier et al. (1982) reported in the previous chapter. It is likely that corresponding to the excitatory OFF center input there must be an inhibitory input from OFF center LGN cells overlapping with the excitatory ON center input.

Finally an HS1 cell would have inputs very similar to the S1 cell, except that the rows of LGN centers projecting to the cell would be more restricted in length, as suggested by Rose (1979). In addition the HS1 cell likely receives input from two additional pools of complex cells with the same optimal orientation as the HS1 cell, but with receptive fields offset lengthwise.

The *pairs of inhibitory interneurons can then generate the inhibitions for other cells not involved in the pairs* (Fig. 12/13). S1 cell pairs would provide inhibition for sidebands and orientation selectivity and possibly direction selectivity of other S cells which would then not have to be interneurons. The pair of C cells would provide inhibition causing orientation selectivity of other C cells (according to the Heggelund model), and contributing to orientation selectivity of S cells. Those C cells would also provide the end-zone inhibition and direction-selective inhibition of any family, some of the monocular cell inhibitions and the noise field inhibition of S cells. Except for the hypothetical inhibitory projection of C family cells onto S family cells, the inhibitory connections demonstrated by the correlation technique of Toyama et al. (1981 a, b) support this scheme. This scheme requires that inhibitory cells can project both locally (to the other member of the pair) and at some distance in the cortex (to cells outside the pair). Both physiological (Hess et al., 1975) and anatomical evidence (Fisken et al., 1975) suggests that indeed intracortical inhibition can project horizontally over some distance. According to Hess et al. (1975) inhibitory effects were seen at distances up to 100–200 µ from the source in 18 out of 29 cases and in 4 out of 25 cases at distances up to 300–500 µ. Fisken et al. (1975) showed that although after local intracortical lesions symmetrical (supposedly inhibitory) synapses on degenerating terminals are less numerous than asymmetrical (supposedly excitatory) synapses, they project proportionally further away from their sources than asymmetrical ones.

12.3 The Structural Counterpart of Inhibitions

One of the objectives of physiologists is to link structure and function. In this respect the intracellular injection experiments, in which cells are physiologically studied, injected with a marker (Procion yellow or more recently HRP), and then recovered on sections to study their morphology, seem to represent the ultimate experiments. Those extremely difficult experiments initiated in the visual cortex by Kelly and Van Essen (1974), are only in their first stages (Gilbert and Wiesel, 1979; Lin et al., 1979, Martin and Whitteridge, 1981). Initially, Kelly and Van Essen (1974) suggested a correlation between the two major physiological types (simple and complex) and the two major morphological types (stellate and pyramidal). However, further work has shown *that this correlation does not hold* (Gilbert and Wiesel, 1979). Garey (1971) and LeVay (1973) have suggested that there are in fact two types of stellate cells: spiny stellate and smooth stellate cells. The typology of non-pyramidal cells has been further expanded by Peters and Regidor (1981). They described 12 types of non-pyramidal cells (see Table 12/1). [6] *Pyramidal and spiny stellate cells* produce axon terminals of type 1 (i.e. asymmetrical with round vesicles and pronounced postsynaptic opacity) and are very likely excitatory in nature. These cells are transmitting cells, projecting either at distance (i.e., outside the cortex) or locally onto higher order cells. Only pyramidal cells were supposed to project outside the cortex, but recently it has been found that layer IV spiny stellates can also project outside the cortex (see Fairén and Valverde, 1980 for review and also Meyer and Albus 1981 a).

On the contrary *smooth (or sparsely spiny) stellate cells*, corresponding to the small multipolar cells and the sparsely spinous stellate cells of Peters and Regidor (1981), have type 2 synapses (symmetrical with flat vesicles and slight postsynaptic thickening) on their terminals (LeVay, 1973; Peters and Fairén, 1978) and are likely to be inhibitory in nature. These smooth stellate cells occur throughout the cortical layers (Garey, 1971), being outnumbered by their spiny counterparts in layer IV but not in the other layers. At least in the rat visual cortex it has been shown that smooth stellate cells receive both type 1 and 2 synapses and receive geniculate afferents. In addition they send their type 2 synapses (supposedly inhibitory) to any other type of neuron (pyramidal, smooth and spiny stellate cells, and actually Peters and Fairén (1978) have shown that smooth stellate cells could reciprocally inhibit each other. The layer IV smooth stellate cells A and B in their Fig. 22 have exactly the connections required for the pair of interneurons postulated above on physiological grounds. Furthermore, Ribak (1978) has shown that smooth

---

[6] Davis and Sterling (1979) have described 7 types of neurons in layer IVab using soma size and shape, dendritic branching pattern and synaptic input.

Table 12/1. Non-pyramidal cell types in area 17 of cat visual cortex (Golgi preparation) (Modified from Peters and Regidor 1981)

Dendritic morphology	Frequency of spines	Axonal features	Layers with cell bodies	Proposal simple name
A. Neurons in layers II through V				
1. Multipolar neurons				
Spherical dendritic trees	Smooth	Prolific local arborization	II/III, IV, V	Small multipolar cell
	Sparsely spinous	Local arborization	II/III	Sparsely spinous stellate
	Spinous	Descending recurrent collaterals	IV	Spinous stellate
Elongate dendritic trees	Sparsely spinous or smooth	Horizontal branches or horizontal branches and arcades or arcades	II/III, IV and V	Basket cell
2. Bitufted neurons				
Vertical dendritic trees	Smooth	Chandeliers	II/III, IV	Chandelier cell
	Sparsely spinous	Vertically oriented	II/III	Sparsely spinous bitufted cell (double bouquet cell?)
3. Bipolar neurons				
Vertical dendritic trees	Smooth or sparsely spinous	Vertically oriented	IV, V	Bipolar cell
B. Neurons in layer I				
1. Bitufted neurons				
Horizontal dendritic trees	Smooth	Horizontal	I	Horizontal cell of layer I
C. Neurons in layer VI				
1. Multipolar neurons				
Elongate dendritic trees	Sparsely spinous	Horizontal and ascending	Upper VI	Basket cells of layer VI
Spherical dendritic trees	Sparsely spinous	Descending	Upper VI	Sparsely spinous cell of layer VI
2. Bipolar neurons				
Horizontal dendritic trees	Sparsely spinous or smooth	Descending	Lower VI	Horizontal cell of layer VI

stellates in the rat visual cortex contain glutamate decarboxylase (GAD), the enzyme that synthesizes the inhibitory transmitter GABA. It is thus very likely that the *smooth stellates are interneurons using GABA*. This is further corroborated by the observation of Davis and Sterling (1979) that their varicose stellate cells (class 3) which is a kind of smooth stellate (Garey, 1971), selectively takes up exogenous $|^3H|$-gamma aminobutyric acid. It seems thus that the pairs of inhibitory S1 cells in layer IV can be identified as pairs of smooth stellates using GABA and indeed Gilbert and Wiesel (1979) showed in one of their figures a layer IV smooth stellate cell with a S family RF. Whether the pairs of C cell interneurons are also smooth stellates in layer IV or in other layers, remains to be seen. Gilbert and Wiesel (1979) described a layer VI smooth stellate with complex RF. Other hypothetical inhibitory neurons have been described anatomically, as, e.g. the chandelier cell (Szentagothai, 1973), the basket cell (DeFilipe and Fairén, 1982), and double bouquet cells (Somogyi and Cowey, 1981). The chandelier cell makes symmetrical synapses on the axon initial segment of a class of pyramidal cells, possibly the callosal projecting cells (Fairén and Valverde, 1980). Basket cells are thought to project both onto pyramidal and non-pyramidal cells (DeFilipe and Fairén, 1982), while double bouquet cells mainly contact dendritic shifts of pyramidal and non-pyramidal cells (Somogyi and Cowey, 1981). More injection experiments are required to find out to what physiological type these interneurons correspond. At the present stage the correlation between physiology and morphology at least suggests that both S and C families can be interneurons (e.g. smooth stellate cells) as they can be transmitting neurons (pyramidal cells or spiny stellate cells). However most output cells which have been physiologically identified belong to the C or B family, with the exception of some corticothalamic cells and a few cortico-cortical cells projecting to LS (see Chapter 10). One of the big challenges for visual cortical experiments is to find the destination of the exquisitely refined output of the S family cells.

12.4 Conclusion

Intracortical inhibitions determine to a large extent visual cortical cell properties. Intracortical inhibition causes orientation and direction selectivity and to a large extent end-zone inhibition. It also determines to some extent the ocular dominance and velocity of cut-off of cortical cells and the absence of simple cell responses to moving noise fields. This study of the parameter dependence of these inhibitions clearly shows that *excitatory and inhibitory inputs are matched, in that they depend on the same parameters and share similar optimal values of these parameters.* From this "law", the author has deduced the hypothesis that cortical inhibitory interneurons, rahter than being non-oriented cells, are ordinary S or C family cells. Pairs of S1 cells and of C cells could reciprocally inhibit each other and be the source of inhibitory inputs for other cortical cells. A possible anatomical counterpart of the pair of S1 inhibitory interneurons could be a pair of layer IV smooth stellate gabaergic cells reciprocally inhibiting each other.

Chapter 13. Non-Visual Influences on Cat Visual Cortex

First the evidence for non-visual sensory inputs to the visual cortex will be evaluated. Second the neuronal correlates of eye movements in the visual cortex will be discussed. Finally the influence of changes in excitability by sleep and anesthesia will be reviewed.

13.1 Non-Visual Sensory Inputs to the Visual Cortex

Vestibular input is the best documented non-visual sensory input to the visual cortex. Initial experiments using labyrinthine polarization (Grüsser et al., 1959; Grüsser and Grüsser-Cornehls 1960, 1972; Kornhuber and Da Fonseca, 1964) yielded high percentages of visual cortical cells receiving vestibular input. Recent experiments using horizontal rotation (Vanni-Mercier and Magnin, 1982 a) yielded only 13% of area 17 and 18 cells receiving vestibular input and 5% of area 19 cells receiving such an input. The difference in response probability between electrical and natural stimuli might be due to the fact that all cupula and otolith receptors are stimulated with electrical stimulation and not with natural stimulation. Vanni-Mercier and Magnin (1982 a) further showed that about 1/3 of the cells receiving vestibular input showed a specific vestibular response in which the firing rate was periodically modulated by a sinusoidal rotation (see Fig. 13/1). These authors furthermore reported a proportionally larger projection to parts of areas 17 and 18 subserving peripheral vision than to those subserving central vision. A possible anatomical route for the vestibulocortical projections is through the intralaminar nuclei of the thalamus (Vanni-Mercier and Magnin, 1982 a). However, the vestibular responses of visual cortical cells to electrical polarization of the labyrinth might also be correlated with the oculomotor excitation aroused by these stimuli. Indeed Grüsser et al. (1959) and Grüsser and Grüsser-Cornehls (1964) mentioned that before the curarization of encephale isolé cats, electrical polarization of the labyrinth evoked conjugate nystagmus.

While the previous experiments investigated the influence of vestibular stimulation on the spontaneous activity of visual cortical cells, other experimenters have looked for *modification of visual properties* of cortical cells by

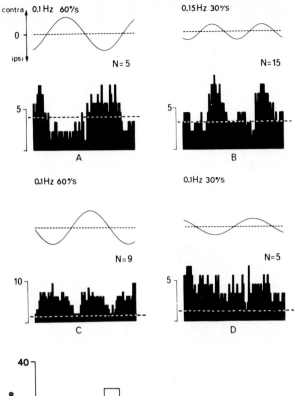

Fig. 13/1. A-D. Examples of cells modulated by vestibular stimulation and recorded in area 17. A-C correspond respectively to specific responses of type 1, 2 and 3. In D, a cell showing a non-specific tonic activation during horizontal vestibular stimulation. Ordinate: number of spikes per bin (bin width = 178 msec); N = number of summations; broken horizontal lines represent the level of spontaneous activity. Upper trace: head velocity. Adapted with permission from Vanni-Mercier and Magnin (1982 a).

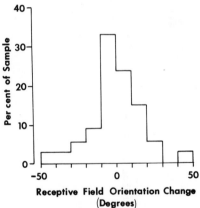

Fig. 13/2. Distribution of receptive field (RF) orientation changes of area 17 simple cells on tilting. Negative or positive values indicate that the RF tilted less (undershoot) or more (overshoot), respectively, than did the animal. Values near zero indicate that there was no change in RF orientation with respect to the animal during the static tilt. Adapted with permission from Tomko et al. (1981).

changing vestibular input. Those experiments chiefly concern the influence of head or body tilt on orientation preferences of area 17 cells. These experiments have produced conflicting results with respect to modification of RF orientations. As shown in Table 13/1, the differences can be largerly accounted for by the differences in methods. A recent study (Tomko et al., 1981) using quantitatively measured orientation tuning curves has shown that 25% of the simple cells in area 17 of paralyzed and unanesthetized cats have their orientation preference changed by body tilt (Fig. 13/2). The differ-

Table 13/1. Effect of tilting on optimal orientation of cortical cells

Authors	Preparation	Cell type	Technique	Amount of tilt	Number of cells	Decision rule	% alterations reported	% cells[+] change RF orientation > 10°
Denney & Adorjani 1972	Unanesthetized Paralyzed	all area 17	hand plotting	20–30° head	33	Any deviation RF orientation from expected orientation	50%	30%
Schwartzkroin 1972	Unanesthetized Paralyzed	all area 17	hand plotting	30° body	33	Deviation or RF orientations from expected orientation not accountable by eye rotation	0%	32%
Horn et al. 1972	Anesthetized Eyes sewed to a ring	all area 17	ORT tuning steps 10°	30–45° body	224	Optimal orientations under tilt outside the expected range (taking into account response variability)	7%	?
Tomko et al. 1981	Unanesthetized Paralyzed	simple cells area 17	ORT tuning steps 5°	45° body	34	Deviation of central tendency of ORT tuning curve from expected value	27%	43%

[+] Uniform criterion applied to all studies, differs from the criteria used by the authors

ent studies agree that the changes in preferred orientation are either compensatory (i.e. making the preferred orientation invariant with the direction of gravity) or anticompensatory. Therefore these changes probably underly more than just orientation perception constancy.

The evidence for *other sensory inputs* to the visual cortex is scant and controversial. Noxious inputs (Murata et al., 1965), auditory inputs (Spinelli et al., 1968; Morrell, 1972; Fishman and Michael, 1973), and proprioceptive inputs (Buisseret and Maffei, 1977) have been reported. A recent study of auditory input to area 17 has failed to substantiate such an input (Bullier and Joseph, personal communication).

13.2 Influence of Eye Movements on Visual Cortical Cells

While all studies agree that eye movements have neuronal correlates in the visual cortex, the proportion of neurons involved vary widely in different reports, the main source of variation being the use of qualitative versus quantitative techniques of analysis (Table 13/2). While from inspection of film records only 7 to 10% cortical cells seem to be influenced by eye movements when the animal is *facing a checkerboard* (Noda et al., 1972; Kasamatsu and Adey, 1973), this proportion rises to 95% when averaging techniques are used (Kimura et al., 1980). It is worth mentioning that Kimura et al. (1980) observed a strong correlation between the type of eye movement effect (excitation or inhibition) and the RF type: all cells excited by eye movements were complex cells, all those inhibited were simple cells, exactly as one would expect from the visual properties of these cells (Orban, 1977). Similarly for cats *in darkness*, single record techniques yield 5% of the cells influenced by saccades (Noda et al., 1972), while averaging raises the proportion to 47% (Kimura et al., 1980) or 25% (Vanni-Mercier and Magnin, 1982 b). Noda et al. (1972) reported both excitation and inhibition after saccades in darkness, while the later studies only report excitation. According to Kimura et al. (1980) all cells activated by saccades in darkness are complex cells. Vanni-Mercier and Magnin (1982 b) showed that about 1/3 of the cells firing after saccades in darkness are directional i.e. fire only for saccades in one direction. The proportion of these directional cells increased with eccentricity of the RF both in areas 17 and 18.

All studies agree that the saccade related influences in darkness have long latencies. As shown in Fig. 13/3, for cells firing both after saccades in light and in darkness, the latency is much longer in the second situation. According to Vanni-Mercier and Magnin (1982 b) the latency of saccades-related excitation in darkness is longer in neurons located in parts of areas 17 and 18 subserving central vision than in those subserving peripheral vision. Both

Table 13/2. Percentages of Visual Cortical Cells Influenced by Eye Movements

Authors	Preparation	Area	Number of cells	Type of eye movements		In darkness	REM or PGO related
				With patterned retinal input			
1) Single record technique							
Noda et al. 1972	awake	17 & 18	357	10%	3/4 excitation & 1/4 inhibition	50% = 5% of total	–
Kasamatsu & Adey 1973	awake	17 & 18	56	7%	3/4 excitation & 1/4 inhibition	–	
	sleep REM	17 & 18	140	–		–	5% excited 45% weak correlation
Hasan & Lehtinen 1981	REM sleep	17 & 18	70	–		–	10% excited 20% weak correlation
Kasamatsu 1976	reserpinized	17 & 18	138	–		–	6,5% excited 19% weak correlation
2) Peristimulus histograms							
Kimura et al. 1980	awake	17	157	95%	2/3 excitation & 1/3 inhibition	75% = 47% of total	–
Vanni-Mercier & Magnin 1982b	awake	17	356	–		0%	–
		18	213	–		27%	–
		19	46	–		24%	–
						2%	–

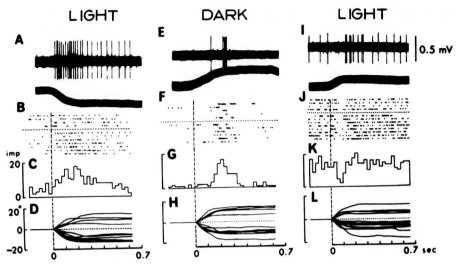

Fig. 13/3. Responses to saccadic eye movements. A-D, responses of a saccade-excited cell during display of a checkerboard. A, upper trace, a specimen record of impulse discharges and lower trace, electrooculogram (EOG) for horizontal eye movement. Upward deflection in EOG represents leftward movement. B, dot displays of impulse discharges. Horizontal dotted line demarcates responses for leftward (upper half) and rightward (lower half) movements. C, an average response histogram for responses shown in B. D, traces of EOG. Time axis is common to A-D. Zero in the axis represents the onset of the saccadic eye movements. E-H, similar to A-D, but in darkness. I-L, similar to A-D, but for a saccade-inhibited cell. Calibration for EOGs is common to A, D, E, H, I and L, and voltage calibration of 0.5 mV to A, E and I. Adapted with permission from Kimura et al. (1980).

in areas 17 and 18 most saccade related excitations occurred with latencies over 100 msec. For comparison it is worth recalling that the latency of visual cortical cell responses to moving stimuli is usually less than 100 ms. Thus *saccadic input latencies are longer than visual input latencies.* This suggests that the saccadic input, which could represent a corollary discharge (Sperry, 1950) is used not for cancellation (von Holst and Mittelstaedt, 1950) but rather for evaluation of the visual input (MacKay, 1973).

Concerning the influence of a third type of rapid eye movement, namely *rapid eye movements* (REM) during deep or paradoxical sleep, there seems to be more consensus although only qualitative techniques were used. Only a small proportion of cells are activated concomitantly with rapid eye movements or their signature, the ponto-geniculo-occipital (PGO) waves. According to Kasamatsu (1976) all these cells are complex cells. A larger proportion of cells are loosely correlated with PGO waves or rapid eye movements. Some of the latter cells were simple cells, others complex cells (Kasamatsu, 1976). Kasamatsu (1976) could further show that cells discharging in tight correlation with PGO waves in reserpinized cats, could also be excited by brain stem stimulation of sites involved in the generation of phasic events during paradoxical sleep (ventral part of locus coeruleus and locus subcoeruleus).

13.3 The Influence of Sleep and Anesthesia

Earlier studies focussed on the changes in spontaneous activity of cortical cells during the waking-sleeping cycle. During waking average spontaneous activity is slightly lower and more widely distributed among neurons than during slow wave sleep (Evarts et al., 1962). Hubel (1959) noted an increase in rythmic bursts during sleep. According to Kasamatsu and Adey (1973) spontaneous activity even further increases during changes from slow wave sleep to paradoxical sleep.

More interesting is the question of how response properties change with changes in arousal level. Livingstone and Hubel (1981) have shown that during sleeping the *signal to noise ratio of cortical cells changes* in the sense that cortical cell activity depends less on stimulus parameters (Fig. 13/4). According to deoxyglucose studies of Livingstone and Hubel (1981) the modulation with sleeping-waking cycle is most marked in the deep cortical layers (V and VI). In this respect it is worth mentioning that Singer et al. (1976) found the largest incidence of facilitatory influences of mesencephalic reticular stimulation among cortical cells with efferents to SC or LGN (100 and 80% respectively), i.e. in the deep layers. It is therefore possible that these

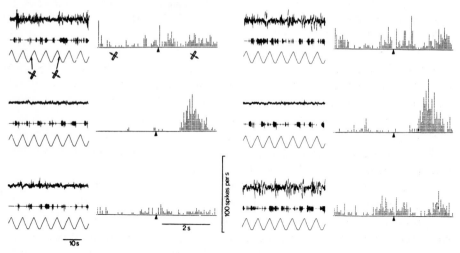

Fig. 13/4. Responses of a cell in the striate cortex of the cat in various levels of arousal. Each record lasts 45 sec and – 3 min elapse between records. As indicated by the EEG (upper trace), the three records on the left side are taken, from above downwards, in slow-wave sleep, awake and slow-wave sleep; those on the right are in slow-wave sleep, awake and slow-wave sleep. The middle trace shows impulse discharges, and lower trace indicates by up-and-down deflections left and right movement of a 1/4° x 2° slit oriented 30° clockwise to vertical. In the alert state the cell responds briskly to rightward movement, but hardly at all to leftward movement. In drowsiness and sleep spontaneous firing is greatly increased, and responses to the moving slit are almost completely absent. Each histogram is the average of 12 responses. Adapted with permission from Livingstone and Hubel (1981).

reticular influences underly the excitability changes during the sleeping and waking cycle.

It seems that anesthesia has about the same influence on response properties as sleep. Ikeda and Wright (1974) have shown that halothane added to a nitrous oxide anesthesia (80% N_2O) reduces the signal to noise ratio of cortical cells and reduces the sustained component of the visual responses. There are some hints that similar changes are induced by barbiturates (Robertson, 1965; Lee, 1970) but no systematic study has been made. By far the most frequently used anesthetic for visual studies is nitrous oxide (usually 70% N_2O and 30% O_2). Mandl et al. (1980) have reported that the properties of some cortical cells are altered by nitrous oxide, although changes in the visual cortex were small compared to those seen in the SC. It remains however to be shown to what extent these effects attributed to nitrous oxide were not due to the pretrigeminal section or to the use of Ketalar, a short acting anesthetic, which in our hands has a disastrous effect on the signal to noise ratio of cortical cells.

Recently it has been shown that nitrous oxide is not an adequate anesthetic for surgical manipulation (Russell, 1973; Steffey et al., 1974). Instead of advocating the use of pentobarbital, of which even the small doses recommended by Hammond (1978) in our experience reduce the tonic component of cortical and LGN responses, we rather suggest *to remove the sources of pain*. If the animal has to be maintained in the stereotaxic apparatus after surgery, a major improvement is the use of a bolt cemented to the skull instead of earbars. Our observations of e.g. the pupillary reflexes suggest that with these precautions nitrous oxide is adequate to maintain a light stable anesthesia in preparations with minimal surgery (venous, tracheal cannula and opening of the skull) as used in visual neurophysiology.

Chapter 14. Response Properties of Monkey Striate Neurons

As pointed out by Hubel and Wiesel (1968) in their pioneering study of monkey striate cortex, response properties of monkey striate neurons are quite similar to those of cat striate neurons. The main differences are the smaller RF size of monkey neurons compared to cat neurons and the greater diversity of response types among monkey striate neurons than among cat striate neurons. Monkey striate neurons can be non-oriented, color specific, and luxotonic. The different aspects of cortical functioning describing for the primary complex of the cat, will now briefly be reviewed for area 17 of the world monkey (chiefly the macaque), highlighting the differences between cat and macaque. While most studies have been conducted in anesthetized and paralyzed monkeys, studies with behaving monkeys (Wurtz, 1969 a; Poggio et al., 1977; Poggio and Fischer, 1977) have shown that neuronal properties are similar in both preparations.

14.1 Retinotopic Organization of Area 17

Area 17 contains a *complete representation of the contralateral hemifield* (Daniel and Whitteridge, 1961; Maunsell, Newsome and Van Essen, personal communication). The vertical meridian is represented at the 17–18 border running about 2 mm behind the lunate sulcus on the lateral side of the hemisphere (Fig. 1/11). The fovea is represented near the lower tip of the lunate sulcus. The lower quadrant is represented in the upper part of area 17 and the upper quadrant in the lower part of area 17. On the lateral or exposed side of the hemisphere the central 9° or 10° of visual field are projected, while the rest of the visual field is represented on the medial side of the hemisphere and in the banks of the calcarine sulcus.

The retinotopic map in monkey striate cortex is a *first order point-to-point transformation* of the visual field with a strong *overrepresentation of the central part of the visual field* (see also Chapter 1). According to Maunsell, Newsome and Van Essen (unpublished) about half of the striate cortex is devoted to the central 7° of the visual field. This is of course reflected in a sharp decrease of cortical magnification with increasing eccentricity. In many studies the inverse magnification factor (deg/mm) is plotted as a function of

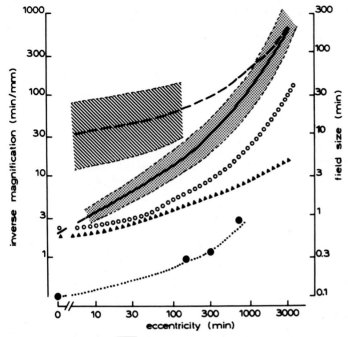

Fig. 14/1. Field size ($\sqrt{\text{area}}$) (stippled line) and inverse magnification (full line) in monkey striate cortex compared to cone separation (filled triangles), minimum angle of resolution (open circles) and hyperacuity (filled circles) in man, all plotted as a function of retinal eccentricity from 0 to 50°. For comparison of spatial performance of human and monkey visual system see Figure 1/18. The mean RF size, indicated by the full line, is from Dow et al. (1981) who used their own data and those of Hubel and Wiesel (1974 b) to calculate the function. The hatching around the mean function indicates the range of field sizes observed by Dow et al. (1981). The mean inverse magnification, indicated by the stippled line, and the range, indicated by hatching, are those calculated by Dow et al. (1981) from their own data and those of Guld and Bertulis (1976), Hubel and Wiesel (1974 b), Daniel and Whitteridge (1961), and Talbot and Marshall (1941). The minimum angle of resolution data are from Weymouth et al. (1928) and Wertheim (1894) reported by Dow et al. (1981). The cone separation data are from Legrand (1967). The hyperacuity data are from Westheimer (1982). Note that a minimum angle of resolution of 1 min corresponds to a grating acuity of 60 cycles/deg (compare with Fig. 1/18A). These relationships illustrate several points: (1) RF size and inverse magnification are not similar functions of eccentricity. (2) RF size exceeds by one log unit the minimum angle of resolution. One could argue that the minimum angle of resolution is achieved by some interpolation process between cells with overlapping RF (see Chapter 5). This may not be required as minimum angle of resolution is of the order of the magnitude of angular resolution of cortical cells. Hence acuity could just reflect the activity of the most finely tuned cortical cells, as the range of spatial frequencies to which primates are sensitive is set by the spatial frequency range of cortical cells. The curves further show (3) that hyperacuity is about one log unit better than ordinary acuity. For this phenomenon the resolution of single cells certainly is inadequate and interpolation processes have to occur; (4) the minimum angle of resolution is close to cone separation at small eccentricities but increases more steeply with eccentricity than cone separation. This probably reflects a limiting step in the receptor ganglion cell connection, which is convergent in the peripheral retina (see Chapter 1).

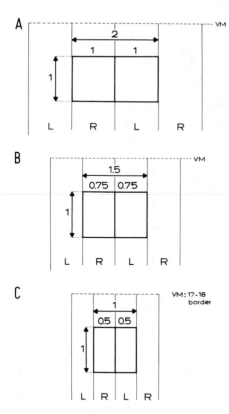

Fig. 14/2. Anisotropy of the cortical magnification factor (CMF). If a square of $1° \times 1°$ in the
visual field gets an isotropic representation in
each ocular dominance column, a grating viewed by each eye separately would be equally well
resolved whether oriented along or across columns. This however requires an anisotropy in
linear CMF of the order 1:2 (A). If the linear
CMF is isotropic (C) this implies that for each
eye separately the magnification is different
whether measured along or across columns. Resolution of a grating oriented along the column
should be twice as low as for a grating oriented
perpendicularly to the columns (Hubel and Wiesel, 1974 b). In fact the anisotropy is of the order
of 1:1.5 (B) (Tootell et al., 1982 a). This implies
that for monocular viewing the ratio of resolution of a grating perpendicular to the columns
and that of a grating parallel to the columns
should be $1:0.75 = 1.36:1$ which was observed
in the periphery of the visual field by Rovamo et
al. (1982).

eccentricity, since this is an approximately linear function (Hubel and Wiesel,
1974 b; Hubel and Freeman, 1977; Tootell et al., 1982 a). In fact Dow et al.
(1981), in a very careful study of the awake monkey, have shown that in the
foveola[1] the MF gets as high as 30 mm/deg (as initially reported by Talbot
and Marshall, 1941), and that the inverse MF is a non-linear function of
eccentricity (Fig. 14/1). There is also some evidence that the cortical magnification factor is *anisotropic*, being larger across ocular dominance columns
than along columns. If each eye has an isotropic representation of a unit
square of visual field, then clearly the unit square in the field would be
mapped on a 1:2 rectangle on the cortex (large dimension going across
columns) (Fig. 14/2). Tootell et al. (1982 a) estimated the ratio to be actually
1:1.5. Since ocular dominance columns run orthogonally to the 17–18
border where the VM is represented, one can expect a greater magnification
along the VM than along the HM. This is also be expected from the shape
of the striate cortex (Sakitt 1982).

---

[1] Central part of the fovea: in humans the diameter of the fovea is 5°, that of the foveola 1.2°
(Bishop, 1981).

14.2 The Input-Output Relations of Monkey Striate Cortex

The geniculate input terminates in layer IV (layer of the spiny stellate cells). In comparison with the cat, layer IV is *more complex* in the monkey (Fig. 14/3): layers IVA and IVC receive LGN afferents, while IVB is an output layer. As in the cat there is a laminar separation of the different types of input (Lund and Boothe 1975; Lund et al., 1975, 1979). The magnocellular afferents, which can be both X and Y (Kaplan and Shapley, 1982), end in layer IVCα. On the contrary, parvocellular afferents which are X like but are less contrast sensitive and more color specific than the magnocellular X cells, terminate in layer IVCβ and IVA. It seems however that the layer IVA input is functionally less important (Mitzdorf and Singer, 1979). There is a reasonably good agreement between the physiological data on successive synaptic activities revealed by current source density analysis and morphological data on termination of different types of geniculate afferents and intralaminar connections (see Fig. 14/4). The electrical stimulation experiments of Bullier and Henry (1980) confirm that the parvocellular afferents end in IVCβ and the magnocellular ones in layer IVCα. As in the cat the supragranular output projects mainly to other cortical areas while infragranular layers project to subcortical structures.

14.3 Receptive Field Organization and Size

In agreement with the first report of Hubel and Wiesel (1968), all subsequent studies (Gouras, 1974; Dow, 1974; Poggio et al., 1975; Schiller et al., 1976a; Bullier and Henry, 1980; Kennedy et al., 1981), have shown that in addition to the RF organizations described in areas 17, 18 and 19 of the cat, monkey striate cortex contains a sizeable proportion of *non-oriented cells* (Table 14/1). Some of these non-oriented cells have concentric RF organization similar to that of ON or OFF center geniculate cells (Hubel and Wiesel, 1968; Poggio et al., 1975; Bullier and Henry, 1980). In many of these cortical cells the surround is more effective than in LGN cells, so that only very small stimuli evoke a response from the cells (Bullier and Henry, 1980). Other non-oriented cells have overlapping ON-OFF subregions and have rather large fields, so that they look like non-oriented complex cells (Kennedy et al., 1981). The latter type of non-oriented cells are especially common in the infragranular layers. Indeed it seems now quite established that, contrary to the initial report of Hubel and Wiesel (1968), non-oriented cells occur outside layer IV, although the bulk of them are found in this layer (Poggio et al., 1975; Dow, 1974; Bullier and Henry, 1980; Schiller et al., 1976a; Kennedy

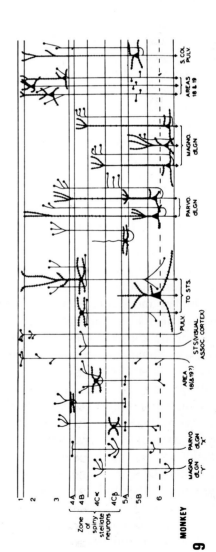

Fig. 14/3. Diagrams summarizing the details of afferent and efferent relationships and intrinsic spinous neuron relays of the cat and monkey striate cortex. With permission from Lund et al. (1979).

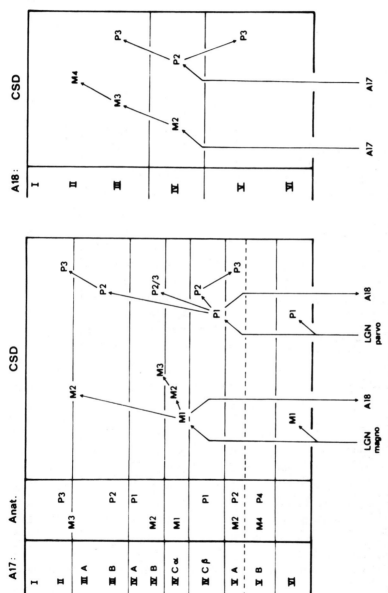

Fig. 14/4. Schematic diagrams of the laminar distribution of successive synaptic activities, as revealed by current source density analysis. The left diagram summarizes the results from area 17, the right diagram sketches the results from the first measurements in area 18. For comparison the analogous conclusions reached by Lund et al. (1975) from anatomical studies are indicated in the central columns of the area 17 diagram. Successive synaptic activities of the fast (magnocellular) group are labelled M1, M2 and successive synaptic activities in the slow (parvocellular) group P1, P2. Physiological and anatomical data are in good agreement with the exception that physiological results put more emphasis on the polysynaptic activity in layer IVC. With permission from Mitzdorf and Singer (1979).

Table 14/1. Proportions of non-oriented and S family cells in two eccentricity classes

	Foveal			Parafoveal	
	% NO	% S		% NO	% S
Gouras (1974) *	46%	5%	Hubel and Wiesel (1968) (0–4°)	6%	9%
Dow (1974) [+]	29%	9 (21%) **	Poggio et al. (1975) * (4–8)	35%	7%
Poggio et al. (1975)*	51%	3%	Schiller et al. (1976 a) (2–8°)	16%	35%
			Bullier and Henry (1980) (2–5°)	31%	49%
			Kennedy et al. (1981)[+] (0–10°)	19%	38%

*   Hypercomplex cells as separate class
** Percentage between brackets is the percentage according to the "Australian criteria"
[+] In the baboon rather the macaque

et al., 1981). According to Hubel and Livingstone (1981), the non-oriented cells outside layer IV, occur in the cytochrome oxydase blobs of layer II–III. There is also good evidence that the proportion of non-oriented cells decrease with eccentricity (see Table 14/1).

Another interesting difference between monkey and cat striate cortex is the *small proportion of simple cells or S family cells* (Table 14/1). Although estimates differ according to the criteria used, it is clear that the proportion of simple like cells is smaller in the monkey than in the cat. Using criteria similar to the initial description of Hubel and Wiesel (1962) the proportion is less than 10%, compared to 30% in the cat. Using the criteria set out in Chapter 4, about 40% the cells belong to the S family compared to 60% in the cat (Table 14/1). As in the cat, corticotectal cells are complex like cells (Finlay et al., 1976 a). In their initial study Hubel and Wiesel (1968) reported 53 out of 272 cells (19%) to be hypercomplex. Subsequent studies have reported much smaller proportions (Gouras, 1974; Poggio et al., 1975; Dow, 1974; Bullier and Henry, 1980) Kennedy et al. (1981) estimated 22% parafoveal striate cells to be end-stopped (including those being only partially end-stopped as defined in Chapter 4). It is not known whether the proportion of end-stopped cells changes with eccentricity as in the primary complex of the cat.

RF sizes of striate neurons in monkey are *smaller* than those in the cat (Hubel and Wiesel, 1968). This is correlated with the spatial discrimination possibilities of both species: acuity of the cat is about 4–6 c/deg (Berkley and Sprague, 1979) compared to 30 or 40 c/deg for the monkey (De Valois et al., 1974 b) (see Fig. 1/18). RF size increases with eccentricity but not exactly linearly as claimed by Hubel and Wiesel (1974 b) and as shown by Dow et al. (1981) the RF size decreases less than inverse magnification factor with decreasing eccentricity (Fig. 14/1). Figure 14/1 also shows that the mean RF size exceeds the minimum angle of resolution (of humans) by a factor of about 10 for small eccentricities.

14.4 Color Specificity in Monkey Striate Cortex

Since the rhesus monkey is a trichromat [2], as are humans (De Valois et al., 1974 a), the macaque is a suitable *animal model* for the study of the neurophysiological basis of color vision. The cat has a very reduced color vision (see Chapter 1) and hence is not a suitable model for the study of color vision mechanisms. Many studies have therefore been directed towards color specificity in the monkey retinogeniculate striate system. There seems to be a remarkable difference between subcortical structures and the striate cortex in that color specificity is much more readily apparent at the subcortical level. Most color specific ganglion and geniculate cells are color *opponent cells*, giving ON responses for one range of wavelengths and OFF responses for another range of wavelengths (Wiesel and Hubel, 1966, de Monasterio and Gouras, 1975). However at the striate level relatively few cells show color opponency (Hubel and Wiesel, 1968). Hence cortical cells are considered as color specific (Hubel and Wiesel, 1968; Dow, 1974; Schiller et al., 1976 a; Kennedy et al., 1981), or narrow band (Gouras, 1974; Bullier and Henry, 1980) or color opponent (Gouras, 1974), not only when they show color opponency as do subcortical cells (spectrally opponent of Poggio et al., 1975), but also when they respond to monochromatic stimuli *over a restricted range of wavelengths* shifted towards one end of the spectrum (spectrally tuned of Poggio et al., 1975) (see Fig. 14/5). The justification for doing so is that with chromatic adaptation spectrally tuned cells show opponent responses (Fig. 14/6) (Dow and Gouras, 1973). Along the same lines it has been shown by Gouras and Krüger (1979) that many cortical cells (over 50% in the foveal region) which do respond to luminosity contrast also respond to pure color contrast when luminosity contrast is eliminated.

As shown in Table 14/2 the *proportions of color specific cells in V1* vary widely among the different studies, although all use the same criteria outlined above. In fact only the studies of which the primary aim was the study of color specific cells come up with high proportions of color specific cells (30–70% in foveal projections). In these studies monochromatic lights were used systematically and action spectra [3] prepared for most cells. The other studies had wider aims and white light was mostly used, monochromatic light being used only when cells responded weakly or not at all to white light. In the latter studies the proportions of color specific cells ranged from 5 to 24%. Probably these proportions are close estimates of what Michael (1978 a) calls color specific cells: cells not responding at all to white light. Among the latter Michael (1978 a, b, c, 1979) distinguishes four types: double opponent non-oriented and simple cells, and color specific complex and hypercomplex cells.

---

[2] Having three different types of cones.
[3] Action spectrum: minimum energy required to activate the cell plotted as a function of wavelength.

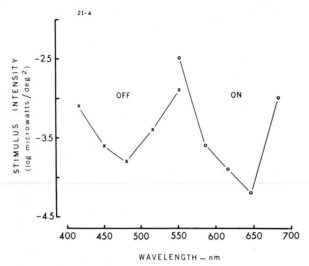

Fig. 14/5 A

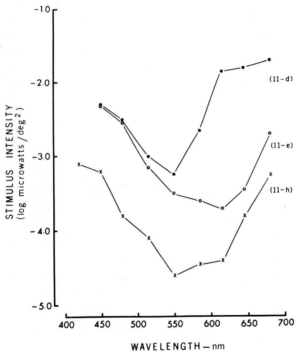

Fig. 14/5 B

Fig. 14/5. Three types of action spectra of cortical cells: (A) spectral opponent neuron, (B) spectrally tuned neurons (11-d and 11-e) and luminosity neurons (11-h). Both spectrally tuned and spectrally opponent cells are considered color specific. The cell in A was a monocular non-uniform oriented cell of layer II. Flashing stimuli were about the size of the RF (0.25° diameter), long wavelengths evoked responses at light ON; short wavelengths at light OFF. The cells in B were all three complex cells: 11-d monocular, layer IVA, 11-e: binocular, layer VI and 11-h monocular, layer VI. All three cells were tested with moving slits, when tested with stationary slits spectrally tuned cells responded uniformly over their whole RF either with ON or OFF and very exceptionally with ON/OFF. With permission from Poggio et al. (1975).

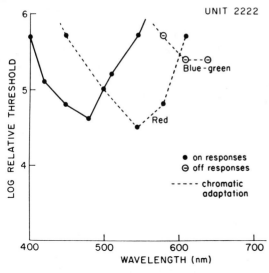

Fig. 14/6. Effect of chromatic adaptation on the action spectrum of a spectrally tuned cell. Stimuli were vertically oriented slits $1/16 \times 2°$ centered in the RF: and presented for 250 msec every 1.6 sec. On a neutral background of 0.0 cd/m^2 the best responses (to light ON) were obtained at $480-500$ nm (full line). The curve of ON response obtained on red background was that of the green sensitive cones. The use of a blue green background brought out OFF responses associated with the red channel. Presumably the inhibition from the red channel caused the narrowing and leftward shift of the green channel action spectrum in the absence of chromatic adaptation. With permission from Dow and Gouras (1973).

The 3 studies in which chromatic properties were systematically investigated (Dow, 1974; Gouras, 1974, Poggio et al., 1975), show several other interesting points: color specificity is more common among non-oriented and simple cells than among complex and hypercomplex cells. Color specific cells occur mainly in layer IV and the supragranular layers. Color specific cells are more numerous in the foveal than parafoveal region (70% compared to 42%). These changes in proportion of color specific cells were recently confirmed and extended by Zeki (1982 a). According to this author the proportion of color specific cells in V1 drops from 40% at an eccentricity of $0-2.5°$ to 2% at $30°$ eccentricity.

Finally it is worth pointing out that what is color specificity in the striate cortex is actually *a wavelength specificity* (Zeki, 1982 b) and that, although

Table 14/2. Percentages of color specific cells

Study	Location cells	Percent
Hubel and Wiesel (1968)	PF	9%
Gouras (1974)	F	41%
Dow (1974)	F	30%
Poggio et al. (1975)	F	70%
	PF	42%
Schiller et al. (1976a)	PF	small
Bullier and Henry (1980)	PF	14%
Kennedy et al. (1981)*	PF	7%

PF = parafoveal region
F = foveal region
* In the baboon rather than the macaque

color perception requires wavelength specificity, the perceived color of an object is not a simple function of the wavelength emitted by the object but of the proportions of long, short, and medium wavelengths emitted by the object and its surroundings (Land, 1977). Secondly it is very possible that many striate color specific cells are not involved in color perception per se, but in the analysis of color contrast, allowing the system to distinguish objects by color (Gouras and Krüger, 1979) thereby increasing the discrimination capabilities of the visual system.

14.5 Influence of Light Intensity and Contrast on Monkey Striate Neurons

Most macaque striate cells respond only to restricted visual stimuli and for these cells "simultaneous"[4] contrast represents the stimulus strength. However, about 24% of monkey striate cells do respond to overall changes in illumination (Kayama et al., 1979). These units have been called *luxotonic cells*. As shown in Fig. 14/7 some of these cells are activated by an increase in overall illumination (photergic), others by a decrease in overall illumination (scotergic). In the cortex photergic cells are more common (ratio photergic/scotergic, 4/1). In the LGN where 28% of the cells were luxotonic, the ratio was 1/1. Cells similar to luxotonic cells have been described among W cells in the cat retina (Stone and Fukuda, 1974) but are reputedly rare in the cat cortex (DeYoe and Bartlett, 1980) although we (Orban and Duysens, unpublished) have seen such cells at the 18–19 border (see Chapter 6). Luxotonic cells are often binocular (2/3 of the cells). They often have non-oriented RFs (corresponding to the T cells of Schiller et al., 1976 a) but can also have other RF organizations such as those of S or B families (Kennedy, Martin, Orban and Whitteridge, unpublished).

As cat striate neurons, monkey striate neurons have contrast-response functions that are best described by an *hyperbolic function* (Albrecht and Hamilton, 1982). In both species, the dynamic range of the cell (i.e. the contrast range over which the cell's response increases with contrast) is independent of the optimal spatial frequency of the cell. Hence, the greater behavioral sensitivity contrast of cat (Bisti and Maffei, 1974) and monkeys (De Valois et al., 1974 b) at middle spatial frequencies is not produced by a greater (average) sensitivity of the individual cells tuned to those spatial frequencies. As shown by De Valois et al. (1982 b), the number of cells preferring those medium spatial frequencies is greater (Fig. 14/9), suggesting that behavioral contrast sensitivity could depend on the number of cells

---

[4] "Simultaneous" contrast refers to a difference in luminance between two adjacent parts of the visual field at a given moment. Contrast was used in this sense in Chapter 6.

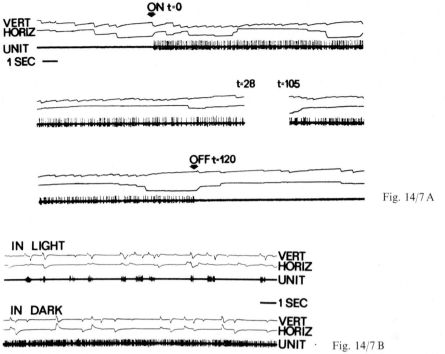

Fig. 14/7 A

Fig. 14/7 B

Fig. 14/7. Luxotonic cells: photergic cell (A); scotergic cell (B). A) Photergic unit with essentially no discharge in the dark (three spikes during 2 min). When light is turned ON, $t = 0$, discharge begins at about 16/sec, which diminishes gradually to 6–9/sec after about 20 sec. The latter rate continues indefinitely until light is turned OFF after 120 sec. Upper trace, vertical EOG, where upward deflection indicates upward eye movement and brief isolated, upward deflection indicates an eye blink. Middle trace is horizontal EOG, upward deflection indicating movement to the right, the EOG, recorded in the DC mode, shows that the monkey has vertical nystagmus in either the light (ganzfeld, 45 cd/m^2) or dark. Analysis showed no correlation between eye movements and unit discharge. Upper set of traces continues with those in middle up to 28 sec; record resumed at 105 sec following light ON and is continuous with lower set of traces. Unit gave no response to illumination of left eye. B) Scotergic unit, in which most of discharge in the light is generated by blinking. Upper set of traces taken about 4 min after light turned ON (188 cd/m^2), and lower set after more than 5 min in darkness. EOG recorded in AC mode; upward deflection signifies upward or rightward eye movement. In most of the instances shown the upward movement probably indicates a slow blink terminated after about 200–300 msec by a downward eye movement. There was no discernible modulation of discharge rate in the dark by eye movements. With permission from Kayama et al. (1979).

tuned to a given spatial frequency.[5] Compared to cat striate cells, monkey cortical cells have a slightly higher threshold and steeper slope in the ascending part of the contrast-response function (Fig. 14/8).

---

[5] Alternatively, the contrast sensitivity could only depend on the most sensitive cortical cells e.g. cells receiving magnocellular input. To exclude this alternative one would have to show that not only the average contrast sensitivty of area 17 cells but also the variance of their sensitivity is invariant with spatial frequency.

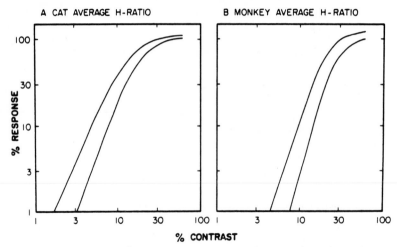

Fig. 14/8. Comparison of contrast-response curves in cat and monkey. The upper and lower bounds (2 SE above and below the parameter means) of the average hyperbolic function (H ratio) are shown for the population of cat and monkey cells separately. The mean exponent and semisaturation contrast are greater for monkey in comparison to cat. With permission from Albrecht and Hamilton (1982). See Chapter 6 for definitions.

14.6 Influence of Spatial Parameters

Contrary to the initial claim of Hubel and Wiesel (1968), monkey striate cells are *not more narrowly tuned for orientation than their cat counterparts* (De Valois et al., 1982 a). As in the cat S cells are more narrowly tuned for orientation than C cells (Schiller et al., 1976 b). As in the cat orientation tuning becomes sharper with increasing stimulus length (Schiller et al., 1976 b). Different authors have reported that in *foveal projection* (0–2° eccentricity) monkey striate neurons prefer vertical and horizontal orientations over oblique ones (Mansfield, 1974; Blakemore et al., 1981; De Valois et al., 1982 a). However, this anisotropy is not present in parafoveal regions (Finlay et al., 1976 b; De Valois et al., 1982 a). If one considers however *only the S cells* and not the overall population of striate cells, then the preference for principal (horizontal and vertical) orientations over obliques is still present in the *parafoveal region* (Kennedy, Martin, Orban and Whitteridge, unpublished). There is no difference in orientation tuning width between cells preferring principal orientations and those preferring oblique ones (De Valois et al., 1982 a). Nor is there a change in orientation tuning width with eccentricity (at least up to 20° eccentricity) (De Valois et al., 1982 a and Schiller et al., 1976 b).

As with the cat cortical cells, cells in striate cortex of the monkey are tuned to different spatial frequencies. The main difference is that the peak

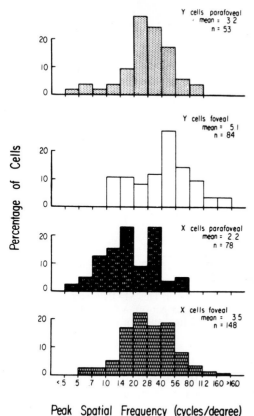

Fig. 14/9. Distributions of optimal spatial frequencies of cortical cells. The total population was segregated into simple and complex cells (unorthodoxically labelled X and Y respectively) recorded from the foveal and parafoveal areas. The foveal samples extend into higher frequencies than the parafoveal samples. Note that the highest optimal spatial frequencies are about a factor 6–8 higher than those in the cat (see Fig. 7/12). This factor 6–8 corresponds grossly to the ratios in grating acuities of cat and monkey (see Fig. 1/17 and 1/18). With permission from De Valois et al. (1982 b).

spatial frequencies are much higher in the monkey than in the cat, in keeping with the smaller RF size mentioned earlier. As shown in Fig. 14/9 the optimal spatial frequency decreases with increasing eccentricity (Schiller et al., 1976 c and De Valois et al., 1982 b). While simple or S cells respond in a modulated way to drifting gratings, complex or C cells respond in an unmodulated way (Schiller et al., 1976 c). This can be used as a criterion of cell classification in the awake behaving monkey (Poggio et al., 1977).

14.7 Influence of Spatio-Temporal Parameters

In their initial study of monkey striate cortex Hubel and Wiesel (1968) reported that about half of the complex cells have a clear preference for one direction of motion over the other. It has been shown by Schiller et al. (1976 a) that C cells can either be directional or not. The overall proportion of direction-selective cells has been estimated at 29% by De Valois et al.

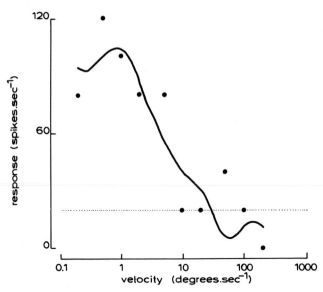

Fig. 14/10. Velocity-response curve of a monkey area 17 cell. This S1 ON center cell recorded in layer VI had a velocity low-pass curve: half height upper cut-off: 4.4°/sec, response to slow movement 88%; response strength 42 sp/sec. Stippled line: spontaneous activity (maximum firing rate) (Kennedy, Orban and Bullier, unpublished).

(1982 a). Our own studies suggest that the proportion of direction-selective cells could be as *low* in monkey striate cortex as in area 17 of the cat (33% cells with clear direction preference with hand plotting). Little information is available about the influence of stimulus velocity on monkey striate neurons. Wurtz (1969 b) has shown that in the behaving monkey some of the cells in the parafoveal region (3–10°) respond up to very high (> 200°/sec) velocities. On the contrary, preliminary results of Van Essen and coworkers (1982) and of Kennedy, Orban and Bullier (unpublished) indicate that in the foveal region all cells have very low upper cut-off velocities. The preliminary results of Kennedy, Orban and Bullier show that the overwhelming majority of striate neurons in the foveal region are of the *velocity low-pass type* (Fig. 14/10).

14.8 Ocular Dominance Distribution and Depth Sensitivity

The ocular dominance distribution of the monkey striate cortex is much more *biased towards monocular cells* than that of the cat area 17 (Hubel and Wiesel, 1968) (compare Fig. 14/11 with Fig. 9/1). This explains why ocular dominance columns are much clearer in the monkey than the cat. As in the cat, simple cells are more monocular than complex cells (Fig. 14/11).

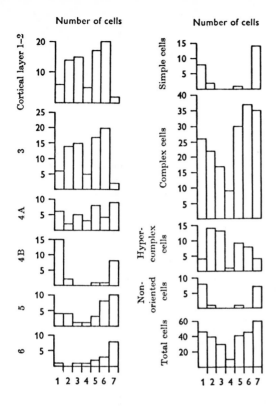

Fig. 14/11. Ocular dominance histogram of monkey area 17 (compare with similar histograms for the cat in Fig. 9/1). Left: ocular dominance distribution of 272 cells among the various layers; right ocular dominance distribution of the same 272 cells among different cell classes. Layer IVA and IVB correspond roughly to IVB and IVC in the more recent terminology (Lund, 1973). With permission from Hubel and Wiesel (1968).

The behaving monkey has proven extremely useful for the study of binocular interactions and depth sensitivity of striate neurons. This preparation is devoid of residual eye movements which plague disparity manipulations in the paralyzed animal. In such a preparation, Poggio and Fisher (1977) have shown that although many cells are monocular, when each eye is tested separately for excitatory drive, almost all cells get a binocular input (195 out of 199 cells). Poggio and Fisher (1977) have described 4 types of depth response curves (Fig. 14/12 and 14/13). *Tuned excitatory and inhibitory neurons* are either activated or inhibited over a small range of depths around the fixation point (Fig. 14/12). *Far or near cells* are activated by a wide range of depths on the far or near side of the fixation point (Fig. 14/12). While tuned excitatory cells had mainly a balanced ocular dominance, the other 3 groups had a rather unbalanced ocular dominance. While tuned excitatory cells could be implicated in fine stereopsis and binocular fusion, far and near cells could contribute to coarse stereopsis and also control vergence eye movements. Pursuing his studies on the neuronal mechanisms of stereopsis, Poggio (personal communication) has shown that striate cells, both simple and complex cells, are sensitive to disparities in Julesz patterns, which are reputed to involve global stereopsis (Julesz, 1971).

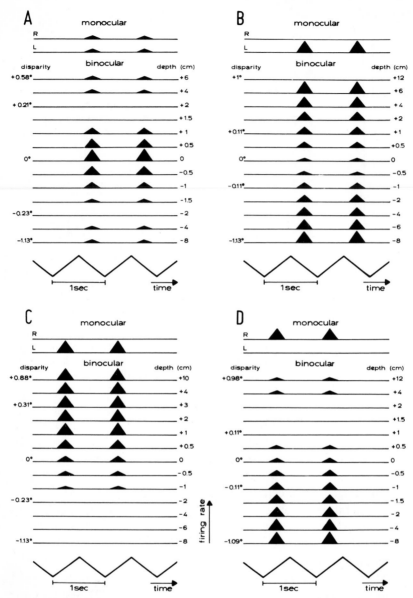

Fig. 14/12. The four types of depth sensitive cells according to Poggio and Fischer (1977): tuned excitatory (A), tuned inhibitory (B), far (C), and near (D) cells. Responses to monocular stimulation and binocular stimulation at different depth are compared. Average firing rate is schematically drawn as a function of time for 2 complete stimulus cycles (forward and backward movement of a slit). Depth is given on the right as deviation (cm) from the fixation distance (38 cm). Corresponding disparities are shown on the left. In A a binocular facilitation is evident over a range of 2.5 cm and inhibitory sidebands occur further and closer (see Chapter 9). In B there is a considerable reduction of response over a range of about 1 cm corresponding to 0.1° disparity. In C the cell responds best to stimuli behind the fixation plane, while inside the fixation plane the responses were suppressed at a distance corresponding to a disparity of −1.13°. In the D the reverse occurred. Note the ocular imbalance in B, C and D.

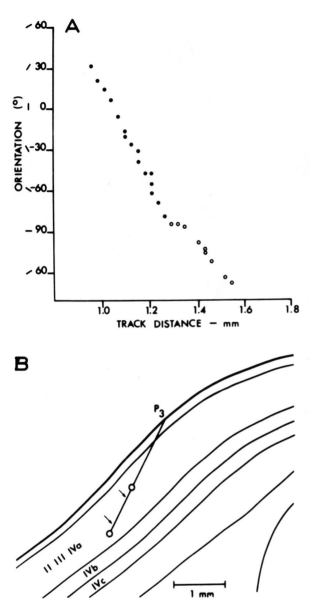

Fig. 14/13. Physiological evidence for orientation columns. A) Plot of preferred orientation of cells or *groups of cells* versus track distance. In plotting orientation, 0° is vertical, angles clockwise up to 90° are positive, counterclockwise to 89° negative. Closed circles: ipsilateral (right eye; open circles, contralateral (left) eye. Track distance is taken from micrometer advances readings. Note the smooth shift in orientation. It should be mentioned that recording from groups of cells rather than from single cells, will tend to produce smoother plots. We have no idea of the proportion of recordings from clusters of cells versus recordings from single cells in this study. However Hubel and Wiesel report in their 1974 paper that they only saw regular sequences when using low impedance electrodes enhancing the chances of recording from clusters. The author's own experience is that when recording only from isolated cells regular orientation sequences are indeed exceptional (but see Fig. 14/15). B) Reconstruction of the electrode track. The electrode entered the striate cortex 8 mm behind the lunate section in the parasagittal plane, 10 mm to the right of the midline, intersecting the surface at 20°. The sequence described in A was recorded between the two arrows. Circles represent electrolytic lesions. Anterior is to the right. With permission from Hubel and Wiesel (1974a).

14.9 Columnar Organization and Functional Architecture of Striate Cortex

The physiological studies of Hubel and Wiesel (1968, 1974a) have suggested that there are at least two independent sets of columns extending vertically from the cortical surface to the white matter: one set of *orientation columns* and one set of *ocular dominance columns* (Fig. 14/14). Recently Dow et al. (1982) have disputed the view that the optimal orientation is constant

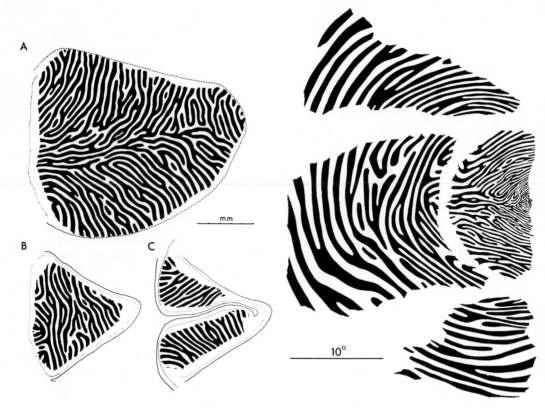

Fig. 14/14. Ocular dominance columns in monkey striate cortex in anatomical reconstruction (left) and visual field reconstruction (right). Left side: A reconstruction of ocular dominance columns from a macaque monkey right occipital lobe, prepared from a set of serial sections roughly tangential to the exposed surface of the occipital lobe, and stained by the reduced silver method of Liesegang (LeVay et al., 1975). In the diagram every other column has been inked in; thus the dark stripes in the figure correspond to one eye and the light stripes to the other. A: stripes on the exposed surface of the occipital lobe. Lateral is to the right; anterior is up. The dashed-shaped line represents the 17–18 border (vertical meridian); at the extreme right, where this line curves around sharply, is the foveal representation. The dotted line at the medial edge (left, in the figure) indicates where the cortex bends over abruptly to continue as a buried fold. The region of cortex shown represents visual field from fovea out to about 9°. B: the continuation of A as a buried fold, one level deeper. This is in reality positioned below A, with the medial parts of the dotted lines superimposed. The more lateral-shaped part of this dotted line suggests the position of another pair of folds, where the cortex continues into a third, still deeper pair of shelves. These are shown in C, B and C together continue the visual-field representation, from 9° out to about 25°. Right side: Visual field reconstruction out to about 25° including all 3 parts shown on the left. Since the reconstructed parts are from the right hemisphere, the projection is into the left visual hemifield. Anterior areas in front of the horizontal meridian projection, project to the inferior visual field, posterior areas project to the superior field. With permission from Hubel and Freeman (1977).

in vertical penetrations extending from supra- to infragranular layers. One of the reasons for discrepancies could be that the Hubel and Wiesel (1974 a) study was done in cortex representing 2 to 10° from the fixation point while the study of Dow et al. (1982) was done in the foveal region. In the latter there is a strong meridional anisotropy in preferred orientations which according to Blakemore et al. (1981) is due to frequent reversals in the sequences of preferred orientations. It could thus well be that orientation columns are less well ordered in the foveal region. The existence of ocular dominance columns (Fig. 14/15) was confirmed by a variety of histological techniques: degenerating axons (Hubel and Wiesel, 1972), transneuronal transport (Wiesel et al., 1974) and reduced silver method (LeVay et al., 1975). These studies have shown that ocular dominance columns are 0.2 to 0.5 mm wide. In their physiological study of orientation columns, Hubel and Wiesel (1974 a) showed that a total orientation shift of 180° also took about 0.5 to 1 mm. Thus 1 mm of cortex is about the cortical distance corresponding to a full range of orientations and of ocular dominance. As this is also about the distance to cross before reaching a cortical region analyzing a different point in visual space (Hubel and Wiesel, 1974 b) and since both sets of columns are independent, Hubel and Wiesel have considered a 1 × 1 mm block of cortex as the functional unit of cortex (*hypercolumn*) containing the necessary machinery for the analysis of one point in visual space (Hubel and Wiesel, 1977) (see Fig. 15/1). Subsequently both orientation and ocular dominance columns have been demonstrated by 2-deoxyglucose labelling experiments (Hubel et al., 1977; Horton and Hubel, 1981; Tootell et al., 1982 b). Such experiments have also been claimed to reveal *spatial frequency columns* (Tootell et al., 1981).

From his physiological studies of color specific cells, defined as cells not responding at all to white light, Michael (1981) has concluded that *color specific cells are aggregated in columns* which seem to be independent of orientation and ocular dominance columns. Within one column the preferred wavelength is constant (Fig. 14/15). It remains to be seen how this system could be related to the system of cytochrome oxidase (Wong-Riley, 1979) blobs (Horton and Hubel, 1981; Humphrey and Hendrickson, 1980) in the supragranular layers, which have been shown by Hubel and Livingstone (1982) to contain non-oriented, color specific cells (see Fig. 15/1).

14.10 Correlation Between Response Properties and Afferent Input

Very few studies have been directed towards the mechanisms underlying striate response properties in monkey. In a study analogous to the one done in the cat (see Chapter 11), Bullier and Henry (1980) have studied the afferent

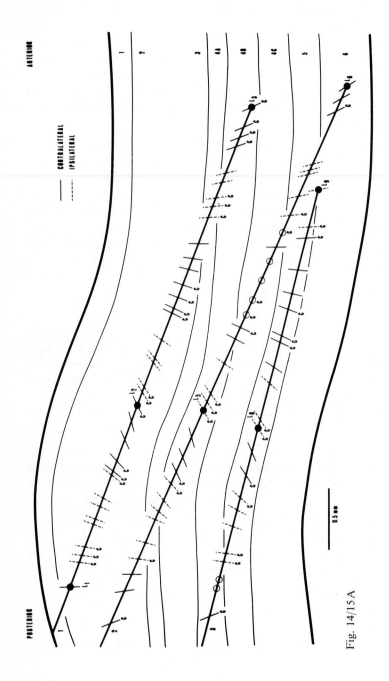

Fig. 14/15 A

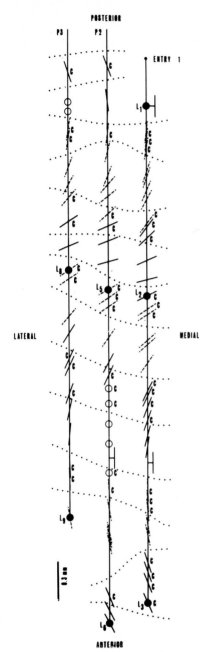

Fig. 14/15 B

Fig. 14/15. Physiological identification of color co-lumns. A) Reconstruction of three oblique electrode penetrations made from posterior to anterior. They were not in the same plane but are depicted so here (see B). Tracks in some places were nearly parallel to layers, particularly in penetration 3. Six color clusters were seen in both tracks 1 and 3; track 2 contained seven. In the beginning of all three tracks the field axes of the cells rotated clockwise; at lesions 2, 5 and 8 the axes reversed direction by 10° and then continued to turn counterclockwise to ends of tracks. Scale, 0.5 mm. B) Surface reconstruction of the color columns in the three electrode tracks of A. Tracks have been projected onto the plane of the cortical surface and viewed from above. Penetrations were in three parallel planes about 300 μm apart. The entry point of track 1 is indicated by a small black dot; tracks 2 and 3 entered the cortex at points off the figure. Color cells are marked by the letter C; areas containing only color cells are bounded by dotted lines. The color columns are actually sheets or slabs of cells. Walls of some of the color columns vary in width along their length. Patterns of eye preference and axis orientation columns can also be seen. Scale, 0.3 mm. With permission from Michael (1981).

input to the different RF types of monkey striate cortex with the electrical stimulation paradigm. All RF types, except B cells and end-stopped S cells, can receive monosynaptic LGN input. Color specific non-oriented cells, all have parvocellular input, while S cells with multiple subregions and C cells have magnocellular input. Non-color specific, non-oriented cells and S cells with one subregion could have either parvo or magnocellular input.

A similar question has been addressed by Malpeli et al. (1981) who assessed response properties of cortical cells before, during and after reversible anesthetic blocks of retinotopically corresponding parts of parvo- and magnocellular LGN layers. These experiments have shown that the dorsal parvocellular LGN layers (layers V and VI) contribute to ON responses of cortical cells, while the ventral ones (layers III and IV) contribute to OFF responses. They have also shown that S cells with a single subregion receive either magno- or parvocellular input. On the contrary, most S cells with multiple subregions and about 2/3 of the C cells receive convergent parvo- *and* magnocellular input. Comparison of these results with those of Bullier and Henry (1980) show that electrical stimulation experiments cannot distinguish between cells which get exclusively magnocellular input and those receiving a convergent magno- and parvocellular input.

14.11 Conclusion

The monkey striate cortex differs most from the cat striate cortex in its color specificity which apparently is subserved by a separate input (parvocellular afferents) and a separate processing system (possibly color columns and cytochrome blobs). The other differences are the larger spatial acuity of the RFs (high peak spatial frequency and tight depth sensitivity) and the luxotonic responses. The functional architecture of the monkey cortex seems highly orderly, although the principles of organization are those already present in the cat striate cortex (except for color systems).

Chapter 15. Conclusion: Signification of Visual Cortical Function in Perception

Present knowledge allows us to formulate a number of principles according to which the cat and monkey visual cortex function. The relevance of these functional principles for human visual perception is considered in the second section. In the final section the role of the primary visual cortex in visual perception is discussed.

15.1 Operating Principles in Cat Visual Cortex

15.1.1 Retinotopic Organization

This organization principle, common to other visual structures, has been known for a long time. It implies that the different parts of the visual field are analyzed in parallel. The high magnification of the projections subserving the central visual field is related to the density of receptors in the area centralis.

15.1.2 Filtering

It is now quite clear that cortical cells, rather than being feature detectors, are filters for certain parameters of the spatio-temporal light distribution on the retina. Until now the list of parameters for which filtering has been demonstrated, includes: orientation, spatial frequency, (length and width), direction and velocity of movement, position disparity, orientation disparity, direction in depth for bandpass filtering; length, velocity and position disparity for low-pass filtering; contrast, length, width, velocity of movement, position disparity, for high-pass filtering. It is likely that not all of these filterings are involved in coding for a parameter (see the two questions concerning velocity in Chapter 8). Indeed in order to be able to code for a parameter, a set of cells must not only filter this parameter but sample some continuum. This means that for bandpass filtering the optima must span a fair range of the parameter, for high-pass filtering that the dynamic range of the cells must be different, and for low-pass filtering that the cut-off values must span some range. It seems that at least low-pass filtering does not imply coding. Velocity low-pass cells provide very little information in stimulus velocity (Orban et al., 1981 a) and low-pass cells for position disparity (near cells) only provide crude information on a stimulus being in front of the horopter. It seems that, except for contrast, high-pass filtering does not imply coding either. Indeed high-pass cells for position disparity (far cells) only indicate depths greater than the horopter. Also velocity discrimination experiments (Orban et al., 1983 a) suggest that little velocity discrimination is done by velocity high-pass cells. It seems therefore that in most cases low- and high-pass filtering only provide a crude information on a parameter, as do far and near cells underlying coarse stereopsis. Only *bandpass filtering seems to subserve coding* for a parameter and to allow fine perceptual discriminations as disparity tuned excitatory cells allow fine stereopsis.

It is also evident that one cell is involved in the filtering of many different parameters. Therefore a parameter is not coded by the activity of 1 cell, but by the activity of a set of cells, most frequently, with bandpass filtering, in a multichannel system: the difference in activity of the cells represents the value of the parameter. Such a differential coding will be insensitive to other visual parameters provided all the cells of the set are affected in a similar way and in general will be insensitive to other influences (e.g. attention) unless they change the filter characteristics (as e.g. the bandwidth). Filtering implies selectivity and hence relies mainly on inhibitory intracortical mechanisms, which however operate on an appropriate geniculate input.[1] At least for spatial frequency filtering, we have introduced the concept of a working range over which a filter is linear. It is possible that other filterings also have such a working range.

15.1.3 "Columnar" Organization

For a number of properties, such as orientation and ocular dominance, but possibly also for other ones (direction, spatial frequency), cells with similar preferences tend to be grouped together in vertical (i.e. orthogonal to cortical surface) slab-like structures, called columns. This ensures a complete and independent representation of different parameters at each retinal locus and favors interactions between cells with similar preferences (e.g. in most inhibitory interactions, orientation preference of inhibitory and inhibited cells are similar).

Hubel and Wiesel (1974 b) noted that one has to move about 1 mm over the cortical surface in V1 of the monkey to encounter all possible orientations

---

[1] One could consider that the weak orientation bias of LGN cells (Vidyasagar and Urbas, 1982) prepares cortical cell orientation selectivity and that the preference of LGN cells for short slits (Cleland et al., 1983) prepares cortical end-stopping.

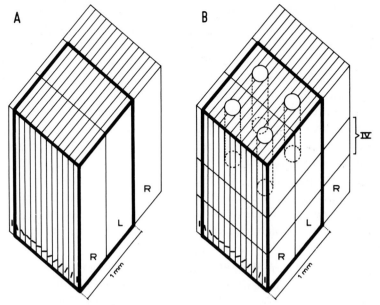

Fig. 15/1. Schematic representation of hypercolumns. A: initial Hubel and Wiesel (1977) proposal. B: latest Hubel and Livingstone (1982) proposal. IV: fourth cortical layer, R, L: right and left eye ocular dominance columns; orientation columns are indicated by lines corresponding to the preferred orientations of the neurons inside the columns. Two ocular dominance columns covering the range of ocular dominance and 12 orientation columns representing the range of preferred orientations correspond to a slab of cortex 1 mm wide. A 1 square mm bloc of cortex containing all ocular dominances and orientations is a hypercolumn. In the latest version of the hypercolumn, 4 subcolumns (extending only in the superficial layers) contain non-oriented, color specific cells and correspond to the cytochrome oxidase blobs (Hubel and Livingstone, 1982). There is strong evidence that the blobs occur in the middle of ocular dominance columns (Horton and Hubel, 1981; Tootell et al., 1982 b). The position of the subcolumns in the oblique orientation columns is suggested by the findings of Horton and Hubel (1981) that the cytochrome oxidase blobs lie along the lattice formed by the deoxyglucose label corresponding to principal orientations. Such a scheme could explain the preference of monkey cortical cells (RFs within 2° from fixation point) for horizontal and vertical orientations. This possible correlation between cytochrome oxidase blobs containing poorly oriented cells and meridional anisotropy in orientation preference of the overall population in area 17 is further strengthened by two additional observations: firstly, blobs are absent in area 17 of the cat (Horton and Hubel, 1981) as is the meridional anisotropy (Chapter 5) and secondly, the anisotropy is limited to RFs close to the fixation point (Chapter 14) and the blobs decrease in size with eccentricity (Hubel, personal communication).

and dominance for both eyes (Fig. 15/1). The distance over which one has to move to shift the RFs to a completely different retinal locus is also 1 mm. From these two observations, Hubel and Wiesel (1974 b) derived the idea that a vertical cortical unit with a surface of 1 by 1 mm contains all the necessary machinery for the analysis of one retinal locus. They called this functional unit of the primary visual cortex the *hypercolumn*. According to Albus (1975 b) hypercolumns have similar dimensions in the cat area 17.

15.1.4 Distributed Processing in the Primary Complex

The concept of distributed processing, involves 2 ideas: that the areas operate in parallel and that they are specialized. There is little left of the arguments used by Hubel and Wiesel (1965) to postulate a serial processing between areas 17, 18 and 19. Overwhelming physiological and anatomical evidence shows that areas 17, 18 and 19 receive direct geniculate input of different types: while area 17 receives X, Y and to a lesser extent W afferents, area 18 receives almost exclusively Y afferents and area 19 mostly W afferents and, especially in the parts subserving the peripheral visual field, Y afferents. The three cortical areas have similar RF organization, although the proportion of S family cells is smaller in area 19 than in the other 2 areas. It seems thus that *areas 17, 18 and 19 operate essentially in parallel* with each other.

Although a single cell of each area (17, 18 or 19) can be very similar in its properties to a cell of the other 2 areas, *the cell popoulations of these three areas*, which are what matters from a functional point of view, show marked differences in functional characteristics. This, together with the similarity in RF organization of the three areas, underlines the necessity of distinguishing between RF organization and functional properties. While there is a good correlation between these two types of neuronal attributes (see Table 4/2, Chapter 4), it is a relative correlation rather than an absolute one. If one were to use functional properties (e.g. velocity preference or narrowness of orientation tuning) as defining characteristics of a RF type, generalization to other areas would be very difficult. Indeed S cells in area 17 subserving central vision all have half-height upper cut-off velocities below 25°/sec. If one were to include this in the definition of a S cell, virtually none of the area 18 cells could be a S cell.

Area 17 cells have small RFs, have optimal spatial frequencies covering a wide range of spatial frequencies, have a narrow orientation tuning, often show a tuned excitatory binocular interaction, and respond better to slowly moving stimuli. Area 17 (especially the part subserving central vision) is thus ideally suited for the analysis of the spatial structure of a stationary object (or an object seen during smooth pursuit). However some area 17 cells are direction selective and a few are even tuned to velocity. While these properties can be used to outline objects (Marr, 1982), it may also indicate that area 17 can contribute to the analysis of moving objects at least when they move at low velocities. Area 18 cells have large RFs, are tuned to coarse spatial frequencies, have wide orientation tuning, but are often direction selective and tuned for velocity and selective for direction in depth. Thus area 18 is ideally suited for the analysis of moving objects both with respect to their movement and spatial structure, although the latter analysis will be less refined than the one performed by area 17 for stationary objects. It seems thus that distinction should *not be made between spatial vision and movement perception* to which both areas can contribute, but *between analysis of different types of objects* (stationary versus moving). It is also noteworthy that an object may be recognized not only by its spatial structure (a given association of spatial parameter values) but also by its movement structure or pattern (i.e., systematic association of movement parameter values). Visual cortical areas can doubtless contribute to these functions, area 17 more to the former and area 18 more to the latter.

Area 19 cells have wide RFs, wide orientation tuning, and little direction or velocity tuning, but they are more often binocular and end-stopped. Whether area 19 performs a specialized function or not is still not clear. It could be that it is important in binocular interactions (binocular end-stopped cells seem to be important in this respect), or rather than filtering the image according to parameters, it could also subserve a sort of lower level function, namely to detect the presence of an object in a given position. Whatever its function, area 19 can to some extent contribute to the analysis of stationary and moving objects performed by the two other areas.

It seems thus that from the cat LGN, the information is distributed to different areas according to its nature. However, the specialization of the 3 primary visual areas is not complete. Each area can to some extent supplement the other two. This may be simply the reflection of a common origin, or reflect the redundancy built into the nervous system as a protective mechanism or may even serve to coordinate the activities in the different areas related to the same visual object.

15.1.5 Changes with Eccentricity

Hubel and Wiesel left us with the idea that area 17 of the cat and the monkey is *very stereotyped and uniform* (Hubel and Wiesel, 1974 b). The only effect of the magnification factor was to increase or decrease the number of hypercolumns per visual degree, but each hypercolumn was essentially similar to all the others. This seems to be at best a partial view. Of course the RFs increase in size with eccentricity and more so in areas 18 and 19 than in 17. Consequently the optimal spatial frequencies decrease with eccentricity. At least for S cells in area 17 the width of orientation tuning increases slightly with eccentricity and the preference for vertical and horizontal orientation fades with eccentricity. Furthermore the proportions of end-stopped cells and of S family cells decrease with eccentricity. The proportion of monocular cells decreases with eccentricity in areas 17 and 18, but increases in area 19. At least in area 18, the contrast threshold decreases with eccentricity. Direction selectivity decreases with eccentricity mainly in area 18 as does the proportion of velocity tuned cells. With increasing eccentricity the response to slow movement decreases, while the velocity upper cut-off increases, as

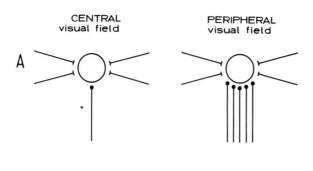

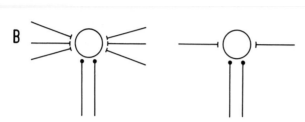

Fig. 15/2. Two models accounting for changes in efficiency of intracotical inhibition with eccentricity: A, change in excitatory (afferent) convergence; B, change in inhibitory (lateral) connections. The latter model is less likely. Dots indicate excitatory inputs, short lines inhibitory inputs.

does the response strength. Finally the latency of responses decreases with eccentricity. Thus *virtually every aspect of visual cortical cells we have looked at, changes with eccentricity*. Using the Hubel and Wiesel terminology one can say that not only the number of hypercolumns per visual degree changes but that the machinery within the hypercolumns also changes.

Most of the changes with eccentricity can be interpreted very simply as a *decrease in efficiency of the inhibitory interactions*. Most notable exceptions are the decrease in contrast threshold which may be simply a reflection of the increase in RF width and possibly the increase in upper cut-off velocity. The hypothetized decrease in efficiency of inhibitory interactions with increasing eccentricity can either be due to a decrease in inhibitory (lateral) inputs or an increase in excitatory (vertical) inputs or both (Fig. 15/2). The former is unlikely given the structural uniformity of the cortex and the indications that, at least in the monkey, the proportion of GAD (enzyme involved in GABA synthesis) does not notably change with eccentricity (Hendrickson, personal communication). On the contrary there are some arguments which postulate that the excitatory inputs increase with eccentricity, due to the larger convergence of geniculocortical afferents in cortex subserving peripheral vision (for review see Myerson et al., 1977). This increase in convergence with eccentricity is also demonstrated by the steeper increase in RF dimension at the cortical level than at the geniculate level. It is noteworthy that these changes with eccentricity can be abolished, at least in area 18, by rearing cats in a stroboscopically illuminated environment (Kennedy and Orban, 1983).

15.1.6 Parallel Streams Within each Area

It is now clear that almost every cell type and especially S and C families can be monosynaptically driven from the LGN. There is good evidence that within each *area there are several streams of information processing*, the major ones being the S and C families. Indeed S and C families differ in some important respects: C family cells have usually cruder selectivities (at least in orientation, direction, velocity domain), more often receive binocular input and respond to large textured patterns and sometimes to diffuse illumination changes, while S family cells only respond to better defined visual patterns such as bars or gratings. It seems, therefore, that the S family cell will be activated by small localized objects, while C family cells will also be activated by the visual background. [2] It could well be that *S family cells are mainly involved in egocentric perception* (objects in relation to the subject), while *C family cells are more devoted to exocentric perception* (the subject related to the surroundings). This is fully in keeping with the projections of C family cells to subcortical structures involved in visuomotor tasks. While C family cells seem to have the required way out of the cortex, this is at present not the case for S family cells: it is unclear what happens to the sophisticated message of S family cells. The available evidence suggests that the area 17-18-19 information is routed to the lateral suprasylvian areas for further intracortical processing (which is probably important for perception). This seems, at first glance, an uninteresting proposal since suprasylvian RFs seem much less sophisticated than those of areas 17, 18 and 19 (Spear and Baumann, 1975), although recently a concealed orientation tuning has been demonstrated for LS cells (Gizzi et al., 1981). It could be that investigation of suprasylvian RFs with more complex and multiple stimuli reveal more specificites and sophistication (see e.g. the recent results of von Grünau and Frost, 1983).

15.2 The Cat and Monkey Visual Cortex as a Model: The Question of the Relationship Between Animal Physiology and Human Visual Perception

As shown in Chapter 14, area 17 (V1) of old world monkeys is remarkably similar to that of the cat if one excepts the presence of non-oriented cells (mainly in layer IVC) and of color specific cells and the smaller dimension of the RFs linked to the greater magnification factor and larger brain volume in the monkey. Many of the filter properties described for cat cortical cells have been demonstrated in the monkey. It also seems that the principle of

---

[2] Collection of unresolved visual objects.

distributed processing will apply to the visual cortical areas of the macaque, although the branching occurs not between the LGN and the cortex as in the cat, but between V1 and the higher order extrastriate areas. It seems that the area called MT or STS, which receives direct input from layer IV of V1, could be the homologue of area 18 in the cat [3]: it has a heavy myelinization, and many direction selective (Zeki, 1978) and velocity tuned cells (Felleman et al., 1981). Some of the extrastriate areas described in area 19 of the owl monkey (DL and DM), have properties reminiscent of area 19 of the cat, mainly the requirements in dimension of the stimuli (Baker et al., 1981). Columnar organization is even clearer in V1 of the monkey (Hubel and Wiesel, 1977) than in the primary cortical areas of the cat. Similar RF types, including S and C family streams, have been described in V1 of the monkey (Bullier and Henry, 1980; Kennedy et al., 1981). It seems thus that although anatomically differently organized, the visual cortical system of the monkey shares many organizational principles with those found in that of the cat. One is therefore tempted to extrapolate and believe that the same may be true for the human visual cortex.

It is thus no wonder that many investigators have observed correlations between *animal cortical physiology* and *human perception*. The most notable examples are the psychophysical demonstration of the existence of orientation and spatial frequency filters in the human visual system by a variety of techniques, initiated by the Cambridge group. In the same vein much of the work in Sekuler's lab is devoted to the demonstration of direction selective filters. The correlation between physiology and psychophysics can be more than just the demonstration of filter processes in human vision. The properties and distribution of these filters can also explain some psychophysical observations. For example the fact that most cells in area 17 subserving central vision, where spatial vision is at its best, are velocity low-pass cells, makes it very understandable that human acuity is equally good for stationary and slowly moving objects but decreases once stimulus velocity exceeds $2-3°/sec$ (Westheimer and Mckee, 1975). On the contrary, if velocity judgements depend on velocity tuned cells, then these judgements should be difficult below some velocity, since in the cat we found no such cell tuned to a velocity lower than $2°/sec$. [4] And indeed differential velocity thresholds decrease for velocities over 1 or $2°/sec$ (McKee, 1981; Orban et al., 1983 a). If judgements of direction of movement rely on direction selective cells, then their tuned velocity profile would suggest that this mechanism is most sensitive at a medium velocity. This is indeed the case for human direction judgements at low contrasts (van der Glas et al., 1981). If judgements of orienta-

---

[3] Others have suggested that MT is the homologue of the suprasylvian areas, more precisely PMLS.
[4] Preliminary observations indicate that the same may be true for the monkey (Kennedy, Orban and Bullier, unpublished).

tion depend on the activity of the most narrowly orientation tuned group of cells in V1 of the cat and the monkey, namely S cells, then given the over-representation of horizontal and vertical orientations among those cells, one would expect better judgements of orientation around horizontal and vertical. This is in fact what one observes for humans (Orban et al., 1983 b).

While the very existence of such correlations is a validation on its own, these correlations can be considerably strengthened by the study of *animal psychophysics*. Only if one can demonstrate that visual perception of a species is in certain aspects similar to that of humans, does it make sense to correlate cortical physiology of that species and human perception for those aspects. For example, since it has been demonstrated that both cats and monkeys have stereopsis (Packwood and Gordon, 1975), it makes sense to look for underlying cortical mechanisms in both species. Conversely, it seems that color perception of the cat is at best very crude (Loop et al., 1979), therefore the cat is not a good model for human color perception while the macaque is a good one. It has been recently shown that the cat can make finer orientation discriminations around vertical and horizontal orientations than around oblique ones (Vandenbussche and Orban, 1983). Furthermore this superiority of horizontal and vertical orientation decreases with decreasing line length (Orban et al., 1984). It seems thus that orientation discrimination is similar in cat and human. Hence it makes sense to explain the superiority of horizontal and vertical orientations in terms of cells similar to S cells of the cat, which are the only RF type in the primary complex of the cat, to have meridional anisometries in orientation preference.

In addition animal psychophysics allows us also to *verify* some of the hypotheses put forward by physiologists. For example the cortical physiology suggests that area 17 in the cat because of its small RFs, fine spatial frequency and orientation tunings is important in spatial vision and especially in acuity functions. One would therefore expect important deficits in this respect when area 17 is removed. This is exactly what Berkley and Sprague (1979) observed. It seems thus that by comparing psychophysical thresholds before and after ablations, one can test some of the predictions made from the cortical physiology. Therefore in order to increase our understanding of the human visual perception, visual cortical physiology should not only be correlated with morphology but also with behavioral studies.

15.3 The Role of the Primary Visual Cortex in Visual Perception: The Significance of Parameter Specificities for Object Recognition

The role attributed to the primary visual cortex depends largely upon the interpretation of the *parameter specificities of cortical cells*. These interpretations are largely centered on the question of how visual objects are represented in the visual system and can be identified and recognized.

The first theory evolved from the description of cortical RFs given by Hubel and Wiesel (1962, 1965) and has been referred to as *feature detection theory*. Hubel and Wiesel described the different RFs (simple, complex, lower and higher order hypercomplex cells) as a chain of information processing, in which the cells became progressively more specific (i.e. responded to smaller and smaller categories of stimuli or conversely to more and more specific configurations of inputs) and more general (i.e. more invariant with position in the visual field). Extrapolating this view one had to reach a neuron that was so specific that it responds only to one object and so general that it responds to this object anywhere in the visual field. This hypothetical neuron has been called the "grand mother" cell. In this theory each single visual object is represented by the activity of a given neuron (this is a theory of labelled lines in its extreme form). This is of course not feasible, as the number of cells in the visual cortex would be too small to signal all the objects we can recognize. Also the loss of a cell would mean that we could no longer recognize the corresponding object.

In a second theory, a version of which was given by myself in (1977), a visual object is *represented in the visual system by its attributes*. The visual cortex functions as a multidimensional hyperspace (each dimension corresponding to an attribute analyzed by the visual system) in which the visual objects are represented as points or small clusters of points.

Both theories have as a principal weakness the fact that they take the segregation of the different objects and the separation of objects and background for granted. In fact as noted by Marr (1982), there is only a light distribution on the retina and the task of the visual system is to extract knowledge about the visual objects from this spatio-temporal light distribution. The *main task, therefore, is to segregate the different objects*. According to Marr (1982) this is done in three steps: the raw primal sketch, the $2\frac{1}{2}$ D model and the 3 D model (Fig. 15/3). According to the same author the raw primal sketch, i.e. the first representation of the visual scene, could result from the processing in area 17 of the monkey (and probably also in the primary complex of the cat). The primitives of this representation are edges, bars, blobs and terminations and these have attributes of orientation, contrast, width, length and position. The primitives are derived from the detection of zero crossing segments which would be the main function of simple cells. The raw primal sketch is a very rich description of an image, since it contains virtually all the information represented by the zero crossings from several differently sized channels. Its importance is that it is the first representation from the retinal image whose primitives have a high probability of reflecting physical reality directly (Marr, 1982).

Upon this raw primal sketch different grouping algorithms operate in order to detect borders and surfaces separating objects. This could be the function of the different retinal representations in areas 18 and 19 of the

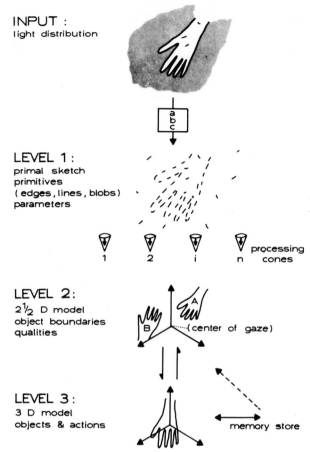

INPUT :
light distribution

LEVEL 1 :
primal sketch
primitives
(edges , lines , blobs)
parameters

processing
cones

LEVEL 2 :
2½ D model
object boundaries
qualities

(center of gaze)

LEVEL 3 :
3 D model
objects & actions

memory store

Fig. 15/3. The 3 levels of representation in the visual system according to Marr (1982). While the first two levels of representation are viewer centered, the last level is object centered. The difference between the $2\frac{1}{2}$ D and 3 D representation is that the $2\frac{1}{2}$ D representation is changing and represents the wealth of our perception, while the 3 D representation is permanent and allows recognition of objects. In order to flow from the input to the different levels the information has to be processed. Between the input and level 1 this processing includes: filtering (∇^2 G) with differently sized filters, zero crossing detection and selection and combination of zero crossings. Between levels 1 and 2 different processing cones operate using e.g. stereo, color, structure from motion, motion parallax, texture etc .... The nature of the processing between levels 2 and 3 is still largely conjectural but must include a change in coordinates.

macaque (and of the LS areas in the cat) to which the information of V1 is dispatched. In a final step the $2\frac{1}{2}$ D model is made into a full 3 D (three-dimensional) model representation. Marr (1982) has given a description of the 3 D model representation for objects and this has been extended to actions by Marr and Vaina (1982). It may well be that these symbolic functions are performed by the infero-temporal visual regions of primates (and by areas 20 and 21 in the cat).

This exciting new theory then puts a double challenge onto the visual physiologist: first there is the question of how the primal sketch is worked out in the primary visual cortex, and second there is the question concerning the algorithms used by the extrastriate areas to achieve objects segregation and the way in which the 3 D model representation is reached in the visual system. Meeting these challenges is the immense task awaiting visual neurophysiologists in the coming decade.

References

Albrecht DG, De Valois RL (1981) Striate cortex responses to periodic patterns with and without the fundamental harmonics. J Physiol (Lond) 319:497–514

Albrecht DG, De Valois RL, Thorell LG (1980) Visual cortical neurons: are bars or gratings the optimal stimuli? Science 207:88–90

Albrecht DG, Hamilton DB (1982) Striate cortex of monkey and cat: contrast response function. J Neurophysiol 48:217–237

Albus K (1975a) A quantitative study of the projection area of the central and the paracentral visual field in area 17 of the cat. I. The precision of the topography. Exp Brain Res 24:159–179

Albus K (1975b) A quantitative study of the projection area of the central and the paracentral visual field in area 17 of the cat. II. The spatial organization of the orientation domain. Exp Brain Res 24:181–202

Albus K (1975c) Predominance of monocularly driven cells in the projection area of the central visual field in cat's striate cortex. Brain Res 89:341–347

Albus K (1979) ^{14}C-Deoxyglucose mapping of orientation subunits in the cats visual cortical areas. Exp Brain Res 37:609–613

Albus K (1980) The detection of movement direction and effects of contrast reversal in the cat's striate cortex. Vision Res 20:289–293

Albus K (1981) Hypothalamic and basal forebrain afferents to the cat's visual cortex: a study with horseradish peroxidase. Neurosci Lett 24:117–121

Albus K, Beckmann R (1980) Second and third visual areas of the cat: interindividual variability in retinotopic arrangement and cortical location. J Physiol (Lond) 299:247–276

Albus K, Donate-Oliver F (1977) Cells of origin of the occipito-pontine projection in the cat: functional properties and intracortical location. Exp Brain Res 28:167–174

Albus K, Donate-Oliver F, Sanides D, Fries W (1981) The distribution of pontine projection cells in visual and association cortex of the cat: an experimental study with horseradish peroxidase. J Comp Neurol 201:175–189

Albus K, Fries W (1980) Inhibitory sidebands of complex receptive fields in the cat's striate cortex. Vision Res 20:369–372

Albus K, Meyer G (1981) Anatomical mapping of representations of the visual field in afferent projections to the visual cortex. Soc Neurosci Abstr 7:761

Allman J (1977) Evolution of the visual system in the early primates. In: Sprague JM, Epstein AN (eds) Progress in psychobiology and physiological psychology. Academic, New York, pp 1–54

Allman JM, Kaas JH (1971a) A representation of the visual field in the caudal third of the middle temporal gyrus of the owl monkey (Aotus trivirgatus). Brain Res 31:85–105

Allman JM, Kaas JH (1971b) Representation of the visual field in striate and adjoining cortex of the owl monkey (Aotus trivirgatus). Brain Res 35:89–106

Allman JM, Kaas JH (1974a) The organization of the second visual area (V II) in the owl monkey: a second order transformation of the visual hemifield. Brain Res 76:247–265

Allman JM, Kaas JH (1974b) A crescent-shaped cortical visual area surrounding the middle temporal area (MT) in the owl monkey (Aotus trivirgatus). Brain Res 81:199–213

Allman JM, Kaas JH (1975) The dorsomedial cortical visual area: a third tier area in the occipial lobe of the owl monkey (Aotus trivirgatus). Brain Res 100:473–487

Allman JM, Kaas JH (1976) Representation of the visual field on the medial wall of occipital-parietal cortex in the owl monkey. Science 191:572–575

Allman JM, Kaas JH, Lane RH, Miezin FM (1972) A representation of the visual field in the inferior nucleus of the pulvinar in the owl monkey (Aotus trivirgatus). Brain Res 40:291–302

Andrews BW, Pollen DA (1979) Relationship between spatial frequency selectivity and receptive field profile of simple cells. J Physiol (Lond) 287:163–176

Baker JF, Petersen SE, Newsome WT, Allman JM (1981) Visual response properties of neurons in four extrastriate visual areas of the owl monkey (Aotus trivirgatus): a quantitative comparison of medial, dorsomedial, dorsolateral, and middle temporal areas. J Neurophysiol 45:397–416

Barlow HB (1981) Critical limiting factors in the design of the eye and visual cortex. Proc R Soc Lond (Biol) 212:1–34

Barlow HB, Levick WR (1969) Three factors limiting the reliable detection of light by retinal ganglion cells of the cat. J Physiol (Lond) 200:1–24

Barlow HB, Blakemore C, Pettigrew JD (1967) The neural mechanism of binocular depth discrimination. J Physiol 193:327–342

Bauer R (1982) A high probability of an orientation shift between layers 4 and 5 in central parts of the cat striate cortex. Exp Brain Res 48:245–255

Bender DB (1981) Retinotopic organization of macique pulvinar. J Neurophysiol 46:672–693

Benevento LA, Davis B (1977) Topographical projections of the prestriate cortex to the pulvinar nuclei in the macaque monkey: an autoradiographic study. Exp Brain Res 30:405–424

Benevento LA, Fallon JH (1975) The ascending projections of the superior colliculus in the rhesus monkey (Macaca mulatta). J Comp Neurol 160:339–362

Benevento LA, Yoshida K (1981) The afferent and efferent organization of the lateral geniculo-prestriate pathways in the macaque monkey. J Comp Neurol 203:455–474

Berardi N, Bisti S, Cattaneo A, Fiorentini A, Maffei L (1979) Spatial frequency rows in area 18 of the cat. J Physiol (Lond) 292:29P

Berardi N, Bisti S, Cattaneo A, Fiorentini A, Maffei L (1982) Correlation between the preferred orientation and spatial frequency of neurones in visual areas 17 and 18 of the cat. J Physiol (Lond) 323:603–618

Berkley MA, Sprague JM (1979) Striate cortex and visual acuity functions in the cat. J Comp Neurol 187:679–702

Berlucchi G, Sprague JM (1980) The cerebral cortex in visual learning and memory, and in inter-hemispheric transfer in the cat. In: Schmitt FO, Worden FG, Adelman G, Dennis JG (eds) The organization of the cerebral cortex. The MIT Press, Cambridge, pp 415–440

Berman N, Jones EG (1977) A retino-pulvinar projection in the cat. Brain Res 134:237–248

Berman N, Payne BR (1982) Contralateral cortifugal projections from the lateral suprasylvian and ectosylvian gyri in the cat. Exp Brain Res 47:234–238

Berman N, Payne BR, Garcia-Kennedy R, Murphy EH (1981) Orientation anisotropy in cat visual cortex. Suppl Invest Ophthalmol Vis Sci 20:147

Berman N, Payne BR, Labar DR, Murphy EH (1982) Functional organization of neurons in cat striate cortex: variations in ocular dominance and receptive-filed type with cortical laminae and location in visual field. J Neurophysiol 48:1362–1377

Beverley KI, Regan D (1973) Evidence for the existence of neural mechanisms selectively sensitive to the direction of movement in space. J Physiol (Lond) 235:17–29

Beverley KI, Regan D (1975) The relation between discrimination and sensitivity in the perception of motion in depth. J Physiol (Lond) 249:387–398

Bilge M, Bingle A, Seneviratne KN, Whitteridge D (1967) A map of the visual cortex in the cat. J Physiol (Lond) 191:116–118P

Bishop PO (1979) Stereopsis and the random element in the organization of the striate cortex. Proc R Soc Lond (Biol) 204:415–434

Bishop PO (1981) Binocular vision. In: Moses RA (ed) Adler's physiology of the eye: Clinical application, 7th edition. CV Mosby, St Louis, pp 575–649

Bishop PO (to be published) Processing of visual information within the retinostriate system. In: Handbook of physiology, section neurophysiology. American Physiological Society, Washington

Bishop PO, Kozak W, Vakkur GJ (1962) Some quantitative aspects of the cat's eye: axis and plane of reference, visual field co-ordinates and optics. J PHysiol (Lond) 163:466–502

Bishop PO, Coombs JS, Henry GH (1971a) Responses to visual contours: spatio-temporal aspects of excitation in the receptive fields of simple striate neurones. J Physiol (Lond) 219:625–657

Bishop PO, Coombs JS, Henry GH (1971b) Interaction effects of visual contours on the discharge frequency of simple striate neurones. J Physiol (Lond) 219:659–687

Bishop PO, Henry GH, Smith CJ (1971c) Binocular interaction fields of single units in the cat striate cortex. J Physiol (Lond) 216:39–68

Bishop PO, Coombs JS, Henry GH (1973) Receptive fields of simple cells in the cat striate cortex. J Physiol (Lond) 231:31–60

Bishop PO, Kato H, Orban GA (1980) Direction-selective cells in complex family in cat striate cortex. J Neurophysiol 43:1266–1283

Bisti S, Maffei L (1974) Behavioural contrast sensitivity of the cat in various visual meridians. J Physiol (Lond) 241:201–210

Bisti S, Clement R, Maffei L, Mecacci L (1977) Spatial frequency and orientation tuning curves of visual neurones in the cat: effects of mean luminance. Exp Brain Res 27:335–345

Blakemore C (1970) The representation of three-dimensional visual space in the cat's striate cortex. J Physiol (Lond) 209:155–178

Blakemore C, Tobin EA (1972) Lateral inhibition between orientation detectors in the cat's visual cortex. Exp Brain Res 15:439–440

Blakemore C, Fiorentini A, Maffei L (1972) A second neural mechanism of binocular depth discrimination. J Physiol (Lond) 226:725–749

Blakemore CB, Garey LJ, Vital-Durand F (1981) Orientation preferences in the monkey's visual cortex. J Physiol (Lond) 319:78P

Blasdel GG, Mitchell DE, Muir DW, Pettigrew JD (1977) A physiological and behavioural study in cats of the effect of early visual experience with contours of a single orientation. J Physiol (Lond) 265:615–636

Bodis-Wollner IG, Pollen DA, Ronner SF (1976) Responses of complex cells in the visual cortex of the cat as a function of the length of moving slits. Brain Res 116:205–216

Bowling DB, Michael CR (1981) Termination patterns of single optic tract axons of different physiological types. Soc Neurosci Abstr 7:25

Boycott BB, Wässle H (1974) The morphological types of ganglion cells of the domestic cat's retina. J Physiol (Lond) 240:397–419

Breitmeyer BG (1973) A relationship between the detection of size, rate, orientation and direction in the human visual system. Vision Res 13:41–58

Brodal P (1972a) The corticopontine projection from the visual cortex in the cat. I. The total projection and the projection from area 17. Brain Res 39:297–317

Brodal P (1972b) The corticopontine projection from the visual cortex in the cat. II. The projection from areas 18 and 19. Brain Res 39:319–335

Buisseret P, Maffei L (1977) Extraocular proprioceptive projections to the visual cortex. Exp Brain Res 28:421–425

Bullier J, Henry GH (1979a) Ordinal position of neurons in cat striate cortex. J Neurophysiol 42: 1251–1263

Bullier J, Henry GH (1979b) Neural path taken by afferent streams in striate cortex of the cat. J Neurophysiol 42:1264–1270

Bullier J, Henry GH (1979c) Laminar distribution of first-order neurons and afferent terminals in cat striate cortex. J Neurophysiol 42:1271–1281

Bullier J, Henry GH (1980) Ordinal position and afferent input of neurons in monkey striate cortex. J Comp Neurol 193:913–935

Bullier J, Kennedy H (1983) Branching axons to V1 and V2 areas of the monkey cortex. Abstracts Third European Winter Conference on Brain Research. Les Arcs, France

Bullier J, Norton TT (1979a) X and Y relay cells in cat lateral geniculate nucleus: quantitative analysis of receptive-field properties and classification. J Neurophysiol 42:244–273

Bullier J, Norton TT (1979b) Comparison of receptive-field properties of X and Y ganglion cells with X and Y lateral geniculate cells in the cat. J Neurophysiol 42:274–291

Bullier J, Mustari MJ, Henry GH (1982) Transformation of receptive field properties between LGN neurons and first order S cells in cat striate cortex. J Neurophysiol 47:417–438

Bunt AH, Hendrickson AE, Lund JS, Lund RD, Fuchs AF (1975) Monkey retinal ganglion cells: morphometric analysis and tracing of axonal projections, with a consideration of the peroxidase technique. J Comp Neurol 164:265–286

Bunt AH, Minckler DS, Johanson GW (1977) Demonstration of bilateral projection of the central retina of the monkey with horseradish peroxidase neuronography. J Comp Neurol 171:619–630

Burr D, Morrone C, Maffei L (1981) Intra-cortical inhibition prevents simple cells from responding to textured visual patterns. Exp Brain Res 43:455–458

Camarda RM (1979) Hypercomplex cell types in area 18 of the cat. Exp Brain Res 36:191–194

Campbell FW, Kulikowski JJ (1966) Orientational selectivity of the human visual system. J Physiol (Lond) 187:437–445

Campbell FW, Robson JG (1968) Application of Fourier analysis to the visibility of gratings. J Physiol (Lond) 197:551–566

Campbell FW, Cleland BG, Cooper GF, Enroth-Cugell C (1968) The angular selectivity of visual cortical cells to moving gratings. J Physiol (Lond) 198:237–250

Campbell FW, Cooper GF, Enroth-Cugell C (1969) The spatial selectivity of the visual cells of the cat. J Physiol (Lond) 203:223–235

Chow KL, Blum JS, Blum RA (1950) Cell ratios in the thalamo-cortical visual system of macaca mulatta. J Comp Neurol 92:227–239

Citron MC, Emerson RC, Ide LS (1981) Spatial and temporal receptive-field analysis of the cat's geniculocortical pathway. Vision Res 21:385–397

Clare MS, Bishop GH (1954) Responses from an association area secondarily activated from optic cortex. J Neurophysiol 17:271–277

Cleland BG, Levick WR (1974a) Brisk and sluggish concentrically organized ganglion cells in the cat's retina. J Physiol (Lond) 240:421–456

Cleland BG, Levick WR (1974b) Properties of rarely encountered types of ganglion cells in the cat's retina and an overall classification. J Physiol (Lond) 240:457–492

Cleland BG, Dubin MW, Levick WR (1971) Sustained and transient neurones in the cat's retina and lateral geniculate nucelus. J Physiol (Lond) 217:473–496

Cleland BG, Levick WR, Wässle H (1975) Physiological identification of a morphological class of cat retinal ganglion cells. J Physiol (Lond) 248:151–171

Cleland BG, Levick WR, Morstyn R, Wagner HG (1976) Lateral geniculate relay of slowly conducting retinal afferents to cat visual cortex. J Physiol (Lond) 255:299–320

Cleland BG, Lee BB, Vidyasagar TR (1983) Response of neurons in the cat's lateral geniculate nucleus to moving bars of different length. J Neurosci 3:108–116

Colonnier M, O'Kusky J (1981) Le nombre de neurones et de synapses dans le cortex visuel de différentes espèces. Rev Can Biol 40:91–99

Cooper ML, Pettigrew JD (1979a) A neurophysiological determination of the vertical horopter in the cat and owl. J Comp Neurol 184:1–26

Cooper ML, Pettigrew JD (1979b) The decussation of the retinothalamic pathway in the cat, with a note on the major meridians of the cat's eye. J Comp Neurol 187:285–312

Cremieux J, Orban GA, Duysens J (to be published) Responses of cat visual cortical cells to continuously and stroboscopically illuminated moving light slits compared. Vision Res

Creutzfeldt OD, Kuhnt U, Benevento LA (1974) An intracellular analysis of visual cortical neurones to moving stimuli: responses in a co-operative neuronal network. Exp Brain Res 21:251–274

Cynader M, Regan D (1978) Neurones in cat parastriate cortex sensitive to the direction of motion in three-dimensional space. J Physiol (Lond) 274:549–569

Cynader M, Regan D (1982) Neurons in cat visual cortex tuned to the direction of motion in depth: effect of positional disparity. Vision Res 22:967–982

Daniel P, Whitteridge D (1961) The representation of the visual field on the cerebral cortex in monkeys. J Physiol (Lond) 159:203–221

Daugman JG (1980) Two-dimensional spectral analysis of cortical receptive field profiles. Vision Res 20:847–856

Davis TL, Sterling P (1979) Microcircuitry of cat visual cortex: classification of neurons in layer IV of area 17, and identification of the patterns of lateral geniculate input. J Comp Neurol 188: 599–628

Daw NW, Pearlman AL (1969) Cat colour vision: one cone process or several. J Physiol (Lond) 201:745–764

Dean AF (1981) The relationship between response amplitude and contrast for cat striate cortical neurones. J Physiol (Lond) 318:413–427

DeFelipe J, Fairén A (1982) A type of basket cell in superficial layers of the cat visual cortex. A Golgi-electron microscope study. Brain Res 244:9–16

De Monasterio FM (1978) Properties of concentrically organized X and Y ganglion cells of macaque retina. J Neurophysiol 41:1394–1417

De Monasterio FM, Gouras P (1975) Functional properties of ganglion cells of the rhesus monkey retina. J Physiol (Lond) 251:167–195

Denney D, Adorjani C (1972) Orientation specificity of visual cortical neurons after head tilt. Exp Brain Res 14:312–317

Desimone R (1982) Contribution to symposium on functions of extra-striate visual cortex. Soc Neurosci Abstr 8:503

De Valois RL, Morgan HC, Polson MC, Mead WR, Hull EM (1974a) Psychophysical studies of monkey vision. I. Macaque luminosity and color vision tests. Vision Res 14:53–67

De Valois RL, Morgan H, Snodderly DM (1974b) Psychophysical studies of monkey vision. III. Spatial luminance contrast sensitivity tests of macaque and human observers. Vision Res 14: 75–81

De Valois KK, De Valois RL, Yund EW (1979) Responses of striate cortex cells to grating and checkerboard patterns. J Physiol (Lond) 291:483–505

De Valois RL, Yund EW, Hepler N (1982a) The orientation and direction selectivity of cells in macaque visual cortex. Vision Res 22:531–544

De Valois RL, Albrecht DG, Thorell LG (1982b) Spatial frequency selectivity of cells in macaque visual cortex. Vision Res 22:545–560

DeYoe EA, Bartlett JR (1980) Rarity of luxotonic responses in cortical visual areas of the cat. Exp Brain Res 39:125–132

Dinse HRO, von Seelen W (1981a) On the function of cell systems in area 18. Part I. Biol Cybern 41:47–58

Dinse HRO, von Seelen W (1981b) On the functionof cell systems in area 18. Part II. Biol Cybern 41:59–69

Donaldson IML, Nash JRG (1975a) Variability of the relative preference for stimulus orientation and direction of movement in some units of the cat visual cortex. J Physiol (Lond) 215:305–324

Donaldson IML, Nash JRG (1975b) The effect of a chronic lesion in cortical area 17 on the visual responses of units in area 18 of the cat. J Physiol (Lond) 245:325–332

Donaldson IML, Whitteridge FRS (1977) The nature of the boundary between cortical visual areas II and III in the cat. Proc R Soc Lond (Biol) 199:445–462

Dow BM (1974) Functional classes of cells and their laminar distribution in monkey visual cortex. J Neurophysiol 37:927–946

Dow BM, Dubner R (1971) Single-unit responses to moving visual stimuli in middle suprasylvian gyrus of the cat. J Neurophysiol 34:47–55

Dow BM, Gouras P (1973) Color and spatial specificity of single units in rhesus monkey foveal striate cortex. J Neurophysiol 36:79–100

Dow BM, Bauer R, Snyder AZ, Vautin R (1982) Orientation shift between upper and lower layers in monkey visual cortex. Soc Neurosci Abstr 8:705

Dow BM, Snyder AZ, Vautin RG, Bauer R (1981) Magnification factor and receptive field size in foveal striate cortex of the monkey. Exp Brain Res 44:213–228

Dreher B (1972) Hypercomplex cells in the cat's striate cortex. Invest Ophthalmol Vis Sci 11: 355–356

Dreher B, Cottee LJ (1975) Visual receptive-field properties of cells in area 18 of cat's cerebral cortex before and after acute lesions in area 17. J Neurophysiol 38:735–750

Dreher B, Sanderson KJ (1973) Receptive field analysis: responses to moving visual contours by single lateral geniculate neurones in the cat. J Physiol (Lond) 234:95–118

Dreher B, Sefton AJ (1979) Properties of neurons in cat's dorsal lateral geniculate nucleus: a comparison between medial interlaminar and laminated parts of the nucleus. J Comp Neurol 183:47–64

Dreher B, Fukuda Y, Rodieck RW (1976) Identification, classification and anatomical segregation of cells with X-like and Y-like properties in the lateral geniculate nucleus of old-world primates. J Physiol (Lond) 258:433–452

Dreher B, Leventhal A, Hale PT (1980) Geniculate input to cat visual cortex: a comparison of area 19 with areas 17 and 18. J Neurophysiol 44:804–826

Duysens J, Orban GA (1981) Is stimulus movement of particular importance in the functioning of cat visual cortex? Brain Res 220:184–187

Duysens J, Orban GA, van der Glas HW, de Zegher FE (1982a) Functional properties of area 19 as compared to area 17 of the cat. Brain Res 231:279–291

Duysens J, Orban GA, van der Glas HW, Maes H (1982b) Receptive field structure of area 19 as compared to area 17 of the cat. Brain Res 231:293–308

Duysens J, Orban GA, Verbeke O (1982c) Velocity sensitivity mechanisms in cat visual cortex. Exp Brain Res 45:285–294

Duysens J, Orban GA, Cremieux J (to be published) Functional basis for the preference for slow movement in area 17 of the cat. Vision Res

Elberger AJ (1982) The functional role of the corpus callosum in the developing visual system: a review. Progress Neurobiol 18:15–79

Emerson RC, Coleman L (1981) Does image movement have a special nature for neurons in the cat's striate cortex? Invest Ophthalmol Vis Sci 20:766–783

Emerson RC, Gerstein GL (1977a) Simple striate neurons in the cat. I. Comparison of responses to moving and stationary stimuli. J Neurophysiol 40:119–135

Emerson RC, Gerstein GL (1977b) Simple striate neurons in the cat. II. Mechanisms underlying directional asymmetry and directional selectivity. J Neurophysiol 40:136–155

Enroth-Cugell C, Robson JG (1966) The contrast sensitivity of retinal ganglion cells of the cat. J Physiol (Lond) 187:517–552

Enroth-Cugell C, Hertz BF, Lennie P (1977) Cone signals in the cat's retina. J Physiol (Lond) 269:273–296

Evarts EV, Bental E, Bihari B, Huttenlocher PR (1962) Spontaneous discharge of single neurons during sleep and waking. Science 135:726–728

Eysel UTh, Grüsser O-J, Hoffmann K-P (1979) Monocular deprivation and the signal transmission by X- and Y-neurons of the cat lateral geniculate nucleus. Exp Brain Res 34:521–539

Famigletti EV Jr (1975) Another look at lateral geniculate lamination in the cat. Soc Neurosci Abstr 1:41

Fairén A, Valverde F (1980) A specialized type of neuron in the visual cortex of cat: a Golgi and electron microscope study of chandelier cells. J Comp Neurol 194:761–779

Felleman DJ, Jones JP, Kaas JH (1981) Some response properties of neurons in the middle temporal visual area (MT) of owl monkeys. Suppl Invest Ophthalmol Vis Sci 20:148

Ferster D (1981) A comparison of binocular depth mechanisms in areas 17 and 18 of the cat visual cortex. J Physiol (Lond) 311:623–655

Ferster D, LeVay S (1978) The axonal arborizations of lateral geniculate neurons in the striate cortex of the cat. J Comp Neurol 182:923–944

Ferster D, Lindström S (1981) An intracellular study of geniculo-cortical connectivity in area 17 of the cat. Soc Neurosci Abstr 7:355

Filiminoff IN (1932) Über die Variabilität der Grosshirnstruktur. Regio occipitalis beim erwachsenen Menschen. J für Psychol und Neurol 55:1–96

Finlay BL, Schiller PH, Volman SF (1976a) Quantitative studies of single-cell properties in monkey striate cortex. IV. Corticotectal cells. J Neurophysiol 39:1352–1361

Finlay BL, Schiller PH, Volman SF (1976b) Meridional differences in orientation sensitivity in monkey striate cortex. Brain Res 105:350–352

Fischer B, Krüger J (1979) Disparity tuning and binocularity of single neurons in cat visual cortex. Exp Brain Res 35:1–8

Fishman MC, Michael CR (1973) Integration of auditory information in the cat's visual cortex. Vision Res 13:1415–1419

Fisken RA, Garey LJ, Powell TPS (1975) The intrinsic, association and commissural connections of area 17 of the visual cortex. Philos Trans R Soc Lond (Biol) 272:487–536

Freeman RD, Robson JG (1982) A new approach to the study of binocular interaction in visual cortex: normal and monocularly deprived cats. Exp Brain Res 48:296–300

Friedlander MJ, Lin CS, Stanford LR, Sherman SM (1981) Morphology of functionally identified neurons in lateral geniculate nucleus of the cat. J Neurophysiol 46:80–129

Fries W, Albus K (1980) Responses of pontine nuclei cells to electrical stimulation of the lateral and suprasylvian gyrus in the cat. Brain Res 188:255–260

Fries W, Albus K, Creutzfeldt OD (1977) Effects of interacting visual patterns on single cell responses in cat's striate cortex. Vision Res 17:1001–1008

Gabor D (1946) Theory of communication. J IEE (Lond) 93:429–457

Galletti C, Maioli MG, Squatrito S, Riva Sanseverino E (1979) Single unit responses to visual stimuli in cat cortical areas 17 and 18. I. Responses to stationary stimuli of variable intensity. Arch Ital Biol 117:208–230

Galletti C, Squatrito S, Battaglini PP, Maioli MG (1981) Contralateral tectal projections from single areas of the visual cortex in the cat. Arch Ital Biol 119:43–51

Garey LJ (1971) A light and electron microscopic study of the visual cortex of the cat and monkey. Proc R Soc Lond (Biol) 179:21–40

Garey LJ, Jones EG, Powell TPS (1968) Interrelationships of striate and extrastriate cortex with the primary relay sites of the visual pathway. J Neurol Neurosurg Psychiat 31:135–157

Gattass R, Gross CG (1981) Visual topography of striate projection zone (MT) in posterior superior temporal sulcus of the macaque. J Neurophysiol 46:621–638

Geisert EE Jr (1980) Cortical projections of the lateral geniculate nucleus in the cat. J Comp Neurol 190:793–812

Gibson A, Baker J, Mower G, Glickstein M (1978) Corticopontine cells in area 18 of the cat. J Neurophysiol 41:484–495

Gilbert CD (1977) Laminar differences in receptive field properties of cells in cat primary visual cortex. J Physiol (Lond) 268:391–421

Gilbert CD, Kelly JP (1975) The projections of cells in different layers of the cat's visual cortex. J Comp Neurol 163:81–106

Gilbert CD, Wiesel TN (1979) Morphology and intracortical projections of cuntionally characterised neurones in the cat visual cortex. Nature 280:120–125

Gilbert CD, Wiesel TN (1980) Interleaving projection bands in cortico-cortical connections. Soc Neurosci Abstr 6:315

Ginsburg AP (1981) Spatial filtering and vision: implications for normal and abnormal vision. In: Proenza M, Enoch M, Jampolsky A (eds) Clinical applications of visual psychophysics. Cambridge, Cambridge University Press, pp 70–106

Gizzi MS, Katz E, Movshon JA (1981) Spatial properties of neurons in the cat's lateral suprasylvian visual cortex. Soc Neurosci Abstr 7:831

Glezer VD, Ivanoff VA, Tscherbach TA (1973) Investigation of complex and hypercomplex receptive fields of visual cortex of the cat as spatial frequency filters. Vision Res 13:1875–1904

Goodwin AW, Henry GH (1975) Direction selectivity of complex cells in a comparison with simple cells. J Neurophysiol 38:1524–1540

Goodwin AW, Henry GH (1978) The influence of stimulus velocity on the responses of single neurones in the striate cortex. J Physiol (Lond) 277:467–482

Goodwin AW, Henry GH, Bishop PO (1975) Direction selectivity of simple striate cells: properties and mechanism. J Neurophysiol 38:1500–1523

Gouras P (1969) Antidromic responses of orthodromically identified ganglion cells in monkey retina. J Physiol (Lond) 264:407–419

Gouras P (1974) Opponent-colour cells in different layers of foveal striate cortex. J Physiol (Lond) 238:583–602

Gouras P, Krüger J (1979) Responses of cells in foveal visual cortex of the monkey to pure color contrast. J Neurophysiol 42:850–860

Graybiel AM, Berson DM (1980) Autoradiographic evidence for a projection from the pretectal nucleus of the optic tract to the dorsal lateral geniculate complex in the cat. Brain Res 195:1–12

Grüsser O-J, Grüsser-Cornehls U (1960) Mikroelektrodenuntersuchungen zur Konvergenz vestibulärer und retinaler Afferenzen an einzelnen Neuronen des optischen Cortex der Katze. Pflügers Arch Ges Physiol 270:227–238

Grüsser O-J, Grüsser-Cornehls U (1972) Interactions of vestibular and visual inputs in the visual system. Prog Brain Res 37:582–583

Grüsser O-J, Grüsser-Cornehls U (1973) Neuronal mechanisms of visual movement perception and some psychophysical and behavioral correlations. In: Jung R (ed) Central visual information. Springer, Berlin Heidelberg New York (Handbook of sensory physiology, vol VII/3A, pp 333–429)

Grüsser O-J, Grüsser-Cornehls U, Saur G (1959) Reaktionen einzelner Neurone im optischen Cortex der Katze nach elektrischer Polarisation des Labyrinths. Pflügers Arch 269:593–612

Guedes R, Watanabe S, Creutzfeldt OD (1983) Functional role of association fibres for a visual association area: the posterior suprasylvian sulcus of the cat. Exp Brain Res 49:13–27

Guillery RW (1966) A study of Golgi preparations from the dorsal lateral geniculate nucleus of the adult cat. J Comp Neurol 128:21–50

Guillery RW (1970) The laminar distribution of retinal fibers in the dorsal lateral geniculate nucleus of the cat: a new interpretation. J Comp Neurol 138:339–368

Guillery RW, Geisert EE Jr, Polley EH, Mason CA (1980) An analysis of the retinal afferents to the cat's medial interlaminar nucleus and to its rostral thalamic extension, the "geniculate wing". J Comp Neurol 194:117–142

Guld C, Bertulis A (1976) Representation of fovea in the striate cortex of vervet monkey, cercopithecus aethiops pygerythrus. Vision Res 16:629–631

Hammond P (1978a) On the use of nitrous oxide/oxygen mixtures for anaesthesia in cats. J Physiol (Lond) 275:64P

Hammond P (1978b) Directional tuning of complex cells in area 17 of the feline visual cortex. J Physiol (Lond) 285:479–491

Hammond P (1979) Stimulus dependence of ocular dominance of complex cells in area 17 of the feline visual cortex. Exp Brain Res 35:583–589

Hammond P (1981a) Simultaneous determination of directional tuning of complex cells in cat striate cortex for bar and for texture motion. Exp Brain Res 41:364–369

Hammond P (1981b) Non-stationarity of ocular dominance in cat striate cortex. Exp Brain Res 42:189–195

Hammond P, Andrews DP (1978) Orientation tuning of cells in areas 17 and 18 of the cat's visual cortex. Exp Brain Res 31:341–351

Hammond P, MacKay DM (1975) Differential responses of cat visual cortical cells to textured stimuli. Exp Brain Res 22:427–430

Hammond P, MacKay DM (1977) Differential responsiveness of simple and complex cells in cat striate cortex to visual texture. Exp Brain Res 30:275–296

Hammond P, MacKay DM (1981) Modulatory influences of moving textured backgrounds on responsiveness of simple cells in feline striate cortex. J Physiol (Lond) 319:431–442

Hammond P, Reck J (1980) Influence of velocity on directional tuning of complex cells in cat striate cortex for texture motion. Neurosci Lett 19:309–314

Hammond P, Andrews DP, James CR (1975) Invariance of orientational and directional tuning in visual cortical cells of the adult cat. Brain Res 96:56–59

Hartline HK (1938) The response of single optic nerve fibers of the vertebrate eye to illumination of the retina. Am J Physiol 121:400

Harvey AR (1980a) The afferent connexions and laminar distribution of cells in area 18 of the cat. J Physiol (Lond) 302:483–505

Harvey AR (1980b) A physiological analysis of subcortical and commissural projections of areas 17 and 18 of the cat. J Physiol (Lond) 302:507–534

Hasan J, Lehtinen I (1981) Eye movement related cellular activity in the visual cortex of the cat. Acta Physiol Scand 112:97–99

Heath CJ, Jones EG (1970) Connexions of area 19 and the lateral suprasylvian area of the visual cortex of the cat. Brain Res 19:302–305

Heath CJ, Jones EG (1971) The anatomical organization of the suprasylvian gyrus of the cat. Ergebn Anat Entwickl Gesch 45:3–64

Heggelund P (1981a) Receptive field organization of simple cells in cat striate cortex. Exp Brain Res 42:89–98

Heggelund P (1981b) Receptive field orgaization of complex cells in cat striate cortex. Exp Brain Res 42:99–107

Heggelund P, Albus K (1978) Response variability and orientation discrimination of single cells in striate cortex of cat. Exp Brain Res 32:197–211

Henry GH (1977) Receptive field classes of cells in the striate cortex of the cat. Brain Res 133: 1–28

Henry GH, Bishop PO, Coombs JS (1969) Inhibitory and subliminal excitatory receptive fields of simple units in cat striate cortex. Vision Res 9:1289–1296

Henry GH, Bishop PO, Dreher B (1974a) Orientation, axis and direction as stimulus parameters for striate cells. Vision Res 14:767–777

Henry GH, Dreher B, Bishop PO (1974b) Orientation specificity of cells in cat striate cortex. J Neurophysiol 37:1394–1409

Henry GH, Bishop PO, Tupper RM, Dreher B (1973) Orientation specificity and response variability of cells in the striate cortex. Vision Res 13:1771–1779

Henry GH, Goodwin AW, Bishop PO (1978a) Spatial summation of responses in receptive fields of single cells in cat striate cortex. Exp Brain Res 32:245–266

Henry GH, Lund JS, Harvey AR (1978b) Cells of the striate cortex projecting to the Clare-Bishop area of the cat. Brain Res 151:154–158

Henry GH, Harvey AR, Lund JS (1979) The afferent connections and laminar distribution of cells in the cat striate cortex. J Comp Neurol 187:725–744

Hess RF, Lillywhite PG (1980) Effect of luminance on contrast coding in cat visual cortex. J Physiol (Lond) 300:56–57P

Hess R, Wolters W (1979) Responses of single cells in cat's lateral geniculate nucleus and area 17 to the velocity of moving visual stimuli. Exp Brain Res 34:273–286

Hess R, Negishi K, Creutzfeldt O (1975) The horizontal spread of intracortical inhibition in the visual cortex. Exp Brain Res 22:415–419

Hickey TL, Guillery RW (1974) An autoradiographic study of retinogeniculate pathways in the cat and the fox. J Comp Neurol 156:239–254

Hoffmann KP (1973) Conduction velocity in pathways from retina to superior colliculus in the cat: a correlation with receptive-field properties. J Neurophysiol 36:409–424

Hoffmann KP (1982) Cortical versus subcortical contributions to the optokinetic reflex in the cat. In: Lennerstrand G et al. (eds) Functional basis of ocular motility disorders. Pergamon, Oxford, pp 303–310

Hoffmann KP, Stone J (1971) Conduction velocity of afferents to cat visual cortex: a correlation with cortical receptive field properties. Brain Res 32:460–466

Hoffmann KP, von Seelen W (1978) Analysis of neuronal networks in the visual system of the cat using statistical signals – simple and complex cells – Part II. Biol Cybern 31:175–185

Hoffmann KP, Stone J, Sherman SM (1972) Relay of receptive-field properties in dorsal lateral geniculate nucleus of the cat. J Neurophysiol 35:518–531

Hoffmann KP, Morrone CM, Reuter JH (1980) A comparison of the responses of single cells in the LGN and visual cortex to bar and noise stimuli in the cat. Vision Res 20:771–777

Holländer H (1974) On the origin of the corticotectal projections in the cat. Exp Brain Res 21: 433–439

Holländer H, Vanegas H (1977) The projection from the lateral geniculate nucleus onto the visual cortex in the cat. A quantitative study with horseradish-peroxidase. J Comp Neurol 173:519–536

Horn G, Stechler G, Hill RM (1972) Receptive fields of units in the visual cortex of the cat in the presence and absence of bodily tilt. Exp Brain Res 15:113–132

Hornung JP, Garey LJ (1980) A direct pathway from thalamus to visual callosal neurons in the cat. Exp Brain Res 38:121–123

Horton JC, Hubel DH (1980) Cytochrome oxidase stain preferentially labels intersection of ocular dominance and vertical orientation columns in macaque striate cortex. Soc Neurosci Abstr 6: 315

Horton JC, Hubel DH (1981) Regular patchy distribution of cytochrome oxidase staining in primary visual cortex of macaque monkey. Nature 292:762–764

Hubel DH (1959) Single unit activity in striate cortex of unrestrained cats. J Physiol (Lond) 147: 226–238

Hubel DH, Freeman DC (1977) Projection into the visual field of ocular dominance columns in macaque monkey. Brain Res 122:336–343

Hubel DH, Livingstone MS (1981) Regions of poor orientation tuning coincide with patches of cytochrome oxidase staining in monkey striate cortex. Soc Neurosci Abstr 7:357

Hubel DH, Livingstone MS (1982) Cytochrome oxidase blobs in monkey area 17:response properties and afferent connections. Soc Neurosci Abstr. 8:706

Hubel DH, Wiesel TN (1959) Receptive fields of single neurones in the cat's striate cortex. J Physiol (Lond) 148:574–591

Hubel DH, Wiesel TN (1962) Receptive fields, binocular interaction and functional architecture in the cat's visual cortex. J Physiol (Lond) 160:106–154

Hubel DH, Wiesel TN (1963) Shape and arrangement of columns in cat's striate cortex. J Physiol (Lond) 165:559–568

Hubel DH, Wiesel TN (1965) Receptive fields and functional architecture in two nonstriate visual areas (18 and 19) of the cat. J Neurophysiol 28:229–289

Hubel DH, Wiesel TN (1967) Cortical and callosal connections concerned with the vertical meridian of visual fields in the cat. J Neurophysiol 30:1561–1573

Hubel DH, Wiesel TN (1968) Receptive fields and functional architecture of monkey striate cortex. J Physiol (Lond) 195:215–243

Hubel DH, Wiesel TN (1969) Visual area of the lateral suprasylvian gyrus (Clare-Bishop area) of the cat. J Physiol (Lond) 202:251–260

Hubel DH, Wiesel TN (1970) Cells sensitive to binocular depth in area 18 of the macaque monkey cortex. Nature 225:41–42

Hubel DH, Wiesel TN (1972) Laminar and columnar distribution of geniculocortical fibers in the macaque monkey. J Comp Neurol 146:421–450

Hubel DH, Wiesel TN (1973) A re-examination of stereoscopic mechanisms in the cat. J Physiol (Lond) 232:29–30P

Hubel DH, Wiesel TN (1974a) Sequence regularity and geometry of orientation columns in the monkey striate cortex. J Comp Neurol 158:267–294

Hubel DH, Wiesel TN (1974b) Uniformity of monkey striate cortex: a parallel relationship between field size, scatter, and magnification factor. J Comp Neurol 158:295–305

Hubel DH, Wiesel TN (1977) Functional architecture of macaque monkey visual cortex. Proc R Soc Lond (Biol) 198:1–59

Hubel DH, Wiesel TN, Stryker MP (1977) Orientation columns in macaque monkey visual cortex demonstrated by the 2-deoxyglucose autoradiographic technique. Nature 269:328–330

Hughes A (1977) The topography of vision in mammals of contrasting life style: comparative optics and retinal organization. In: Crescitelli F (ed) The visual system in evolution. A Vertebrates. Springer, Berlin Heidelberg New York (Handbook of sensory physiology, pp 615–737)

Hughes A (1981) Population magnitudes and distribution of the major modal classes of cat retinal ganglion cell as estimated from HRP filling and a systematic survey of the soma diameter spectra for classical neurones. J Comp Neurol 197:303–339

Hughes HC (1980) Efferent organization of the cat pulvinar complex, with a note on bilateral claustrocortical and reticulocortical connections. J Comp Neurol 193:937–963

Humphrey AL, Hendrickson AE (1980) Radial zones of high metabolic activity in squirrel monkey striate cortex. Soc Neurosci Abstr 6:315

Ikeda H, Wright MJ (1974) Sensitivity of neurones in visual cortex (area 17) under different levels of anaesthesia. Exp Brain Res 20:471–484

Ikeda H, Wright MJ (1975a) The latency of visual cortical neurones in area 17 in the cat to visual stimuli with reference to the sustained (X) and transient (Y) and 'simple' and 'complex' cell classification. J Physiol (Lond) 245:114–115P

Ikeda H, Wright MJ (1975b) Spatial and temporal properties of "sustained" and "transient" neurones in area 17 of the cat's visual cortex. J Physiol (Lond) 22:363–383

Illing R-B, Wässle H (1981) The retinal projection to the thalamus in the cat: a quantitative investigation and a comparison with the retinotectal pathway. J Comp Neurol 202:265–285

Imig TJ, Morel A (1983) Organization of the thalamocortical auditory system in the cat. Ann Rev Neurosci 6:95−120

Innocenti GM (1980) The primary visual pathway through the corpus callosum: morphological and functional aspects in the cat. Arch Ital Biol 118:124−188

Innocenti GM, Fiore L (1974) Post-synaptic inhibitory components of the responses to moving stimuli in area 17. Brain Res 80:122−126

Ito M, Sanides D, Creutzfeldt OD (1977) A study of binocular convergence in cat visual cortex neurons. Exp Brain Res 28:21−35

Iwai E, Mishkin M (1969) Further evidence on the locus of the visual area in the temporal lobe of the monkey. Exp Neurol 25:585−594

Jacobs GH (1977a) Visual capacities of the owl monkey (Aotus trivirgatus) − I. Spectral sensitivity and color vision. Vision Res 17:811−820

Jacobs GH (1977b) Visual capacities of the owl monkey (Aotus trivirgatus) − II. Spatial contrast sensitivity. Vision Res 17:821−826

Jayaraman A, Updyke BV (1979) Organization of visual cortical projections to the claustrum in the cat. Brain Res 178:107−115

Johansson G (1975) Visual motion perception. Sci Am 232:76−88

Joshua DE, Bishop PO (1970) Binocular single vision and depth discrimination. Receptive field disparities for central and peripheral vision and binocular interaction on peripheral single units in cat striate cortex. Exp Brain Res 10:389−416

Julesz B (1971) Foundations of cyclopean perception. University of Chicago Press, Chicago

Kaas JH, Huerta MF, Weber JT, Harting JK (1978) Patterns of retinal terminations and laminar organization of the lateral geniculate nucleus of primates. J Comp Neurol 182:517−554

Kalia M, Whitteridge D (1973) The visual areas in the splenial sulcus of the cat. J Physiol (Lond) 232:272−283

Kalil R, Worden I (1978) Cytoplasmic laminated bodies in the lateral geniculate nucleus of normal and dark reared cats. J Comp Neurol 178:469−486

Kaplan E, Shapley RM (1982) X and Y cells in the lateral geniculate nucleus of macaque monkeys. J Physiol (Lond) 330:125−143

Kasamatsu T (1976) Visual cortical neurons influenced by the oculomotor input: characterization of their receptive field properties. Brain Res 113:271−292

Kasamatsu T, Adey WR (1973) Visual cortical units associated with phasic activity in REM sleep and wakefulness. Brain Res 55:323−331

Kato H, Bishop PO, Orban GA (1978) Hypercomplex and the simple/complex cell classifications in cat striate cortex. J Neurophysiol 41:1071−1095

Kato H, Bishop PO, Orban GA (1981) Binocular interaction on monocularly-discharged lateral geniculate and striate neurons in the cat. J Neurophysiol 46:932−951

Kawamura K (1973) Corticocortical fiber connections of the cat cerebrum. III. The occipital region. Brain Res 51:41−60

Kawamura K, Chiba M (1979) Cortical neurons projecting to the pontine nuclei in the cat. An experimental study with the horseradish peroxidase technique. Exp Brain Res 35:269−285

Kawamura K, Konno T (1979) Various types of corticotectal neurons of cats as demonstrated by means of retrograde axonal transport of horseradish peroxidase. Exp Brain Res 35:161−175

Kawamura K, Naito J (1980) Corticocortical neurons projecting to the medial and lateral banks of the middle suprasylvian sulcus in the cat: an experimental study with the horseradish peroxidase method. J Comp Neurol 193:1009−1022

Kawamura S, Sprague JM, Niimi K (1974) Corticofugal projections from the visual cortices to the thalamus, pretectum and superior colliculus in the cat. J Comp Neurol 158:339−362

Kayama Y, Riso RR, Bartlett JR, Doty RW (1979) Luxotonic responses of units in macaque striate cortex. J Neurophysiol 42:1495−1517

Keller G, Innocenti GM (1981) Callosal connections of suprasylvian visual areas in the cat. Neuroscience 6:703−712

Kelly JP, Van Essen DC (1974) Cell structure and function in the visual cortex of the cat. J Physiol (Lond) 238:515−547

Kennedy H, Baleydier C (1977) Direct projections from thalamic intralaminar nuclei to extrastriate visual cortex in the cat traced with horseradish peroxidase. Exp Brain Res 28:133−139

Kennedy H, Orban GA (1983) Response properties of visual cortical neurons in cats reared in stroboscopic illumination. J Neurophysiol 49:686−704

Kennedy H, Martin K, Orban GA, Whitteridge D (1980) Neuronal properties in V1 and V2 of the baboon (Papio Ursinus). Exp Brain Res 41:A20

Kennedy H, Martin KAC, Orban GA, Whitteridge D (1981) Receptive field characteristics in V1 and V2 of the cat and monkey. J Physiol (Lond) 319:81P

Kimura M, Shiida T, Tanaka K, Toyama K (1980) Three classes of area 19 cortical cells of the cat classified by their connectivity and photic responsiveness. Vision Res 20:69–77

Kimura M, Komatsu Y, Toxama K (1980) Differential responses of "simple" and "complex" cells of cat's striate cortex during saccadic eye movements. Vision Res 20:553–556

Kornhuber H, Da Fonseca JS (1964) Optovestibular integration in the cat's cortex. A study of sensory convergence on cortical neurons. In: Bender MB (ed) The oculomotor system. Harper and Row, New York, pp 239–276

Kratz KE, Webb SV, Sherman SM (1978) Studies of the cat's medial interlaminar nucleus: a subdivision of the dorsal lateral geniculate nucleus. J Comp Neurol 181:601–614

Kuffler SW (1953) Discharge patterns and functional organization of mammalian retina. J Neurophysiol 16:37–68

Kulikowski JJ, Bishop PO (1981a) Fourier analysis and spatial representation in the visual cortex. Experientia 37:160–162

Kulikowski JJ, Bishop PO (1981b) Linear analysis of the responses of simple cells in the cat visual cortex. Exp Brain Res 44:386–400

Kulikowski JJ, Bishop PO (1982) Silent periodic cells in the cat striate cortex. Vision Res 22:191–200

Kulikowski JJ, Bishop PO, Kato H (1979) Sustained and transient responses by cat striate cells to stationary flashing light and dark bars. Brain Res 170:362–367

Kulikowski JJ, Bishop PO, Kato H (1981) Spatial arrangements of responses by cells in the visual cortex to light and dark bars and edges. Exp Brain Res 44:371–385

Land EH (1977) The retinex theory of colour vision. Sci Am 237:108–129

Lee BB (1970) Effect of anaesthetics upon visual responses of neurones in the cat's striate cortex. J Physiol (Lond) 207:74P

Lee BB, Albus K, Heggelund P, Hulme MJ, Creutzfeldt OD (1977a) The depth distribution of optimal stimulus orientations for neurones in cat area 17. Exp Brain Res 27:301–314

Lee BB, Cleland BG, Creutzfeldt OD (1979b) The retinal input to cells in area 17 of the cat's cortex. Exp Brain Res 30:527–538

Lee BB, Elepfandt A, Virsu V (1981a) Phase of responses to moving sinusoidal gratings in cells of cat retina and lateral geniculate nucleus. J Neurophysiol 45:807–817

Lee BB, Elepfandt A, Virsu V (1981b) Phase of responses to sinusoidal gratings of simple cells in cat striate cortex. J Neurophysiol 45:818–828

LeGrand Y (1967) Form and space vision (translated by Millodot M, Heath GG) Indian University Press, Bloomington

Lehmkuhle S, Kratz KE, Mangel SC, Sherman SM (1980) Spatial and temporal sensitivity of X- and Y-cells in dorsal lateral geniculate nucleus of the cat. J Neurophysiol 43:520–541

Leicester J (1968) Projection of the visual vertical meridian to cerebral cortex of the cat. J Neurophysiol 31:371–382

Lennie P (1980) Parallel visual pathways: a review. Vision Res 20:561–594

LeVay S (1973) Synaptic patterns in the visual cortex of the cat and monkey. Electron microscopy of Golgi preparations. J Comp Neurol 150:53–86

LeVay S, Ferster D (1977) Relay cell classes in the lateral geniculate nucleus of the cat and the effects of visual deprivation. J Comp Neurol 172:563–584

LeVay S, Gilbert CD (1976) Laminar patterns of geniculocortical projection in the cat. Brain Res 113:1–19

LeVay S, Sherk H (1981) The visual claustrum of the cat. I. Structure and connections. J Neurosci 1:956–980

Le Vay S, Hubel DH, Wiesel TN (1975) The pattern of ocular dominance columns in macaque visual cortex revealed by a reduced silver stain. J Comp Neurol 159:559–576

LeVay S, Stryker MP, Shatz CJ (1978) Ocular dominance columns and their development in layer IV of the cat's visual cortex: a quantitative study. J Comp Neurol 179:223–244

Leventhal AG (1979) Evidence that the different classes of relay cells of the cat's lateral geniculate nucleus terminate in different layers of the striate cortex. Exp Brain Res 37:349–372

Leventhal AG, Hirsch HVB (1978) Receptive-field properties of neurons in different laminae of visual cortex of the cat. J Neurophysiol 41:948–962

Leventhal AG, Hirsch HVB (1980) Receptive-field properties of different classes of neurons in visual cortex of normal and dark-reared cats. J Neurophysiol 43:1111–1132

Leventhal AG, Keens J, Törk I (1980) The afferent ganglion cells and cortical projections of the retinal recipient zone (RRZ) of the cat's 'pulvinar complex'. J Comp Neurol 194:535–554

Levick WR, Thibos LN (1980) X/Y analysis of sluggish-concentric retinal ganglion cells of the cat. Exp Brain Res 41:A5–A6

Lin CS, Kaas JH (1979) The inferior pulvinar complex in owl monkeys: architectonic subdivisions and patterns of input from the superior colliculus and subdivisions of visual cortex. J Comp Neurol 187:655–678

Lin CS, Wagor E, Kaas JH (1974) Projections from the pulvinar to the middle temporal visual area (MT) in the owl monkey, Aotus trivirgatus. Brain Res 76:145–149

Lin CS, Kratz KE, Sherman SM (1977) Percentage of relay cells in the cat's lateral geniculate nucleus. Brain Res 131:167–173

Lin CS, Friedlander MJ, Sherman SM (1979) Morphology of physiologically identified neurons in the visual cortex of the cat. Brain Res 172:344–345

Lin CS, Weller RE, Kaas JH (1982) Cortical connections of striate cortex in the owl monkey. J Comp Neurol 211:165–176

Livingstone MS, Hubel DH (1981) Effects of sleep and arousal on the processing of issual information in the cat. Nature 291:554–561

Loop MS, Bruce LL, Petuchowski S (1979) Cat color vision: the effect of stimulus size, shape and viewing distance. Vision Res 19:507–513

Lund JS (1973) Organization of neurons in the visual cortex, area 17, of the monkey (Macaca mulatta). J Comp Neurol 147:455–495

Lund JS, Boothe RG (1975) Interlaminar connections and pyramidal neuron organisation in the visual cortex, area 17, of the macaque monkey. J Comp Neurol 159:305–334

Lund JS, Lund RD, Hendrickson AE, Bunt AH, Fuchs AF (1975) The origin of efferent pathways from the primary visual cortex, area 17, of the macaque monkey as shown by retrograde transport of horseradish peroxidase. J Comp Neurol 164:287–304

Lund JS, Henry GH, Macqueen CL, Harvey AR (1979) Anatomical organization of the primary visual cortex (area 17) of the cat. A comparison with area 17 of the macaque monkey. J Comp Neurol 184:599–618

Lund JS, Hendrickson AE, Ogren MP, Tobin EA (1981) Anatomical organization of primate visual cortex area VII. J Comp Neurol 202:19–45

Maciewicz RJ (1975) Thalamic afferents to areas 17, 18 and 19 of cat cortex traced with horseradish peroxidase. Brain Res 84:308–312

MacKay DM (1973) Visual stability and voluntary eye movements. In: Jung R (ed) Handbook of sensory physiology, vol VII/3A. Springer, Berlin Heidelberg New York, pp 307–331

MacKay DM (1981) Strife over visual cortical function. Nature 289:117–118

Macko KA, Jarvis CD, Kennedy C, Miyaoka M, Shinohara M, Sokoloff L, Mishkin M (1982) Mapping the primate visual system with $[2\text{-}^{14}C]$deoxyglucose. Science 218:394–396

Macy A, Ohzawa I, Freeman RD (1982) A quantitative study of the classification and stability of ocular dominance in the cat's visual cortex. Exp Brain Res 48:401–408

Maffei L, Fiorentini A (1973) The visual cortex as a spatial frequency analyser. Vision Res 13:1255–1267

Maffei L, Fiorentini A (1976) The unresponsive regions of visual cortical receptive fields. Vision Res 16:1131–1139

Maffei L, Fiorentini A (1977) Spatial frequency rows in the striate visual cortex. Vision Res 17:257–264

Maffei L, Morrone C, Pirchio M, Sandini G (1979) Responses of visual cortical cells to periodic and non-periodic stimuli. J Physiol (Lond) 296:27–47

Magalhães-Castro HH, Saraiva PES, Magalhães-Castro B (1975) Identification of corticotectal cells of the visual cortex of cats by means of horseradish peroxidase. Brain Res 83:474–479

Malpeli JG (1981) Effects of blocking A-layer geniculate input on cat area 17. Soc Neurosci Abstr 7:355

Malpeli JG, Baker FH (1975) The representation of the visual field in the lateral geniculate nucleus of Macaca mulatta. J Comp Neurol 161:569–594

Malpeli JG, Schiller PH, Colby CL (1981) Response properties of single cells in monkey striate cortex during reversible inactivation of individual lateral geniculate laminae. J Neurophysiol 46:1102–1119

Mandl G, Desai N, Capaday C (1980) Nitrous oxide modifies visual responses in the cat retina, striate cortex and superior colliculus. Brain Res 193:401–414

Mansfield RJW (1974) Neural basis of orientation perception in primate vision. Science 186:1133–1135

Marr D (1982) Vision. Freeman WH and Company, San Francisco, 397 p

Marr D, Ullman S (1981) Directional selectivity and its use in early visual processing. Proc R Soc Lond (Biol) 211:151–180

Marr D, Vaina L (1982) Representation and recognition of the movements of shapes. Proc R Soc Lond (Biol) 214:501–524

Marrocco RT, McClurkin JW, Young RA (1982) Spatial summation and conduction latency classification of cells in the lateral geniculate nucleus of macaques. J Neurosc 2:1275–1291

Marshall WH, Talbot SA, Ades HW (1943) Cortical responses of the anesthetized cat to gross photic and electrical afferent stimulation. J Neurophysiol 6:1–15

Martin KM, Whitteridge D (1981) Morphological identification of cells of the cat's visual cortex, classified with regard to their afferent input and receptive field type. J Physiol (Lond) 320: 14–15P

Mason R (1978) Functional organization in the cat's pulvinar complex. Exp Brain Res 31:51–66

McIlwain JT (1973) Topographic relationships in projection from striate cortex to superior colliculus of the cat. J Neurophysiol 36:690–701

McIlwain JT (1977) Topographic organization and convergence in corticotectal projections from areas 17, 18, and 19 in the cat. J Neurophysiol 40:189–198

McKee SP (1981) A local mechanism for differential velocity detection. Vision Res 21:491–500

Meyer G, Albus K (1981a) Spiny stellates as cells of origin of association fibres from area 17 to area 18 in the cat's neocortex. Brain Res 210:335–341

Meyer G, Albus K (1981b) Topography and cortical projections of morphologically identified neurons in the visual thalamus of the cat. J Comp Neurol 201:353–374

Michael CR (1978a) Color vision mechanisms in monkey striate cortex: dual-opponent cells with concentric receptive fields. J Neurophysiol 41:572–588

Michael CR (1978b) Color vision mechanisms in monkey striate cortex: simple cells with dual opponent-color receptive fields. J Neurophysiol 41:1233–1249

Michael CR (1978c) Color-sensitive complex cells in monkey striate cortex. J Neurophysiol 41: 1250–1266

Michael CR (1979) Color-sensitive hypercomplex cells in monkey striate cortex. J Neurophysiol 42:726–744

Michael CR (1981) Columnar organization of color cells in monkey's striate cortex. J Neurophysiol 46:587–604

Miller JW, Buschmann MBT, Benevento LA (1980) Extrageniculate thalamic projections to the primary visual cortex. Brain Res 189:221–227

Mishkin M (1980) Two cortical visual systems. Exp Brain Res 41:A17–A18

Missotten L (1974) Estimation of the ratio of cones to neurons in the fovea of the human retina. Invest Ophthalmol Vis Sci 13:1045–1049

Mitzdorf U, Singer W (1977) Laminar segregation of afferents to lateral geniculate nucleus of the cat: an analysis of current source density. J Neurophysiol 40:1227–1244

Mitzdorf U, Singer W (1979) Excitatory synaptic ensemble properties in the visual cortex of the macaque monkey: a current source density analysis of electrically evoked potentials. J Comp Neurol 17:71–84

Mize BR, Murphy EH (1976) Alterations in receptive field properties of superior colliculus cells produced by visual cortex ablation in infant and adult cats. J Comp Neurol 168:393–424

Montero VM (1981) Topography of the cortico-cortical connections from the striate cortex in the cat. Brain Behav Evol 18:194–218

Morrell F (1972) Visual system's view of acoustic space. Nature 238:44–46

Morrone MC, Burr DC, Maffei L (1982) Functional implications of cross-orientation inhibition of cortical visual cells. I. Neurophysiological evidence. Proc Roy Soc Lond (Biol) 216:335–354

Mountcastle VB (1957) Modality and topographic properties of single neurons of cat's somatic sensory cortex. J Neurophysiol 20:408–434

Movshon JA (1975) The velocity tuning of single units in cat striate cortex. J Physiol (Lond) 249: 445–468

Movshon JA, Thompson ID, Tolhurst DJ (1978a) Spatial summation in the receptive fields of simple cells in the cat's striate cortex. J Physiol (Lond) 283:53–77

Movshon JA, Thompson ID, Tolhurst DJ (1978b) Receptive field organization of complex cells in the cat's striate cortex. J Physiol (Lond) 283:79–99

Movshon JA, Thompson ID, Tolhurst DJ (1978c) Spatial and temporal contrast sensitivity of neurones in areas 17 and 18 of the cat's visual cortex. J Physiol (Lond) 283:101–120

Movshon JA, Davis ET, Adelson EH (1980) Directional movement selectivity in cortical complex cells. IIIrd European Conference on Visual Perception, Brighton

Mucke L, Norita M, Benedek G, Creutzfeldt O (1982) Physiologic and anatomic investigation of a visual cortical area situated in the ventral bank of the anterior ectosylvian sulcus of the cat. Exp Brain Res 46:1–11

Mullikin WH, Jones JP, Palmer LA (1981) Receptive fields and laminar distribution of X-like and Y-like simple cells. Soc Neurosci Abstr 7:356

Murata K, Cramer H, Bach y Rita P (1965) Neuronal convergence of noxious, acoustic and visual stimuli in the visual cortex of the cat. J Neurophysiol 28:1223–1240

Mustari MJ, Bullier J, Henry GH (1982) Comparison of the response properties of three types of monosynaptic S cell in cat striate cortex. J Neurophysiol 47:439–454

Myerson J, Manis P, Miezin F, Allman J (1977) Magnification in striate cortex and retinal ganglion cell layer of owl monkey: a quantitative comparison. Science 198:855–857

Nelson JI, Frost BJ (1978) Orientation-selective inhibition from beyond the classic visual receptive field. Brain Res 139:359–364

Nelson JI, Kato H, Bishop PO (1977) Discrimination of orientation and position disparities by binocularly activated neurons in cat striate cortex. J Neurophysiol 40:260–283

Newsome WT, Allman JM (1980) Interhemispheric connections of visual cortex in the owl monkey, Aotus trivirgatus, and the bushbaby, Galago senegalensis. J Comp Neurol 194:209–233

Niimi K, Kuwahara E (1973) The dorsal thalamus of the cat and comparison with monkey and man. J Hirnforsch 14:303–325

Niimi K, Sprague JM (1970) Thalamo-cortical organization of the visual system in the cat. J Comp Neurol 138:219–250

Niimi K, Matsuoka H, Yamazaki Y, Matsumoto H (1981) Thalamic afferents to the visual cortex in the cat studied by retrograde axonal transport of horseradish peroxidase. Brain Behav Evol 18:114–139

Nikara T, Bishop PO, Pettigrew JD (1968) Analysis of retinal correspondence by studying receptive fields of binocular single units in cat striate cortex. Exp Brain Res 6:353–372

Noda H, Freeman RB Jr, Gies B, Creutzfeldt OD (1971) Neuronal responses in the visual cortex of awake cats to stationary and moving targets. Exp Brain Res 12:389–405

Noda H, Freeman RB Jr, Creitzfeldt OD (1972) Neuronal correlates of eye movements in the visual cortex of the cat. Science 175:661–664

Norton TT, Casagrande VA (1982) Laminar organization of receptive-field properties in lateral geniculate nucleus of bush baby (Galago crassicaudatus). J Neurophysiol 47:715–741

Ogden TE (1975) The receptor mosaic of aotus trivirgatus: distribution of rods and cones. J Comp Neurol 163:193–202

Ogren M, Hendrickson A (1976) Pathways between striate cortex and subcortical regions in Macaca mulatta and Saimiri sciureus: evidence for a reciprocal pulvinar connection. Exp Neurol 53:780–800

Ohzawa I, Sclar G, Freeman RD (1982) Contrast gain control in the cat visual cortex. Nature 298:266–268

O'Kusky J, Colonnier M (1982) A laminar analysis of the number of neurons, glia and synapses in the visual cortex (area 17) of adult macaque monkeys. J Comp Neurol 210:278–290

O'Leary J (1941) Structure of area striata of the cat. J Comp Neurol 75:131–164

Olson CR, Graybiel AM (1981) A visual area in the anterior ectosylvian sulcus of the cat. Soc Neurosci Abstr 7:831

Orban GA (1975) Movement-sensitive neurones in the peripheral projections of area 18 of the cat. Brain Res 85:181–182

Orban GA (1977) Area 18 of the cat: the first step in processing visual movement information. Perception 6:501–511

Orban GA, Callens M (1977a) Recpetive field types of area 18 neurones in the cat. Exp Brain Res 30:107–123

Orban GA, Callens M (1977b) Influence of movement parameters on area 18 neurones in the cat. Exp Brain Res 30:125–140

Orban GA, Kennedy H (1981) The influence of eccentricity on receptive field types and orientation selectivity in areas 17 and 18 of the cat. Brain Res 208:203–208

Orban GA, Callens M, Colle J (1975) Unit responses to moving stimuli in area 18 of the cat. Brain Res 90:205–219

Orban GA, Kennedy H, Maes H (1978) Influence of eccentricity on velocity characteristics of area 18 neurones in the cat. Brain Res 159:391–395

Orban GA, Kato H, Bishop PO (1979a) End-zone region in receptive fields of hypercomplex and other striate neurons in the cat. J Neurophysiol 42:818–832

Orban GA, Kato H, Bishop PO (1979b) Dimensions and properties of end-zone inhibitory areas in receptive fields of hypercomplex cells in cat striate cortex. J Neurophysiol 42:833–849

Orban GA, Kennedy H, Maes H (1980) Functional changes across the 17-18 border in the cat. Exp Brain Res 39:177–186

Orban GA, Kennedy H, Maes H (1981a) Response to movement of neurons in areas 17 and 18 of the cat: velocity sensitivity. J Neurophysiol 45:1043–1058

Orban GA, Kennedy H, Maes H (1981b) Response to movement of neurons in areas 17 and 18 of the cat: direction selectivity. J Neurophysiol 45:1059–1073

Orban GA, Hoffmann KP, Duysens J (1981c) Influence of stimulus velocity on LGN neurons. Soc Neurosci Abstr 7:24

Orban GA, Duysens J, Cremieux J (to be published) Contribution des interactions spatio-temporelles au codage par les neurones corticaux visuel de la vitesse et de la direction du mouvement. J Physiol (Paris)

Orban GA, Duysens J, Cremieux J (1982a) Spatio-temporal interactions determining the velocity sensitivity of cat visual cortical neurones. Invest Ophthalmol Vis Sci 22:118

Orban GA, Duysens J, Kennedy H (1982b) Possible contribution of the cortical areas 17, 18, and 19 to the optokinetic response in the cat. In: Roucoux A, Crommelinck M (eds) Physiological and pathological aspects of eye movement. Junk Publishers, The Hague, pp 187–192

Orban GA, Kennedy H, Duysens J (1982c) The primary visual cortical complex of the cat (areas 17, 18, and 19): changes with eccentricity. Arch Int Physiol Biochim 90:11–12P

Orban GA, De Wolf J, Maes H (to be published 1983a) Factors influencing velocity coding in the human visual system. Vision Res

Orban GA, Vandenbussche E, Vogels R (to be published 1983b) Human orientation discrimination tested with long stimuli. Vision Res

Orban GA, Vandenbussche E, Vogels R (1984) Meridional variations and other properties, suggesting that acuity and orientation discrimination rely on different neuronal mechanisms. Ophthal Physiol Optics (in press)

Østerberg G (1935) Topography of the layer of rods and cones in the human retina. Acta Ophthalmol (Suppl) (Copenh) 6

Otsuka R, Hassler R (1962) Über Aufbau und Gliederung der corticalen Sehsphäre bei der Katze. Arch Psychiat und Z ges Neurol 203:212–234

Packwood J, Gordon B (1975) Stereopsis in normal domestic cat, Siamese cat, and cat raised with alternating monocular occlusions. J Neurophysiol 38:1485

Palmer LA, Davis TL (1981a) Receptive-field structure in cat striate cortex. J Neurophysiol 46: 260–276

Palmer LA, Davis TL (1981b) Comparison of responses to moving and stationary stimuli in cat striate cortex. J Neurophysiol 46:277–295

Palmer LA, Rosenquist AC (1974) Visual receptive fields of single striate cortical units projecting to the superior colliculus in the cat. Brain Res 67:27–42

Palmer LA, Rosenquist AC, Tusa RJ (1978) The retinotopic organization of lateral suprasylvian visual areas in the cat. J Comp Neurol 177:237–256

Pasternak T, Merigan WH (1981) The luminance dependence of spatial vision in the cat. Vision Res 21:1333–1340

Payne BR, Berman N, Murphy EH (1981) Organization of direction preferences in cat visual cortex. Brain Res 211:445–450

Perry VH, Cowey A (1981) The morphological correlates of X- and Y-like retinal ganglion cells in the retina of monkeys. Exp Brain Res 43:226–228

Perry VH, Cowey A (1983) The retinal ganglion cells of monkeys and their cerebral targets. Abstracts Third European Winter Conference on Brain Research. Les Arcs, France

Peters A, Fairén A (1978) Smooth and sparsely-spined stellate cells in the visual cortex of the rat: a study using a combined Golgi-electron microscope technique. J Comp Neurol 181:129–172

Peters A, Rigidor J (1981) A reassessment of the forms of nonpyramidal neurons in area 17 of cat visual cortex. J Comp Neurol 203:685–716

Petersen SE, Baker JF, Allman JM (1980) Dimensional selectivity of neurons in the dorsolateral visual area of the owl monkey. Brain Res 197:507–511

Petr R, Holden LB, Jirout J (1949) The efferent intercortical connections of the superficial cortex of the temporal lobe (Macaca mulatta). J Neuropathol Expt Neurol 8:100–103

Petrov AP, Pigarev IN, Zenkin GM (1980) Some evidence against Fourier analysis as a function of the receptive fields in cat's striate cortex. Vision Res 20:1023–1025

Pettigrew JD, Nikara T, Bishop PO (1968a) Responses to moving slits by single units in cat striate cortex. Exp Brain Res 6:373–390

Pettigrew JD, Nikara T, Bishop PO (1968b) Binocular interaction on single units in cat striate cortex: simultaneous stimulation by single moving slit with receptive fields in correspondence. Exp Brain Res 6:391–410

Poggio GF, Fischer B (1977) Binocular interaction and depth sensitivity in striate and prestriate cortex of behaving rhesus monkey. J Neurophysiol 40:1392–1405

Poggio GF, Baker FH, Mansfield RJW, Sillito A, Grigg P (1975) Spatial and chromatic properties of neurons subserving foveal and parafoveal vision in rhesus monkey. Brain Res 100:25–59

Poggio GF, Doty RW Jr, Talbot WH (1977) Foveal striate cortex of behaving monkey: single-neuron responses to square-wave gratings during fixation of gaze. J Neurophysiol 40:1369–1391

Pollen D, Ronner SF (1975) Periodic excitability changes across the receptive feilds of complex cells in the striate and parastriate cortex of the cat. J Physiol (Lond) 245:667–697

Pollen DA, Ronner SF (1981) Phase relationships between adjacent simple cells in the visual cortex. Science 212:1409–1411

Pollen DA, Ronner SF (1982) Spatial computation performed by simple and complex cells in the visual cortex of the cat. Vision Res 22:101–118

Pollen DA, Lee JR, Taylor JH (1971) How does the striate cortex begin the reconstruction of the visual world? Science 173:74–77

Polyak SD (1941) The retina. University of Chicago Press, Chicago, Illinois

Polyak SD (1957) The vertebrate visual System. University of Chicago Press, Chicago, Illinois

Popoff I (1927) Zur Kenntnis der Grösseder Area striate und die Methodik ihrer Ausmessung. J für Psychol und Neurol 34:238–242

Popoff I (1929) Über einige Grössenverhältnisse der Affenhirne. J für Psychol und Neurol 38:82–90

Powell TPS (1976) Bilateral cortico-tectal projection from the visual cortex in the cat. Nature 260:526–527

Raczkowski D, Rosenquist AC (1980) Connections of the parvocellular C laminae of the dorsal lateral geniculate nucleus with the visual cortex in the cat. Brain Res 199:447–451

Raczkowski D, Rosenquist AC (1981) Retinotopic organization in the cat lateral posterior-pulvinar complex. Brain Res 221:185–191

Regan D (1982) Visual information channeling in normal and disordered vision. Psychol Rev 89:407

Regan D, Beverley KI (1978a) Looming detectors in the human visual pathway. Vision Res 18:415–421

Regan D, Beverley KI (1978b) Illusory motion in depth: aftereffect of adaptation to changing size. Vision Res 18:209–212

Regan D, Cynader M (1979) Neurons in area 18 of cat visual cortex selectively sensitive to changing size: nonlinear interactions between responses to two edges. Vision Res 19:699–711

Regan D, Cynader M (1981) Motion-in-depth neurons: effects of speed and disparity. Invest Ophthalmol Vis Sci 20:148

Rezak M, Benevento LA (1979) A comparison of the organization of the projections of the dorsal lateral geniculate nucleus, the inferior pulvinar and adjacent lateral pulvinar to primary visual cortex (area 17) in the macaque monkey. Brain Res 167:19–40

Ribak CE (1978) Aspinous and sparsely-spinous stellate neurons in the visual cortex of rats contain glutamic acid decarboxylase. J Neurocytol 7:461–478

Riche D, Lanoir J (1978) Some claustro-cortical connections in the cat and baboon as studied by retrograde horseradish peroxidase transport. J Comp Neurol 177:435–444

Riva Sanseverino E, Galletti C, Maioli MG, Squatrito S (1979) Single unit responses to visual stimuli in cat cortical areas 17 and 18. III. Responses to moving stimuli of variable velocity. Arch Ital Biol 117:248–267

Rizzolatti G, Tradardi V, Camarda R (1970) Unit responses to visual stimuli in the cat's superior colliculus after removal of the visual cortex. Brain Res 24:336–339

Robertson ADJ (1965) Anaesthesia and receptive fields. Nature 205:80

Robson JG (1975) Receptive fields: neural representation of the spatial and intensive attributes of the visual image. In: Carterette EC, Friedman MP (eds) Handbook of perception. New York: Academic, vol 5, pp 81–112

Robson JG, Campbell FW (1964) A threshold contrast function for the visual system. Symposium on the physiological basis for form discrimination, pp 44–48. Hunter Laboratory of Psychology, Brown University, Providence, RI

Rockland KS, Pandya DN (1979) Laminar origins and terminations of cortical connections of the occipital lobe in the rhesus monkey. Brain Res 179:3–20

Rockland KS, Randya DN (1981) Cortical connections of the occipital lobe in the rhesus monkey: interconnections between areas 17, 18, 19 and the superior temporal sulcus. Brain Res 212:249–270

Rodieck RW (1979) Visual pathways. Ann Rev Neurosci 2:193–225

Rolls ET, Cowey A (1970) Topography of the retina and striate cortex and its relationship to visual acuity in rhesus monkeys and squirrel monkeys. Exp Brain Res 10:298–310

Rose D (1977) Responses of single units in cat visual cortex to moving bars of light as a function of bar length. J Physiol (Lond) 271:1–23

Rose D (1979) Mechanisms underlying the receptive field properties of neurons in cat visual cortex. Vision Res 19:533–544

Rose D, Blakemore C (1974) An analysis of orientation selectivity in the cat's visual cortex. Exp Brain Res 20:1–17

Rosenquist AC, Palmer LA (1971) Visual receptive field properties of cells of the superior colliculus after cortical lesions in the cat. Exp Neurol 33:629–652

Rosenquist AC, Edwards SB, Palmer LA (1974) An autoradiographic study of the projections of the dorsal lateral geniculate nucleus and the posterior nucleus in the cat. Brain Res 80:71–93

Rovamo J, Virsu V (1979) An estimation and application of the human cortical magnification factor. Exp Brain Res 37:495–510

Rovamo J, Virsu V, Laurinen P, Hyvärinen L (1982) Resolution of gratings oriented along and across meridians in peripheral vision. Invest Ophthalmol Vis Sci 23:666–670

Rowe MH, Dreher B (1982) Functional morphology of beta cells in the area centralis of the cat's retina: a model for the evolution of central retinal specializations. Brain Behav Evol 21:1–23

Rowe MH, Stone J (1976) Properties of ganglion cells in the visual streak of the cat's retina. J Comp Neurol 169:99–125

Russell WJ (1973) Nitrous oxide – is it an adequate anaesthetic? J Physiol (Lond) 231:20–21P

Sakitt B (1982) Why the cortical magnification factor in rhesus can not be isotropic. Vision Res 22:417–421

Sandell JH, Schiller PH (1982) Effect of cooling area 18 on striate cortex cells in the squirrel monkey. J Neurophysiol 48:38–48

Sanderson KJ (1971a) The projection of the visual field to the lateral geniculate and medial interlaminar nuclei in the cat. J Comp Neurol 143:101–118

Sanderson KJ (1971b) Visual field projection columns and magnification factors in the lateral geniculate nucleus of the cat. Exp Brain Res 13:159–177

Sanderson KJ, Sherman SM (1971) Nasotemporal overlap in visual field projected to lateral geniculate nucleus in the cat. J Neurophysiol 34:453–466

Sanides D (1978) The retinotopic distribution of visual callosal projections in the suprasylvian visual areas compared to the classical visual areas (17, 18, 19) in the cat. Exp Brain Res 33:435–443

Sanides D, Albus K (1980) The distribution of interhemispheric projections in area 18 of the cat: coincidence with discontinuities of the representation of the visual field in the second visual area (V2). Exp Brain Res 38:237–240

Sanides D, Buchholtz CS (1979) Identification of the projection from the visual cortex to the claustrum by anterograde axonal transport in the cat. Exp Brain Res 34:197–200

Sanides F, Hoffmann J (1969) Cyto- and myelo-architecture of the visual cortex of the cat and of the surrounding integration cortices. J Hirnforsch 11:79–104

Sanides D, Fries W, Albus K (1978) The corticopontine projection from the visual cortex of the cat: an autoradiographic investigation. J Comp Neurol 179:77–88

Sawyer CE, Palmer LA (1982) Receptive field organization of area 18 neurons. Soc Neurosci Abstr 8:810

Schiller PH, Malpeli JG (1977) Properties and tectal projections of monkey retinal ganglion cells. J Neurophysiol 40:428–445

Schiller PH, Finlay BL, Volman SF (1976a) Quantitative studies of single-cell properties in monkey striate cortex. I. Spatiotemporal organization of receptive fields. J Neurophysiol 39:1288–1319

Schiller PH, Finlay BL, Volman SF (1976b) Quantitative studies of single-cell properties in monkey striate cortex. II. Orientation specificity and ocular dominance. J Neurophysiol 39:1320–1333

Schiller PH, Finlay BL, Volman SF (1976c) Quantitative studies of single-cell properties in monkey striate cortex. III. Spatial frequency. J Neurophysiol 39:1334–1351

Schmidt ML, Hirsch HVB (1980) A quantitative study of the occurrence and distribution of cytoplasmic laminated bodies in the lateral geniculate nucleus of the normal adult cat. J Comp Neurol 189:235–247

Schmielau F, Singer W (1977) The role of visual cortex for binocular interactions in the cat lateral geniculate nucleus. Brain Res 120:354–361

Schneider GE (1969) Two visual systems. Science 163:895–902

Schoppmann A (1981) Projection from areas 17 and 18 of the visual cortex to the nucleus of the optic tract. Brain Res 223:1–18

Schoppmann A, Stryker MP (1981) Physiological evidence that 2-deoxyglucose method reveals orientation columns in cat visual cortex. Nature 293:574–576

Schwartzkroin PA (1972) The effect of body tilt on the directionality of units in cat visual cortex. Exp Neurol 36:498–506

Sclar G, Freeman RD (1982) Orientation selectivity in the cats striate cortex in invariant with stimulus contrast. Exp Brain Res 46:457–462

Segraves MA, Rosenquist AC (1982a) The distribution of the cells of origin of callosal projections in cat visual cortex. J Neurosci 2:1079–1089

Segraves MA, Rosenquist AC (1982b) The afferent and efferent callosal connections of retinotopically defined areas in cat cortex. J Neurosci 2:1090–1107

Shatz CJ (1977a) A comparison of visual pathways in Boston and Midwestern Siamese cats. J Comp Neurol 171:205–228

Shatz CJ (1977b) Abnormal interhemispheric connections in the visual system of Boston Siamese cats: a physiological study. J Comp Neurol 171:229–245

Shatz CJ (1977c) Anatomy of interhemispheric connections in the visual system of Boston Siamese and ordinary cats. J Comp Neurol 173:497–518

Shatz CJ, Stryker MP (1978) Ocular dominance in layer IV of the cat's visual cortex and the effects of monocular deprivation. J Physiol (Lond) 281:267–283

Shatz CJ, Lindström S, Wiesel TN (1977) The distribution of afferents representing the right and left eyes in the cat's visual cortex. Brain Res 131:103–116

Sherk H (1978) Area 18 cell responses in cat during reversible inactivation of area 17. J Neurophysiol 41:204–215

Sherk H, LeVay S (1981a) Visual claustrum: topography and receptive field properties in the cat. Science 212:87–89

Sherk H, LeVay S (1981b) The visual claustrum of the cat. III. Receptive field properties. J Neurosci 1:993–1002

Sherk H, LeVay S (1982) The cortico-claustral loop contributes to end-inhibition of neurons in area 17 of the cat. Soc Neurosci Abstr 8:677

Sherman SM, Watkins DW, Wilson JR (1976a) Further differences in receptive field properties of simple and complex cells in cat striate cortex. Vision Res 16:919–927

Sherman SM, Wilson JR, Kaas JH, Webb SV (1976b) X- and Y-cells in the dorsal lateral geniculate nucleus of the owl monkey (Aotus trivirgatus). Science 192:475–477

Shoumura K (1972) Patterns of fiber degeneration in the lateral wall of the suprasylvian gyrus (Clare-Bishop area) following lesions in the visual cortex in cats. Brain Res 43:264–267

Shoumura K (1974) An attempt to relate the origin and distribution of commissural fibers to the presence of large and medium pyramids in layer III in the cat's visual cortex. Brain Res 67:13–26

Shoumura K, Itoh K (1972) Intercortical projections from the lateral wall of the suprasylvian gyrus, the Clare-Bishop area, of the cat. Brain Res 39:536–539

Sillito AM (1975) The contribution of inhibitory mechanisms to the receptive field properties of neurones in the striate cortex of the cat. J Physiol (Lond) 250:305–329

Sillito AM (1977a) Inhibitory processes underlying the directional specificity of simple, complex and hypercomplex cells in the cat's visual cortex. J Physiol (Lond) 271:699–720

Sillito AM (1977b) The spatial extent of excitatory and inhibitory zones in the receptive field of superficial layer hypercomplex cells. J Physiol (Lond) 273:791–803

Sillito AM (1979) Inhibitory mechanisms influencing complex cell orientation selectivity and their modification at high resting discharge levels. J Physiol (Lond) 289:33–53

Sillito AM, Versiani V (1977) The contribution of excitatory and inhibitory inputs to the length preference of hypercomplex cells in layers II and III of the cat's striate cortex. J Physiol (Lond) 273:775–790

Sillito AM, Kemp JA, Patel H (1980a) Inhibitory interactions contributing to the ocular dominance of monocularly dominated cells in the normal cat striate cortex. Exp Brain Res 41:1–10

Sillito AM, Kemp JA, Milson JA, Berardi N (1980b) A re-evaluation of the mechanisms underlying simple cell orientation selectivity. Brain Res 194:517–520

Silverman MS, Tootell RBH, De Valois RL (1981) Electrophysiological verification of deoxyglucose spatial frequency columns in cat striate cortex. Soc Neurosci Abstr 7:356

Singer W (1977) Control of thalamic transmission by corticofugal and ascending reticular pathways in the visual system. Physiol Rev 57:386–420

Singer W, Tretter F, Cynader M (1975) Organization of cat striate cortex: a correlation of receptive-field properties with afferent and efferent connections. J Neurophysiol 38:1080–1098

Singer W, Tretter F, Cynader M (1976) The effect of reticular stimulation on spontaneous and evoked activity in the cat visual cortex. Brain Res 102:71–90

Sireteanu R, Hoffmann KP (1979) Relative frequency and visual resolution on X- and Y-cells in the LGN of normal and monocularly deprived cats: interlaminar differences. Exp Brain Res 34:591–603

So YT, Shapley R (1981) Spatial tuning of cells in and around lateral geniculate nucleus of the cat: X and Y relay cells and perigeniculate interneurons. J Neurophysiol 45:107–120

Somogyi P, Cowey A (1981) Combined Golgi and electron microscopic study on the synapses formed by double bouquet cells in the visual cortex of the cat and monkey. J Comp Neurol 195:547–566

Spear PD, Baumann TP (1975) Receptive-field characteristics of single neurons in lateral supra-sylvian visual area of the cat. J Neurophysiol 38:1403–1420

Spear PD, Baumann TP (1979) Effects of visual cortex removal on receptive-field properties of neurons in lateral suprasylvian visual area of the cat. J Neurophysiol 42:31–56

Spear PD, Tong L (1980) Effects of monocular deprivation of neurons in cat's lateral suprasylvian visual area. I. Comparison of binocular and monocular segments. J Neurophysiol 44:568–584

Sperry RW (1950) Neural basis of the spontaneous optokinetic response produced by visual inversion. J Comp Physiol Psychol 43:482–489

Spinelli DN, Starr A, Barrett TW (1968) Auditory specificity in unit recordings from cat's visual cortex. Exp Neurol 22:75–84

Sprague JM, Levy J, DiBerardino A, Berlucchi G (1977) Visual cortical areas mediating form dis-crimination in the cat. J Comp Neurol 172:441–488

Squatrito S, Battaglini PP, Galletti C, Riva Sanseverino E (1980a) Autoradiographic evidence for projections from cortical visual areas 17, 18, 19 and the Clare-Bishop area to the ipsilateral claustrum in the cat. Neurosci Lett 19:265–269

Squatrito S, Battaglini PP, Galletti C, Riva Sanseverino E (1980b) Projections from the visual cortex to the contralateral claustrum of the cat revealed by an anterograde axonal transport method. Neurosci Lett 19:271–275

Squatrito S, Galletti C, Battaglini PP, Riva Sanseverino E (1981a) Bilateral cortical projections from cat visual areas 17 and 18. An autoradiographic study. Arch Ital Biol 119:1–20

Squatrito S, Galletti C, Battaglini PP, Riva Sanseverino E (1981b) An autoradiographic study of bilateral cortical projections from cat area 19 and lateral suprasylvian visual area. Arch Ital Biol 119:21–42

Stanford LR, Friedlander MJ, Sherman SM (1981) Morphology of physiologically identified W cells in the C laminae of the cat's lateral geniculate nucleus. J Neurosci 1:578–584

Steffey EP, Gillespie JR, Berry JD, Eger EI II, Munson ES (1974) Anesthetic potency (MAC) of nitrous oxide in the dog, cat, and stump-tail monkey. J Appl Physiol 36:530–532

Steinberg RH, Reid M, Lacy PL (1973) The distribution of rods and cones in the retina of the cat (Felis domesticus). J Comp Neurol 148:229–248

Sterling P (1983) Microcircuitry of the cat retina. Annu Rev Neurosci 6:149–185

Stevens JK, Gerstein GL (1976) Spatiotemporal organization of cat lateral geniculate receptive fields. J Neurophysiol 39:213–238

Stone J (1965) A quantitative analysis of the distribution of ganglion cells in the cat's retina. J Comp Neurol 124:337–352

Stone J (1966) The naso-temporal division of the cat's retina. J Comp Neurol 126:585–600

Stone J (1973) Sampling properties of microelectrodes assessed in the cat's retina. J Neurophysiol 36:1071–1080

Stone J (1978) The number and distribution of ganglion cells in the cat's retina. J Comp Neurol 180:753–772

Stone J, Clarke R (1980) Correlation between soma size and dendritic morphology in cat retinal ganglion cells: evidence of further variation in the γ-cell class. J Comp Neurol 192:211–217

Stone J, Dreher B (1973) Projection of X- and Y-cells of the cat's lateral geniculate nucleus to areas 17 and 18 of visual cortex. J Neurophysiol 36:551–567

Stone J, Fukuda Y (1974) Properties of cat retinal ganglion cells: a comparison of W-cells with X- and Y-cells. J Neurophysiol 37:722–748

Stone J, Hoffmann KP (1971) Conduction velocity as a parameter in the organisation of the affer-ent relay in the cat's lateral geniculate nucleus. Brain Res 32:454–459

Stone J, Hoffmann KP (1972) Very slow-conducting ganglion cells in the cat's retina: a major new functional type? Brain Res 43:610–616

Stone J, Johnston E (1981) The topography of primate retina: a study of the human bushbaby, and new- and old-world monkeys. J Comp Neurol 196:205–223

Stone J, Leicester J, Sherman SM (1973) The nasotemporal division of the monkey retina. J Comp Neurol 150:333–348

Stone J, Dreher B, Leventhal A (1979) Hierarchical and parallel mechanisms in the organization of visual cortex. Brain Res Rev 1:345–394

Sur M, Sherman SM (1982) Linear and nonlinear W-cells in C laminae of the cat's lateral geniculate nucleus. J Neurophysiol 47:869–884

Sur M, Stanford LR, Sherman SM (1981) W-cells in the C laminae of the cat's lateral geniculate nucleus: contrast sensitivity and other response measures. Soc Neurosci Abstr 7:25

Sugiyama M (1979) The projection of the visual cortex on the Clare-Bishop area in the cat. Exp Brain Res 36:433–443

Symonds L, Rosenquist AC (1979) Visual cortical input to area 20 of the cat: anatomical evidence for subdivision of this region into two areas. Soc Neurosci Abstr 5:809

Szentagothai J (1973) Synaptology of the visual cortex. In: Jung R (ed) Central visual information B. Springer, Berlin Heidelberg New York (Handbook of sensory physiology, vol VII/3, pp 269–324)

Talbot SA, Marshall WH (1941) Physiological studies on neural mechanisms of visual localization and discrimination. Am J Ophthalmol 24:1255–1263

Thompson ID, Tolhurst DJ (1979) Variation in the spatial frequency selectivity of neurones in the cat visual cortex. J Physiol (Lond) 295:33P

Thompson ID, Tolhurst DJ (1980a) Optimal spatial frequencies of neighbouring neurones in the cat's visual cortex. J Physiol (Lond) 300:57–58P

Thompson ID, Tolhurst DJ (1980b) The representation of spatial frequency in cat visual cortex: a ^{14}C-2-deoxyglucose study. J Physiol (Lond) 300:58P

Thompson ID, Kossut M, Blakemore C (1983) A 2-deoxyglucose study of the development of orientation columns in cat striate cortex. Abstracts third european winter conference on brain research. Les Arcs, France

Thompson P (1982) Perceived rate of movement depends on contrast. Vis Res 22:377–380

Thuma BD (1928) Studies on the diencephalon of the cat. I. The cytoarchitecture of the corpus geniculatum laterale. J Comp Neurol 46:173–200

Tigges J, Tigges M, Anschel S, Cross NA, Letbetter WD, McBride RL (1981) Areal and laminar distribution of neurons interconnecting the central visual cortical areas 17, 18, 19, and MT in squirrel monkey (Saimiri). J Comp Neurol 202:539–560

Tolhurst DJ, Movshon JA (1975) Spatial and temporal contrast sensitivity of striate cortical neurones. Nature 257:674–675

Tolhurst DJ, Movshon JA, Thompson ID (1981) The dependence of response amplitude and variance of cat visual cortical neurones on stimulus contrast. Exp Brain Res 41:414–419

Tömböl T, Hajdu F, Somogyi Gy (1975) Identification of the Golgi picture of the layer VI cortico-geniculate projection neurons. Exp Brain Res 24:107–110

Tomko DL, Barbaro NM, Ali FN (1981) Effect of body tilt on receptive field orientation of simple visual cortical neurons in unanesthetized cats. Exp Brain Res 43:309–314

Tootell RBH, Silverman MS, De Valois RL (1981) Spatial frequency columns in primary visual cortex. Science 214:813–815

Tootell RBH, Silverman MS, Switkes E, De Valois RL (1982a) Deoxyglucose analysis of retinotopic organization in primate striate cortex. Science 218:902–904

Tootell RBH, Silverman MS, Switkes E, De Valois RL (1982b) The organization of cortical modules in primate striate cortex. Soc Neurosci Abstr 8:707

Torrealba F, Partlow GD, Guillery RW (1981) Organization of the projection from the superior colliculus to the dorsal lateral geniculate nucleus of the cat. Neurosci 6:1341–1360

Toyama K, Takeda T (1974) A unique class of cat's visual cortical cells that exhibit either ON or OFF excitation for stationary light slit and are responsive to moving edge patterns. Brain Res 73:350–355

Toyama, K, Matsunami K, Ohno T (1969a) Antidromic identification of association, commissural and corticofugal efferent cells in cat visual cortex. Brain Res 14:513–517

Toyama K, Tokashiki S, Matsunami K (1969b) Synaptic action of commissural impulses upon association efferent cells in cat visual cortex. Brain Res 14:518–520

Toyama K, Matsunami K, Ohno T, Tokashiki S (1974) An intracellular study of neuronal organization in the visual cortex. Exp Brain Res 21:45–66

Toyama K, Kimura M, Shiida T, Takeda T (1977a) Convergence of retinal inputs onto visual cortical cells: II. A study of the cells disynaptically excited from the lateral geniculate body. Brain Res 137:221–231

Toyama K, Maekawa K, Takeda T (1977b) Convergence of retinal inputs onto visual cortical cells: I. A study of the cells monosynaptically excited from the lateral geniculate body. Brain Res 137:207–220

Toyama K, Kimura M, Tanaka K (1981a) Cross-correlation analysis of interneuronal connectivity in cat visual cortex. J Neurophysiol 46:191–201

Toyama K, Kimura M, Tanaka K (1981b) Organization of cat visual cortex as investigated by cross-correlation technique. J Neurophysiol 46:202–214

Tretter F, Cynader M, Singer W (1975) Cat parastriate cortex: a primary or secondary visual area? J Neurophysiol 38:1099–1113

Trevarthen CB (1968) Two mechanisms of vision in primates. Psychol Forsch 31:299–337

Tsumoto T (1978) Inhibitory and excitatory binocular convergence to visual cortical neurons of the cat. Brain Res 159:85–97

Tsumoto T, Suda K (1980) Three groups of cortico-geniculate neurons and their distribution in binocular and monocular segments of cat striate cortex. J Comp Neurol 193:223–236

Tsumoto T, Creutzfeldt OD, Legendy CR (1978) Functional organization of the corticofugal system from visual cortex to lateral geniculate nucleus in the cat (with an appendix on geniculo-cortical monosynaptic connections). Exp Brain Res 32:345–364

Tsumoto T, Eckart W, Creutzfeldt OD (1979) Modification of orientation sensitivity of cat visual cortex neurons by removal of GABA-mediated inhibition. Exp Brain Res 34:351–363

Tusa RJ, Palmer LA (1980) Retinotopic organization of areas 20 and 21 in the cat. J Comp Neurol 193:147–164

Tusa RJ, Palmer LA, Rosenquist AC (1978) The retinotopic organization of area 17 (striate cortex) in the cat. J Comp Neurol 177:213–236

Tusa RJ, Rosenquist AC, Palmer LA (1979) Retinotopic organization of areas 18 and 19 in the cat. J Comp Neurol 185:657–678

Ullman S (1979) The interpretation of structure from motion. Proc Roy Soc Lond (Biol) 203: 405–426

Updyke BV (1975) The patterns of projection of cortical areas 17, 18, and 19 onto the laminae of the dorsal lateral geniculate nucleus in the cat. J Comp Neurol 163:377–396

Updyke BV (1977) Topographic organization of the projections from cortical areas 17, 18, and 19 onto the thalamus, pretectum and superior colliculus in the cat. J Comp Neurol 173:81–122

Updyke BV (1981) Projections from visual areas of the middle suprasylvian sulcus onto the lateral posterior complex and adjacent thalamic nuclei in cat. J Comp Neurol 201:477–506

Vandenbussche E, Orban GA, Vogels R, Van Horenbeeck R (1980) The orientation acuity in human: evidence for an oblique effect. Arch Int Physiol Biochim 88:34–35

Vandenbussche E, Orban GA (1983) Meridional variations in the line orientation discrimination of the cat. Behav Brain Res 9:237–255

van der Glas HW, Orban GA, Joris PhX, Verhoeven FJ (1981) Direction selectivity in human visual perception, investigated with low contrast gratings. Acta Psychol 48:15–23

Van Essen DC (1979) Visual areas of the mammalian cerebral cortex. Ann Rev Neurosci 2:227–263

Van Essen DC, Maunsell JHR (1980) Two-dimensional maps of the cerebral cortex. J Comp Neurol 191:255–281

Van Essen DC, Zeki SM (1978) The topographic organization of rhesus monkey prestriate cortex. J Physiol (Lond) 277:192–226

Van Essen DC, Maunsell JHR, Bixby JL (1980a) Two visual areas in the macaque cortex involved in the analysis of movement. Exp Brain Res 41:A28

Van Essen DC, Maunsell JHR, Newsome WT, Bixby JL (1980b) The location of extrastriate visual areas in the macaque monkey. Exp Brain Res 41:A24

Van Essen DC, Maunsell JHR, Bixby JL (1981) The middle temporal visual area in the macaque: myeloarchitecture, connections, functional properties and topographic organization. J Comp Neurol 199:293–326

Van Essen DC, Maunsell JHR, Connolly MP, Burkhalter A (1982a) Visual areas involved in motion analysis in the macaque monkey. Perception 11:A3

Van Essen DC, Newsome WT, Bixby JL (1982b) The pattern of interhemispheric connections and its relationship to extrastriate visual areas in the macaque monkey. J Neurosci 2:265–283

Vaney DI, Peichl L, Wässle H, Illing RB (1981) Almost all ganglion cells in the rabbit retina project to the superior colliculus. Brain Res 212:447–453

Vanni-Mercier G, Magnin M (1982a) Single neuron activity related to natural vestibular stimulation in the cat's visual cortex. Exp Brain Res 45:451–455

Vanni-Mercier G, Magnin M (1982b) Retinotopic organization of extra-retinal saccade-related input to the visual cortex in the cat. Exp Brain Res 46:368–376

Vidyasager TR, Urbas JV (1981) Orientation bias of cat geniculate neurones and the role of the visual cortex. Neurosci Lett (Suppl) 7:38

Vidyasagar TR, Urbas JV (1982) Orientation sensitivity of cat LGN neurones with and without inputs from visual cortical areas 17 and 18. Exp Brain Res 46:157–169

von der Heydt R, Adorjani Cs, Hänny P, Baumgartner G (1978) Disparity sensitivity and receptive field incongruity of units in the cat striate cortex. Exp Brain Res 31:523–545

Von Economo C (1929) The cytoarchitectonics of the human cerebral cortex. Oxford University Press

von Grünau M, Frost BJ (1983) Double-opponent-process mechanism underlying RF-structure of directionally specific cells of cat lateral suprasylvian visual area. Exp Brain Res 49:84–92

von Holst E, Mittelstaedt H (1950) Das Reafferenzprinzip. Wechselwirkungen zwischen Zentralnervensystem und Peripherie. Naturwissenschaften 37:464–476

Wässle H, Illing RB (1980) The retinal projection to the superior colliculus in the cat: a quantitative study with HRP. J Comp Neurol 190:333–356

Wässle H, Levick WR, Cleland BG (1975) The distribution of the alpha type of ganglion cells in the cat's retina. J Comp Neurol 159:419–438

Wässle H, Boycott BB, Illing RB (1981a) Morphology and mosaic of on- and off-beta cells in the cat retina and some functional considerations. Proc Roy Soc Lond (Biol) 212:177–195

Wässle H, Peichl L, Boycott BB (1981b) Morphology and topography of on- and off-alpha cells in the cat retina. Proc Roy Soc Lond (Biol) 212:157–175

Watkins DW, Berkley MA (1974) The orientation selectivity of single neurons in cat striate cortex. Exp Brain Res 19:433–446

Webb SV, Kaas JH (1976) The sizes and distribution of ganglion cells in the retina of the owl monkey, Aotus trivirgatus. Vision Res 16:1247–1254

Wertheim T (1894) Über die indirekte Sehschärfe. Z Psychol Physiol Sinnesorg 7:172–189

Westheimer G (1979) Cooperative neural processes involved in stereoscopic acuity. Exp Brain Res 36:585–597

Westheimer G (1981) Visual hyperacuity. In: Progress in sensory physiology, vol 1. Springer, Berlin Heidelberg New York, pp 1–30

Westheimer G (1982) The spatial grain of the perifoveal visual field. Vision Res 22:157–162

Westheimer G, McKee SP (1975) Visual acuity in the presence of retinal-image motion. J Opt Soc Am 65:847

Weymouth FW, Hines DC, Acres LH, Raaf JE, Wheeler MC (1928) Visual acuity within the area centralis and its relation to eye movements and fixation. Am J Ophthalmol 11:947–960

Whitteridge D (1973) Projection of the optic pathway to the visual cortex. In: Jung R (ed) Handbook of sensory physiology, vol VII/3B. Springer, Berlin Heidelberg New York, pp 247–268

Wickelgren BG, Sterling P (1969) Influence of visual cortex on receptive field properties in the superior colliculus of the cat. J Neurophysiol 32:16–23

Wiesel TN, Hubel DH, Lam DMK (1974) Autoradiographic demonstration of ocular-dominance columns in the monkey striate cortex by means of transneuronal transport. Brain Res 79:273–279

Wiesel TN, Hubel DH (1966) Spatial and chromatic interactions in the lateral geniculate body of the rhesus monkey. J Neurophysiol 29:1115–1156

Wilson ME (1968) Cortico-cortical connexions of the cat visual areas. J Anat 102:375–386

Wilson JR, Sherman SM (1976) Receptive-field characteristics of neurons in cat striate cortex: changes with visual field eccentricity. J Neurophysiol 39:512–533

Wilson PD, Rowe MH, Stone J (1976) Properties of relay cells in cat's lateral geniculate nucleus: a comparison of W-cells with X- and Y-cells. J Neurophysiol 39:1193–1209

Wong-Riley M (1979) Changes in the visual system of monocularly sutured or enucleated cats demonstrable with cytochrome oxidase histochemistry. Brain Res 171:11–28

Woolsey CN (1971) Comparative studies on cortical representation of vision. Vision Res Suppl 3:365–382

Wurtz RH (1969a) Visual receptive fields of striate cortex neurons in awake monkeys. J Neurophysiol 32:727–742

Wurtz RH (1969b) Comparison of effects of eye movements and stimulus movements on striate cortex neurons of the monkey. J Neurophysiol 32:987–994

Yamane S, Nikara T, Sugie N (1977) Sustained and transient cortical neurones in area 18 of the cat. Experientia 33:477–479

Yukie M, Iwai E (1981) Direct projection from the dorsal lateral geniculate nucleus to the prestriate cortex in the macaque monkeys. J Comp Neurol 201:81–97

Zeki SM (1969) Representation of central visual fields in prestriate cortex of monkey. Brain Res 14:271–291

Zeki SM (1970) Interhemispheric connections of prestriate cortex in monkey. Brain Res 19:63–75

Zeki SM (1978) Functional specialisation in the visual cortex of the rhesus monkey. Nature 274:423–428

Zeki SM (1982a) A comparison of the distribution of wavelength selective cells at different eccentricities in three visual areas of monkey cortex. J Physiol (Lond) 330:57P

Zeki SM (1982b) Do wavelength selective cells in monkey striate cortex respond to colours? J Physiol (Lond) 330:57–58P

Subject Index

A cells 109, 113
acuity 32, 314
A family cells 101, 103, 106, 109, 113, 198
A laminae 13, 63
amplitude of movement 215
anesthesia 307
animal psychophysics 339
area 17 34, 99, 110, 156, 195, 208, 308
area 18 39, 99, 110, 156, 195, 208
area 19 39, 99, 110, 156, 195, 208
area 20 47
area 21 47
area 17-18 border 57, 143
area 18-19 border 62, 144

bandpass filter 125, 131
B cells 109
B family cells 101, 103, 106, 109, 198
bicuculline 274, 278, 281, 282
binocular fusion 218, 234
binocular interactions 218
binocularity 218

C cells 109
C family cells 101, 103, 106, 109, 198
C laminae 63
claustrum 83, 250
coding 125
color specificity 315
color columns 327
columnar organization 332
complex cells 88
cones 7, 27
contrast 135
contrast adaptation 138
constrast-response curves 135, 142, 318
contrast sensitivity
    behavioral 32
    single cell 165, 320
convergence 25
corpus callosum 23, 85, 250
corticocortical connections 48, 84, 252
corticogeniculate cells 249
corticotectal cells 117, 244
coupling connections 49

depth perception
    static 226, 235

dynamic 239
differencing operations between filters 129
directional tuning 202, 209
direction index 203
direction of movement 201
direction selectivity 202, 321
direction selectivity in depth 239
disparity insensitive cells 233
disparity tuning curves 229
divergence 25

eccentricity
    changes in direction selectivity with 206
    changes in magnification with 38, 46, 308
    changes in ocular dominance with 219
    changes in orientation tuning with 157
    changes in properties with 335
    changes in receptive field size with 99, 103
    changes in receptive field types with 113
    changes in spatial frequency selectivity with
        167
    changes in velocity sensitivity with 187
electrical stimulation experiments 76, 256,
    330
electrophysiological mapping 35
end-stopping 90, 104, 162, 279
extrastriate areas 19
eye movements 184, 303

far cells 232, 323
feature detector 1, 340
feeding connections 48
filter 1, 125, 331
Fourier analyzer: the visual cortex as a 178

GABA 274, 298
ganglion cells 8, 69
geniculate cells
    morphology 65, 72
    physiology 69, 72
geniculocortical projection
    anatomy 66
    physiology 76
geniculate wing 63, 65
gratings 149

HA cells 109, 113
half-height upper cut-off velocity 186, 190, 269

half-width at half-heigth 125, 151
hand-plotting 88, 93, 155, 185, 203
HB cells 109
HC cells 109
hierarchy between areas 21, 47
high-pass filter 132
HS cells 109
hypercomplex cells 90, 104, 107, 314

inhibitory interneurons 284, 289, 296
inhibitory sidebands 91, 100, 230, 284
intracortical inhibition
    role of
    in absence of response to visual noise 283
        in direction selectivity 276
        in end-stopping 279
        in ocular dominance 282
        in orientation selectivity 272
        in velocity upper cut-off 282

lamination
    of efferent projections 244
    of geniculate afferents 80, 311
    of receptive field types 110
    of velocity types 190
lateral suprasylvian areas 42
length-response curves 102, 105, 107, 161
LGN 13, 63
linearity
    linear behaviour 173
    linearity of summation 9, 69, 173
looming 239
luminance 137, 144, 147, 318
luxotonic cells 144, 318

magnification 20
magnification factor 29, 38, 46
magnocellular layers 13, 311, 330
masking: influence of — on direction selectivity
    212
mean direction index 206
meridional variations in orientation preferences
    157, 320
MIN 63, 65
monocular cells 219, 224, 322
monosynaptic input from LGN 256
moving edges 91, 96, 120, 169
moving stimuli 89, 94, 184
multichannel representation of a parameter
    125

naso-temporal overlap 13, 60, 251
near cells 232, 323
non-oriented cells 107, 110, 311
numbers of cells in retinocortical pathway 25

ocular dominance
    columns 82, 222, 325
    distributions 219, 322
    scheme 218
OFF center Input 261
OFF responses 88, 94, 97, 120

ON center input 261
ON responses 88, 94, 97, 120
optic chiasm 11
orientation
    columns 158, 325
    dependence of inhibitions 284
    disparity 235
    selectivity 150
    tuning curves 151
OX-OR latency differences 76, 256

parallel processing 47, 50, 334, 337
parvocellular layers 13, 311, 330
passband 125
pons 247
position disparity 226
position test 97
pretectum 248
primary visual complex 3, 50, 334
pulvinar 21, 83, 248
pyramidal cells 296

raw primal sketch 182, 340
receptive field
    classification criteria 92
    classification schemes 88, 106, 117
    definition 35, 87
    dimensions 97
    organization 87, 311
    scatter 55
    subregions 94
    types and binocularity 111, 222
    types and direction selectivity 111, 209
    types and orientation selectivity 111, 153,
        155
    types and spatial frequency selectivity 167
    types and velocity sensitivity 111, 198
response planes 97, 120, 269
response strength 186, 270
response to slow movement 186
retina 7
retinal cell population 27
retinotopic organization
    definition 11
    principle 331
    types 19, 37, 40, 43, 44, 308
rods 7, 27

S cells 109
S1 subfamily 113
S2 subfamily 113
serial processing 47, 90
S family cells 101, 103, 106, 109, 113, 198,
    209, 314
simple cells 88
single channel representation of a parameter
    132
sleep 306
spatial frequency
    coding 169
    columns 168
    selectivity 165

spots 117
stationnary flashed stimuli 94
stellate cells 296
stereopsis
    coarse 232, 239, 323
    fine 232, 323
superior colliculus 11, 244
sustained 9, 70, 268

temporal frequency 200
threshold
    contrast 135
    firing 162, 295
transformation of visual field 19
transient 9, 70, 268
tuned excitatory cells 229, 323
tuned inhibitory cells 232, 323
tuning curve 125

variability
    of cortical maps 53
    of orientation preferences 152
    of single cell responses 129

velocity
    broad-band cells 190
    high-pass cells 190, 197
    influence on direction selectivity 203
    low-pass cells 190, 193, 322
    response curves 185
    sensitivity profiles 186
    tuned cells 190, 195
vestibular input to visual cortex 300
visual
    areas 17
    cortex 17
    discriminations 2, 338
    field 5, 45
    field islands 41, 62
    noise 116, 149, 181, 283

W cells 9, 16, 70
width of velocity tuning 186
wiring diagram S family cells 292
working range of spatial frequency filter 171

X cells 9, 15, 70, 256

Y cells 9, 15, 70, 256

E. Zrenner

Neurophysiological Aspects of Color Vision in Primates

Comparative Studies on Simian Retinal Ganglion Cells and the Human Visual System

1983. 71 figures. XVI, 218 pages. (Studies of Brain Function, Volume 9). ISBN 3-540-11653-2

Contents: Introduction. – Methods. – Types of Retinal Ganglion Cells and Their Distribution. – Special Properties of Blue-Sentitive Ganglion Cells. – Temporal Properties of Color-Opponent Ganglion Cells. – The Spectral Properties of the Human Visual System as Revealed by Visually Evoked Cortical Potentials (VECP) and Psychophysical Investigations. – Epilogue. – Summary. – References. – Subject Index.

Vision under daylight conditions is based on the neuronal interaction between spectrally different receptor mechanisms and its thereby inextricably linked in all its aspects to the mechanisms of color vision. This book presents the results of research in three different directions: (1) Extensive studies on **single retinal ganglion cells** of Rhesus monkeys are described which stress the optimizing role of variability in color-opponent processing for vision in general. (2) The spectral properties of the various functional groups of cells in the **human visual system** are revealed by the visually evoked cortical potentials and are compared with simultaneously recorded psychophysical data. (3) The application of new methods of selectively testing individual cell functions is described in **clinical studies** on congenital and acquired color vision deficiencies as well as in controlled pharmacological studies.

In a holistic effort to combine the various experimental facts, a search was made for possible contributions of individual physiological mechanisms to more complex perceptual phenomena, such as color contrast enhancement, color coding in the retinal periphery, tritanoptic phenomena, and the flicker-induced colors. The reader is provided with an account of new developments and ideas of neuronal processing of color which are based on numerous experiments and are critically surveyed with extensive references.

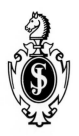

Springer-Verlag
Berlin
Heidelberg
New York
Tokyo

Ocular Size and Shape Regulation During Development

Editors: **S. R. Hilfer, J. B. Sheffield**
1981. 80 figures. XII, 211 pages. (Cell and Developmental Biology of the Eye). ISBN 3-540-90619-3

Contents: The Role of Cell Death and Related Phenomena During Formation of the Optic Pathway. – Mechanisms of Cell Shape Determination in Teleost Retinal Cones. – Intracellular and Extracellular Changes During Early Ocular Development in the Chick Embryo. – The Mechanism of Cell Elongation During Lens Fiber Cell Differentiation. – Cell Surface Differentiation in the Embryonic Chick Retina. – Intercellular Adhesion Among Developing Retional Cells: A Role for Ligatin as a Baseplate. – Topographic Gradient of Cell-Membrane Molecules in Avian Neural Retina Detected with Monoclonal Antibody. – Maturation of the Lens Fiber Cell: Some Morphological and Biochemical Correlates. – Recent Development in Therapy of Cataracts. – Index.

Cellular Communication During Ocular Development

Editors: **J. B. Sheffield, S. R. Hilfer**
1982. 64 figures. XII, 196 pages. (Cell and Developmental Biology of the Eye). ISBN 3-540-90773-4

Contents: The Development of Specificity of Retinal Central Connections: Changing Concepts. – Development of Retinal Synaptic Arrays in Mouse, Chicken, and Xenopus: A Comparative Study. – Physiological Development of Retinal Synapses. – Development of Cholinergic and Amino Acid Neurotransmitter Systems in the Chick Retina. – Control of Intercellular Communication via Gap Junctions. – Transient Dye Coupling Between Developing Neurons Reveals Patterns of Intercellular Communication During Embryogenesis. – Molecular Biology of Lens Induction. – Regulation of Lens Morphogenesis and Cataract Pathogenesis by Pituitary-dependent, Insulin-like Mitogens. – Coordinate Control of Retinal Neovascularization. – Theories of Magnification Relative to the Visually Impaired. – Index.

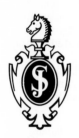

Springer-Verlag
Berlin
Heidelberg
NewYork
Tokyo